Pressure Perturbation Approach in Biochemistry and Structural Biology. In memoriam of Dr. Gaston Hui Bon Hoa

Pressure Perturbation Approach in Biochemistry and Structural Biology. In memoriam of Dr. Gaston Hui Bon Hoa

Editors

Dmitri Davydov
Christiane Jung

MDPI • Basel • Beijing • Wuhan • Barcelona • Belgrade • Manchester • Tokyo • Cluj • Tianjin

Editors
Dmitri Davydov
Department of Chemistry,
Washington State University
USA

Christiane Jung
KKS Ultraschall AG,
Ultrasonic Technology &
Surface Refinement
Switzerland

Editorial Office
MDPI
St. Alban-Anlage 66
4052 Basel, Switzerland

This is a reprint of articles from the Special Issue published online in the open access journal *Biology* (ISSN 2079-7737) (available at: https://www.mdpi.com/journal/biology/special_issues/pressure-perturbation).

For citation purposes, cite each article independently as indicated on the article page online and as indicated below:

LastName, A.A.; LastName, B.B.; LastName, C.C. Article Title. *Journal Name* **Year**, *Volume Number*, Page Range.

ISBN 978-3-0365-4671-1 (Hbk)
ISBN 978-3-0365-4672-8 (PDF)

Contents

About the Editors vii

Preface to "Pressure Perturbation Approach in Biochemistry and Structural Biology. In memoriam of Dr. Gaston Hui Bon Hoa" ix

Dmitri R. Davydov, Christiane Jung, Gregory A. Petsko, Stephen G. Sligar and Jack A. Kornblatt
A Pathfinder in High-Pressure Bioscience: In Memoriam of Gaston Hui Bon Hoa
Reprinted from: *Biology* **2021**, *10*, 778, doi:10.3390/biology10080778 1

Kazuyuki Akasaka and Akihiro Maeno
Proteins in Wonderland: The Magical World of Pressure
Reprinted from: *Biology* **2022**, *11*, 6, doi:10.3390/biology11010006 9

Vincent Van Deuren, Yin-Shan Yang, Karine de Guillen, Cécile Dubois, Catherine Anne Royer, Christian Roumestand and Philippe Barthe
Comparative Assessment of NMR Probes for the Experimental Description of Protein Folding Pathways with High-Pressure NMR
Reprinted from: *Biology* **2021**, *10*, 656, doi:10.3390/biology10070656 19

Bixia Zhang, ChulHee Kang and Dmitri R. Davydov
Conformational Rearrangements in the Redox Cycling of NADPH-Cytochrome P450 Reductase from *Sorghum bicolor* Explored with FRET and Pressure-Perturbation Spectroscopy
Reprinted from: *Biology* **2022**, *11*, 510, doi:10.3390/biology11040510 33

Ryan W. Penhallurick and Toshiko Ichiye
Pressure Adaptations in Deep-Sea *Moritella* Dihydrofolate Reductases: Compressibility versus Stability
Reprinted from: *Biology* **2021**, *10*, 1211, doi:10.3390/biology10111211 61

Nisrine Jahmidi-Azizi, Rosario Oliva, Stewart Gault, Charles S. Cockell and Roland Winter
The Effects of Temperature and Pressure on Protein-Ligand Binding in the Presence of Mars-Relevant Salts
Reprinted from: *Biology* **2021**, *10*, 687, doi:10.3390/biology10070687 73

Hussein Kaddour, Honorine Lucchi, Guy Hervé, Jacques Vergne and Marie-Christine Maurel
Kinetic Study of the Avocado Sunblotch Viroid Self-Cleavage Reaction Reveals Compensatory Effects between High-Pressure and High-Temperature: Implications for Origins of Life on Earth
Reprinted from: *Biology* **2021**, *10*, 720, doi:10.3390/biology10080720 89

Judit Somkuti, Orsolya Réka Molnár, Anna Grád and László Smeller
Pressure Perturbation Studies of Noncanonical Viral Nucleic Acid Structures
Reprinted from: *Biology* **2021**, *10*, 1173, doi:10.3390/biology10111173 101

Tigran V. Chalikian and Robert B. Macgregor, Jr.
Volumetric Properties of Four-Stranded DNA Structures
Reprinted from: *Biology* **2021**, *10*, 813, doi:10.3390/biology10080813 115

Fumiyoshi Abe
Molecular Responses to High Hydrostatic Pressure in Eukaryotes: Genetic Insights from Studies on *Saccharomyces cerevisiae*
Reprinted from: *Biology* **2021**, *10*, 1305, doi:10.3390/biology10121305 133

About the Editors

Dmitri R. Davydov

Dmitri R. Davydov, Ph.D., currently holds an Adjunct position in the Department of Chemistry at Washington State University (Pullman, WA, USA). He is an enzymologist, biophysicist, and biochemist with over 40 years of experience in molecular enzymology, protein biophysics, and high-pressure bioscience. He obtained his Master's degree in 1978 from Moscow State University and Ph.D. in biochemistry in 1982 from Russian State Medical University (Moscow, Russia). During his career, Dr. Davydov has worked in several leading research institutions in Russia, France, and the United States. His research has always been directed towards understanding the mechanisms of protein–protein and enzyme–substrate interactions in cytochromes P450 and exploring protein conformational dynamics related to the mechanisms of their function and regulation. In 1991–1993, during his fellowship in the group of Dr. Gaston Hui Bon Hoa (INSERM Unite 310, Paris, France), Dr. Davydov became involved in the studies of protein transitions with high hydrostatic pressures. Since then, pressure perturbation approaches have remained an essential ingredient of his research strategy. In his current research, Dr. Davydov focuses on the systems biochemistry of drug metabolism and the mechanisms of functional integration in the human cytochrome P450 ensemble.

Christiane Jung

Christiane Jung, PD Dr. habil., is currently the Senior Scientist at KKS Ultraschall AG, Ultrasonic Technology & Surface Refinement; Medical Surface Center, Switzerland. She studied chemistry at the Humboldt University in Berlin, Germany; received a Ph.D. in theoretical chemistry and a habilitation degree in physical biochemistry. She was also a lecturer for theoretical biochemistry at the University of Potsdam, Germany, for 10 years. She did the basic research in cytochrome P450 biophysics for more than 30 years at academic institutes in Germany and has held Visiting Researcher and Associated Professor positions at the University of Illinois, Urbana-Champaign, and at the Institut de Biologie Physico-Chimique, INSERM, U310, Paris. In Paris, in the laboratory of Dr. Gaston Hui Bon Hoa, she performed biophysical studies on cytochromes P450 using the high hydrostatic pressure approach. Since 2005, she has been involved in applied research in the MedTech industry in Switzerland, on the surface treatment of titanium implants. Her general scientific interests are protein biophysics, spectroscopy, cytochromes P450, effects of hydrostatic pressure, and ultrasound on biological materials. Recent research and projects in the industry are focused on surface treatment, functionalizing, and ultrasonic cleaning of medical devices for traumatology, orthopedics, and dentistry.

Preface to "Pressure Perturbation Approach in Biochemistry and Structural Biology. In memoriam of Dr. Gaston Hui Bon Hoa"

This Special Issue is devoted to the effects of hydrostatic pressure on biological systems and the use of these effects for exploring the structure and function of biological macromolecules and their ensembles. Hydrostatic pressure, a fundamental thermodynamic parameter, profoundly affects the conformation of proteins and nucleic acids and biological membrane structure. It is widely used in protein biophysics and mechanistic enzymology as a tool for exploring protein conformational landscapes through displacing protein conformational equilibria and affecting protein–protein and protein–ligand interactions. Pressure perturbation spectroscopy and calorimetry complemented by ultrasound velocity measurements are indispensable for studying protein solvation and its role in enzyme functionality. The effects of hydrostatic pressure on proteins, nucleic acids, and biomembranes are also critical for understanding the mechanisms of piezophilic adaptation that allows deep-sea species (piezophiles) to survive at extreme pressures of ocean depth. In some sense, structural consequences of evolutionary adaptation to high hydrostatic pressure may be viewed as the effects of pressure perturbation imprinted in the structure of pressure-adapted biological systems.

Despite a plethora of experimental papers and a dozen fundamental reviews devoted to the effects of pressure on biological systems, this important field appears to be severely underrepresented in modern literature. This Special Issue has been launched to bring together the most important new findings and concepts in high-pressure biosciences and promote researchers' interest in the unique exploratory potential of the pressure perturbation approach for biochemistry, biophysics, mechanistic enzymology, and evolutionary biology.

We devote this Special Issue to the memory of Gaston Hui Bon Hoa, French biophysicist, our friend and colleague, who passed away in July 2020. Gaston was one of the pioneers studying the effects of hydrostatic pressure on proteins, nucleic acids, and their assemblies. He devoted over 40 years in his scientific career to establishing pressure perturbation approaches and applying them in studies of protein structure and function. Gaston was internationally recognized as a leading expert in high-pressure biophysics.

Dmitri Davydov and Christiane Jung

Editors

biology MDPI

Editorial

A Pathfinder in High-Pressure Bioscience: In Memoriam of Gaston Hui Bon Hoa

Dmitri R. Davydov [1,*], Christiane Jung [2,*], Gregory A. Petsko [3], Stephen G. Sligar [4] and Jack A. Kornblatt [5]

1 Department of Chemistry, Washington State University, Pullman, CA 99164-4630, USA
2 KKS Ultraschall AG, Medical Surface Center, 6422 Steinen, Switzerland
3 Ann Romney Center for Neurologic Diseases, Department of Neurology, Harvard Medical School and Brigham & Women's Hospital, Boston, MA 02115, USA; gpetsko@bwh.harvard.edu
4 Department of Chemistry, University of Illinois, Urbana, IL 61801, USA; s-sligar@illinois.edu
5 Department of Biology, Concordia University, Montréal, QC H4B 1R6, Canada; Jack.Kornblatt@concordia.ca
* Correspondence: d.davydov@wsu.edu (D.R.D.); christiane.jung@kks-ultraschall.ch (C.J.)

On 26 July 2020, our colleague and friend Dr. Gaston Hui Bon Hoa passed away. Gaston was an enthusiastic scientist. He was one of the pioneers studying the effects of hydrostatic pressure on proteins, nucleic acids, and their assemblies. He devoted over 40 years of his scientific career to establishing pressure perturbation approaches and applying them in the study of protein structure and function. We dedicate this Special Issue to the memory of Gaston Hui Bon Hoa.

Gaston Hui Bon Hoa was born on 13 May 1934 in Ku Lang Su, China. Gaston's family originated from the Chinese Fujian province but had French citizenship since 1887 and resided in Vietnam. By the end of the French presence in Indochina, most of his family members had migrated to France. Gaston Hui Bon Hoa arrived in Paris with his parents and brother in August 1951. Here, he attended a state school. In 1956 Gaston enrolled at the Department of Physics at the Faculty of Science, Paris-Sorbonne University. In 1962, he received his license (B.S.) diploma in physics and electronics from the University Paris XI (Orsay).

Citation: Davydov, D.R.; Jung, C.; Petsko, G.A.; Sligar, S.G.; Kornblatt, J.A. A Pathfinder in High-Pressure Bioscience: In Memoriam of Gaston Hui Bon Hoa. *Biology* **2021**, *10*, 778. https://doi.org/10.3390/biology10080778

Received: 9 August 2021
Accepted: 12 August 2021
Published: 16 August 2021

Most of Gaston's scientific carrier was associated with the Institute of Physical-Chemical Biology (Institut de Biologie Physico-Chimique, IBPC, Paris, France). In 1965, he joined the Department of Bio-Spectroscopy at IBPC, headed by Professor Pierre Douzou, as a Research Fellow. In 1974 Gaston obtained his Ph.D. degree from the University Paris XI for the study "Establishing experimental conditions for low-temperature studies of proteins" supervised by Professor Pierre Douzou. Gaston continued his carrier under Prof. Douzou's mentorship as a permanent staff member of the National Institute of Health and Medical Research (INSERM, Unité 310) (Figure 1). During a sabbatical year, 1977–1978, Gaston visited the laboratory of Professor Irvin C. Gunsalus at the University of Illinois Urbana-Champaign, where he became involved in studying cytochrome P450 [1,2]. This enzyme played a central role in his research in the following years. After receiving several promotions, in 1992, Gaston was appointed the INSERM Research Director (Directeur de Research, DR1). After his retirement in 2000, Gaston continued his scientific work as an Emeritus Director of Research in INSERM, Unité 779, Le Kremlin Bicêtre.

The predominant part of Gaston's scientific heritage is devoted to the effects of hydrostatic pressure on proteins and their use in the studies of protein conformational dynamics and function. His first publication in this field, "High-pressure spectrometry at sub-zero temperatures," appeared in 1982 [3]. In this paper, Gaston and his co-authors describe the high-pressure optical cell of their construction and report the results of their pioneering study on the effects of pressure on the spin equilibrium of cytochrome P450. Since then, the idea of using pressure to displace protein conformational equilibria and perturb protein–solvent interactions became the keynote of Gaston's research. Likewise, cytochrome P450 became the main object for Gaston's studies for over 20 years. Gaston's research on the effects of hydrostatic pressure on substrate binding, equilibria of heme iron ligation, and the protein–protein interactions of cytochromes P450 [4–13] has become a part of the golden fund of cytochrome P450 science and has served as a prototype for pressure perturbation studies in other laboratories. Another essential part of Gaston's heritage is a series of studies on cytochrome c oxidase and its interactions with cytochrome c in collaboration with Jack Kornblatt [14–16]. During the most recent years, Gaston applied pressure perturbation to the studies of neuroglobin and other globins [17–19] and viroid RNA [20,21]. Regardless of the subject of Gaston's research, his experimental approaches have always been distinguishable by their inventive design and innovative research strategies. The list of Gaston's scientific publications includes over 150 experimental and review papers in reputable scientific journals. He attended various scientific congresses as a participant and keynote speaker (Figure 2).

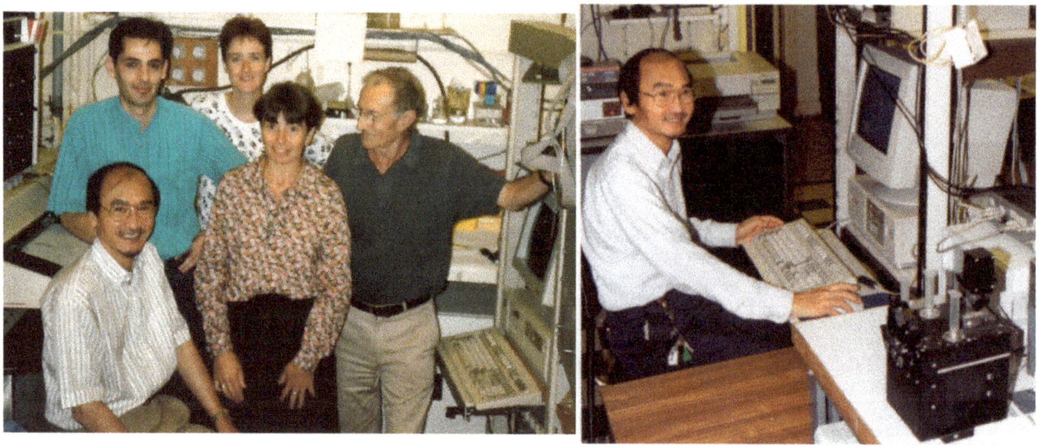

Figure 1. Gaston Hui Bon Hoa at the Institute of Physico-Chemical Biology (Paris, France). **Left**: Laboratory of Prof. Pierre Douzou (INSERM Unité 310). Front row: Gaston Hui Bon Hoa, Pascale Debey, Pierre Douzou. Back row: Carmelo Di Primo, Sylvie Le Bihan. Summer 1992, Paris, France. **Right**: Gaston Hui Bon Hoa at his workplace, November 1996.

Besides being a prominent scientist, Gaston was distinguished by his remarkable engineering skills. Since the experimental equipment that he needed for his innovative studies had not yet been (and remains not to be) commercially available, he designed and built research instruments by himself. The list of unique equipment built by Gaston in his laboratory in Paris includes thermostatically controlled high-pressure optical cells withstanding pressures up to 6 kbar, pressure jump and high-pressure stop-flow devices, and photoacoustic spectrophotometer.

In the European Union Biotechnology Program projects, Gaston collaborated with many laboratories in Germany, France, and the United Kingdom. He also coordinated two multilateral research grants funded by the International Association for Cooperation with Scientists from the former Soviet Union (INTAS). The list of Gaston's collaborators includes such scientists as Gregory A. Petsko (Wayne State University, Detroit, MI, USA), Jack and Judith Kornblatt (Concordia University Montreal, Quebec, QC, Canada); Stephen G. Sligar (University of Illinois, Urbana, IL, USA); Dmitri R. Davydov (Institute of Biomedical Chemistry, Moscow, Russia); Christiane Jung (Max Delbrück Centrum for Molecular Medicine, Berlin, Germany); and many more.

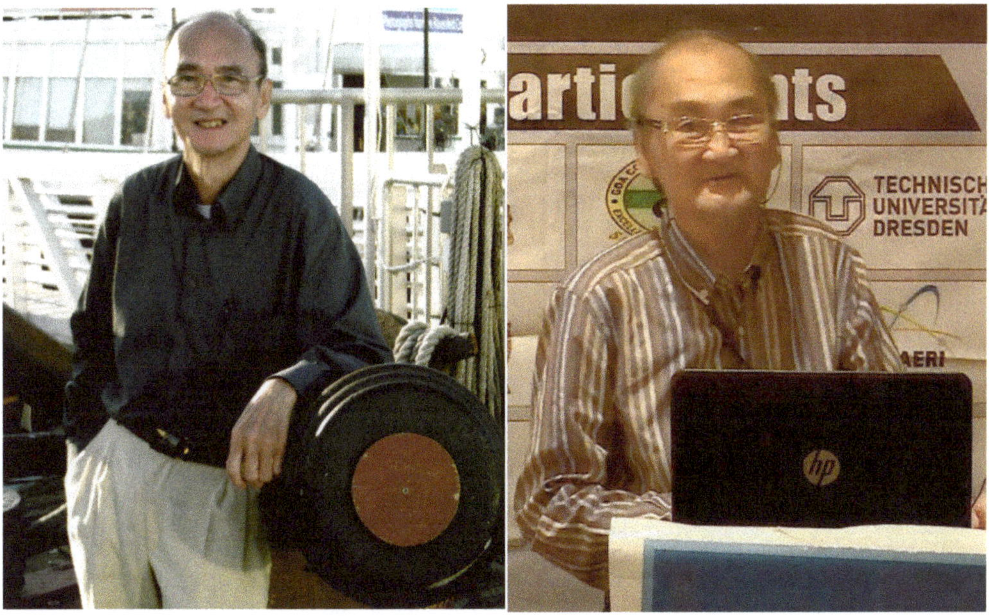

Figure 2. Gaston Hui Bon Hoa at Scientific Meetings. **Left**: A photo taken during the Fifth International Conference on High-Pressure Biosciences and Biotechnology (San Diego, CA, USA, September 2008). **Right**: Gaston presents his talk at the 7th Asia-Pacific Biotech Congress (Beijing, China, July 2015, Available online: https://www.youtube.com/watch?v=-4vs2mvqSGs (accessed on 18 July 2021)).

Below we give the floor to some of Gaston's collaborators and friends to allow them to share their memories about this remarkable scientist.

Gregory A. Petsko

He was one of the nicest human beings I ever knew. He was also a brilliant experimentalist, with some of the best hands I have ever seen and a keen instinct for doing just the right experiment.

When you are a young scientist, it is impossible to overstate the importance of your intellectual growth and self-esteem that come about when an older scientist takes an interest in you, teaches you, and encourages your own ideas. During my time in Prof. Pierre Douzou's lab as an EMBO fellow in 1973, I benefited from just such interest not only from Pierre but also from Gaston. I had been a protein crystallography graduate student, so much of what I know about studying proteins in solution, including enzyme kinetics, I learned at the bench from Gaston. He probably never had a more willing—and more inept—pupil. However, a more patient, generous, and able teacher one could not have asked for.

We were trying to measure enzyme reactions in aqueous–organic media at subzero temperatures so that we could trap kinetically significant intermediates and characterize them spectroscopically [22]. My dream, which he shared, was that, ultimately, I could use these same techniques, pioneered by him and Pierre, to accumulate such intermediates in enzyme crystals so that their structures could be determined at atomic resolution. That dream was fully realized twenty-seven years later, when Steve Sligar, Dagmar Ringe, Ilme Schlichting, and I successfully determined the three-dimensional structures of every kinetically significant intermediate in the very enzyme Gaston had taught me about those many years before, cytochrome P450.

The past never ceases to call to us, and if we heed that call, it can summon up bad memories as well as good ones. I have nothing but the best memories of my time in Paris, my time before striking out on my own as a scientist, and my time with Gaston Hui Bon Hoa. My life is so much better for having known him.

Stephen G. Sligar

In science, it is the interpersonal connections that define opportunities and career paths. When I was a graduate student in physics at the University of Illinois, wandering into the Biochemistry Department led me to meet I. C. Gunsalus or Gunny. A giant in microbiology and biochemistry, he was a close friend with Marianne Grunberg-Manago and Pierre Douzou at the Institute de Biologie Physico Chimique (IBPC). Thus, when I was a tenured professor, I sought Gunny's advice as to where to spend a sabbatical year—and his suggestion was Paris, IPBC, and Pierre's laboratory.

Through some magic of these greats, I received a Fullbright Fellowship in 1989 to support the move of our family to Paris. After arriving, I learned my de jour mentor was a most energetic Gaston Hui Bon Hoa. What a great time scientifically and a most memorable personal life experience. Never, to this day, have I met anyone with such boundless energy and enthusiasm for doing experiments. Gaston would always prefer to do another experiment than write anything up for publication. His filing cabinets were full of so much data that, at any point, if one wanted a manuscript, you just went to the cabinet, pulled out a folder, and started writing. The IBPC was such a motivating place that we returned for several summers after the sabbatical. We formed partnerships with Jack and Judy Kornblatt, Dimitri Davydov, Christiane Jung, and others. This family spawned many discoveries. One memorable idea was hatched at a group wine event on the top floor of the IBPC. We were discussing water under pressure and then the osmotic forces that can act to desolvate. One problem facing molecular biologists was the "star" activity of restriction endonucleases. A list of solutions to avoid to prevent the loss of 6-base pair recognition was at the back of every catalog. After a lot of wine, it occurred to us that these were all osmolytes. Several pioneering papers ensued, showing that osmotic pressure indeed removed bridging hydrogen bonding water between protein and the outer base pairs that could be reversed by applying hydrostatic pressure!

Gaston was unique and a source of motivation and companionship that is missed by all. He continued doing experiments after IBPC, working with Mike Marden, and thinking of new ways to advance biophysics through careful measurement. A real pioneer!

Jack A. Kornblatt

How do I remember our love affair with IBPC, Pierre Douzou, and most especially, with Gaston Hui Bon Hoa? It was in June 1982 when I and Judy, my wife, arrived in Paris from Cap d'Ail after a month at a French-language school. It was cold and raining heavily. We were wet and tired when we eventually came to our apartment and went back down to the bar on the rez de chaussee, where we tried to calm down with a large brandy each. A very inauspicious beginning to a wonderful year!

I went on up the street to IBPC and was introduced to Gaston Hui Bon Hoa, with whom I would work that year and during the summers in subsequent years. I had come to do low-temperature studies on the cytochrome c oxidase. However, Pierre explained that Gaston had just finished building a high-pressure optical cell (la bombe) that could be interfaced with a spectrophotometer or fluorometer. I put the oxidase into Gaston's "la bombe" and was hooked. The world's most exciting data poured out. The influence of high hydrostatic pressure on the oxidase was phenomenal. It allowed the catching and trapping of the intermediates with very large volume changes and helped us point out the energy transduction mechanism. All throughout this, Gaston guided my hands.

Later, when Steve Sligar came into the lab, he brought the beautiful structure of cytochrome P450cam. After staring at it for days, it finally occurred to me that osmolytes worked by reducing the activity of water and that it might be one of the reasons why they aid camphor in gaining access to a water-filled pocket. This realization launched me to finally complete the description of the energy transduction and catalytic cycles of the oxidase. The papers wrote themselves.

Very recently (2008), the team at Cornell developed high-pressure SAXS. Were Gaston with us today, he would be incredibly excited. "I have to try it out on P450cam", he would have said. He was a man with boundless enthusiasm and energy, and he happily shared it.

At the beginning of this overlong appreciation, I used the term love affair. It was just that. Additionally, by the way, 20 years later, I finally got to do the low-temperature work that I had initially planned!

Christiane Jung

During my research stay in the laboratory of Professor Irvin C. Gunsalus at the University of Illinois at Urbana-Champaign in 1982, I heard that there was a talented scientist in the INSERM laboratory of Professor Pierre Douzou at the Institute de Biology Physico-Chimique (IBPC) in Paris who was setting-up subzero-temperature and high-hydrostatic pressure equipment for studying the conformational behavior of cytochrome P450. His name was Gaston Hui Bon Hoa. I met Gaston personally for the first time in 1991 during my two-month stay as a visiting scientist in the laboratory of Professor Pierre Douzou. I was impressed by the enthusiasm with which Gaston built the experimental equipment. Our studies focused on cytochrome P450—the enzyme I had been working on since 1973 in Professor Klaus Ruckpaul's group at the Academy of Sciences in Berlin and which remained the main object of studies in my own laboratory at the Max Delbrück Centrum for Molecular Medicine in Berlin later [11]. The high-pressure approach used by Gaston encouraged me to keep working together. During another seven-month stay in Gaston's laboratory in 1993, we worked together with B. Canny and J.C. Chervin from the Université Pierre et Marie Curie Paris, Laboratoire de Physique des Milieux Condensés, to design a high-pressure cell with sapphire anvils, which we later used in Berlin for FTIR spectroscopic investigations on the carbon monoxide complex of cytochromes P450 [23]. Gaston visited my laboratory in Berlin several times as a participant in the EU project BIO2-942060. Looking back, I have to say that without Gaston, I would not have been able to establish high-pressure technology on my own.

In addition to being an inspiring scientist, Gaston was a good friend and, as I realized, a great family man. I fondly remember a trip with his family in 1991 to the Pont de Normandie near Le Havre and Honfleur, a beautiful little French port town in Normandy near the Seine estuary in the English Channel. In addition, I had the pleasure of attending his 80th birthday party in Paris seven years ago. I will always remember Gaston.

Dmitri R. Davydov

I first met Gaston Hui Bon Hoa at the international conference on Cytochromes P450 in Moscow in 1991. At that moment, the focus of my studies was (and remains to be) on the catalytic mechanisms and the protein–protein interactions of cytochromes P450. I knew very little about the effects of hydrostatic pressure on proteins and their use in biophysical studies. Still, I knew Gaston's name from his publications on the impact of pressure on P450cam [7,24]. My attention was drawn to Gaston's presentation at the meeting. It spurred my interest in the use of pressure perturbation. I got captivated by his enthusiasm and ideas on how pressure perturbation may be used in P450 research. Soon, I joined his research group in the laboratory of Pierre Douzou in IBPC in Paris as an INSERM fellow ("poste verte"). It was a wonderful time. I enjoyed the creative atmosphere in the lab and admired Gaston's engineering ingenuity. Besides researching pressure-induced transitions in P450 2B4 (which I brought from my lab in Moscow) [5,25], I also participated in Gaston's engineering efforts. I designed data acquisition and analysis software for high-pressure spectroscopy, which became a core of my SpectraLab software that I still use in my research. At the end of my fellowship, we were successful in acquiring an INSERM collaborative grant followed by an INTAS multilateral research grant. This funding allowed us to continue our collaboration [9,26,27]. From 1993 to 1999, I enjoyed visiting Gaston's lab several times a year. After my move to the US, our collaboration continued [6], and in 2002, Gaston visited me in the University of Texas Medical Branch (UTMB, Galveston, TX) to install his high-pressure equipment, which I still use in my research. Later, we met several times in San Diego, Paris, and other places. Owing to my collaboration with

Gaston, pressure perturbation became an integral part of my research strategy, and the effects of pressure on proteins became another focus of my scientific interests. I enjoyed our collaboration and friendship a lot. Besides being a talented experimentalist and prominent scientist, he was also a wonderful person and a good friend.

Collaboration with Gaston became momentous and life-defining for many of his colleagues and friends. Gaston's ingenuity and enthusiasm swept them along with him and promoted the development of high-pressure bioscience all over the world. So, let this Special Issue become our tribute to this impassioned pathfinder, a talented scientist, and great friend.

Author Contributions: Writing—original draft preparation, D.R.D., C.J., G.A.P., S.G.S., J.A.K.; writing—review and editing, D.R.D. and C.J. All authors have read and agreed to the published version of the manuscript.

Institutional Review Board Statement: Not applicable.

Informed Consent Statement: Not applicable.

Data Availability Statement: Not applicable.

Acknowledgments: The authors are grateful to Marie Pascale Debey (Museum National d'Histoire Naturelle, Paris, France) and Carmelo Di Primo (L'Institut Européen de Chimie et de Biologie (IECB), Bordeaux, France) for their help with finding illustrative material for this publication.

Conflicts of Interest: The authors declare no conflict of interest.

References

1. Hui Bon Hoa, G.; Begard, E.; Debey, P.; Gunsalus, I.C. Two univalent electron transfers from putidaredoxin to bacterial cytochrome p-450 at subzero temperature. *Biochemistry* **1978**, *17*, 2835–2839. [CrossRef]
2. Lange, R.; Hui Bon Hoa, G.; Debey, P.; Gunsalus, I.C. Spin transition of camphor-bound cytochrome P-450. 2. Kinetics following rapid changes of the local pa_H at sub-zero temperatures. *Eur. J. Biochem.* **1979**, *94*, 491–496. [CrossRef]
3. Hui Bon Hoa, G.; Douzou, P.; Dahan, N.; Balny, C. High-pressure spectrometry at subzero temperatures. *Anal. Biochem.* **1982**, *120*, 125–135. [CrossRef]
4. Martinis, S.A.; Blanke, S.R.; Hager, L.P.; Sligar, S.G.; Hui Bon Hoa, G.; Rux, J.J.; Dawson, J.H. Probing the heme iron coordination structure of pressure-induced cytochrome P420(cam). *Biochemistry* **1996**, *35*, 14530–14536. [CrossRef] [PubMed]
5. Davydov, D.R.; Deprez, E.; Hui Bon Hoa, G.; Knyushko, T.V.; Kuznetsova, G.P.; Koen, Y.M.; Archakov, A.I. High-pressure-induced transitions in microsomal cytochrome P450 2B4 in solution—Evidence for conformational inhomogeneity in the oligomers. *Arch. Biochem. Biophys.* **1995**, *320*, 330–344. [CrossRef]
6. Davydov, D.R.; Halpert, J.R.; Renaud, J.P.; Hui Bon Hoa, G. Conformational heterogeneity of cytochrome P450 3A4 revealed by high pressure spectroscopy. *Biochem. Biophys. Res. Commun.* **2003**, *312*, 121–130. [CrossRef] [PubMed]
7. Hui Bon Hoa, G.; Di Primo, C.; Dondaine, I.; Sligar, S.G.; Gunsalus, I.C.; Douzou, P. Conformational changes of cytochromes P-450cam and P-450lin induced by high pressure. *Biochemistry* **1989**, *28*, 651–656. [CrossRef]
8. Kornblatt, J.A.; Hui Bon Hoa, G.; Eltis, L.; Mauk, A.G. The effects of pressure on porphyrin cytochrome c-cytochrome b5 complex formation. *J. Am. Chem. Soc.* **1988**, *110*, 5909–5911. [CrossRef]
9. Renaud, J.P.; Davydov, D.R.; Heirwegh, K.P.M.; Mansuy, D.; Hui Bon Hoa, G. Thermodynamic studies of substrate binding and spin transitions in human cytochrome P-450 3A4 expressed in yeast microsomes. *Biochem. J.* **1996**, *319*, 675–681. [CrossRef]
10. Diprimo, C.; Deprez, E.; Hui Bon Hoa, G.; Douzou, P. Antagonistic effects of hydrostatic-pressure and osmotic-pressure on cytochrome P-450(cam) spin transition. *Biophys. J.* **1995**, *68*, 2056–2061. [CrossRef]
11. Jung, C.; Hui Bon Hoa, G.; Davydov, D.; Gill, E.; Heremans, K. Compressibility of the heme pocket of substrate-analog complexes of cytochrome P450cam-CO—The effect of hydrostatic-pressure on the Soret band. *Eur. J. Biochem.* **1995**, *233*, 600–606. [CrossRef]
12. Hui Bon Hoa, G.; McLean, M.A.; Sligar, S.G. High pressure, a tool for exploring heme protein active sites. *Biochim. Biophys. Acta* **2002**, *1595*, 297–308. [CrossRef]
13. Tschirret-Guth, R.A.; Koo, L.S.; Hui Bon Hoa, G.; de Montellano, P.R.O. Reversible pressure deformation of a thermophilic cytochrome P450 enzyme (CYP119) and its active-site mutants. *J. Am. Chem. Soc.* **2001**, *123*, 3412–3417. [CrossRef]
14. Kornblatt, J.A.; Hui Bon Hoa, G.; Heremans, K. Pressure-induced effects on cytochrome-oxidase—The aerobic steady-state. *Biochemistry* **1988**, *27*, 5122–5128. [CrossRef]
15. Kornblatt, J.A.; Hui Bon Hoa, G. A nontraditional role for water in the cytochrome c oxidase reaction. *Biochemistry* **1990**, *29*, 9370–9376. [CrossRef]
16. Kornblatt, J.A.; Kornblatt, M.J.; Hui Bon Hoa, G.; Mauk, A.G. Responses of two protein-protein complexes to solvent stress—Does water play a role at the interface. *Biophys. J.* **1993**, *65*, 1059–1065. [CrossRef]

17. Hamdane, D.; Kiger, L.; Hui Bon Hoa, G.; Dewilde, S.; Uzan, J.; Burmester, T.; Hankeln, T.; Moens, L.; Marden, M.C. High pressure enhances hexacoordination in neuroglobin and other globins. *J. Biol. Chem.* **2005**, *280*, 36809–36814. [CrossRef] [PubMed]
18. Hamdane, D.; Kiger, L.; Hui Bon Hoa, G.; Marden, M.C. Kinetics Inside the Protein: Shape of the Geminate Kinetics in Myoglobin. *J. Phys. Chem. B* **2011**, *115*, 3919–3923. [CrossRef]
19. Hamdane, D.; Vasseur-Godbillion, C.; Baudin-Creuza, V.; Hui Bon Hoa, G.; Marden, M.C. Reversible hexacoordination of alpha-hemoglobin-stabilizing protein (AHSP)/alpha-hemoglobin versus pressure—Evidence for protection of the alpha-chains by their chaperone. *J. Biol. Chem.* **2007**, *282*, 6398–6404. [CrossRef]
20. Hui Bon Hoa, G.; Kaddour, H.; Vergne, J.; Kruglik, S.G.; Maurel, M.-C. Raman characterization of Avocado Sunblotch viroid and its response to external perturbations and self-cleavage. *BMC Biophys.* **2014**, *7*, 1–15. [CrossRef]
21. Hui Bon Hoa, G.; Kruglik, S.G.; Maurel, M.-C. Impacts of the Extreme Conditons of Environments on RNA's structure and function from the Avocado Sunblotch Viroid: Applicaton of NIR-Raman Spectroscopy and ad hoc Baro-Bio-Reactor. *Acta Sci. Microbiol.* **2019**, *2*, 167–184.
22. Douzou, P.; Hui Bon Hoa, G.; Petsko, G.A. Protein crystallography at subzero temperatures: Lysozyme substrate complexes in cooled mixed solvents. *J. Mol. Biol.* **1975**, *96*, 367–380. [CrossRef]
23. Jung, C.; Canny, B.; Chervin, J.C.; Hui Bon Hoa, G. Heme pocket compressibility in P450cam-CO high pressure effect on the FTIR CO stretch mode. In *13th International Conference on Cytochromes P450: Biochemistry, Biophysics and Drug Metabolism*; Anzenbacher, P., Hudeček, J., Eds.; Monduzzi Editore—International Proceedings Division: Bologna, Italy, 2003; pp. 195–199.
24. Hui Bon Hoa, G.; Diprimo, C.; Geze, M.; Douzou, P.; Kornblatt, J.A.; Sligar, S.G. The formation of cytochrome P-450 from cytochrome P-420 is promoted by spermine. *Biochemistry* **1990**, *29*, 6810–6815. [CrossRef]
25. Davydov, D.R.; Knyushko, T.V.; Hui Bon Hoa, G. High-pressure induced inactivation of ferrous cytochrome P-450 LM2 (IIB4) CO complex—Evidence for the presence of 2 conformers in the oligomer. *Biochem. Biophys. Res. Commun.* **1992**, *188*, 216–221. [CrossRef]
26. Davydov, D.R.; Hui Bon Hoa, G.; Peterson, J.A. Dynamics of protein-bound water in the heme domain of P450BM3 studied by high-pressure spectroscopy: Comparison with P450cam and P450 2B4. *Biochemistry* **1999**, *38*, 751–761. [CrossRef]
27. Davydov, D.R.; Knyushko, T.V.; Kanaeva, I.P.; Koen, Y.M.; Samenkova, N.F.; Archakov, A.I.; Hui Bon Hoa, G. Interactions of cytochrome P450 2B4 with NADPH-cytochrome P450 reductase studied by fluorescent probe. *Biochimie* **1996**, *78*, 734–743. [CrossRef]

biology

MDPI

Article

Proteins in Wonderland: The Magical World of Pressure

Kazuyuki Akasaka [1,*] and Akihiro Maeno [2]

[1] Keihanna Academy of Science & Culture, Kansai Science City, Keihanna Interaction Plaza, Lab. Wing, Kyoto 619-0237, Japan

[2] Lab of Medical Chemistry, Kansai Medical University, 2-5-1 Shin-machi, Osaka 573-1010, Japan; maenoak@hirakata.kmu.ac.jp

* Correspondence: akasaka.kazuyuki.o06@kyoto-u.jp

Simple Summary: Unlike temperature, pH or chemical reagent, the effect of hydrostatic pressure on proteins is unique in that it controls selectively the equilibrium populations among different conformational states, without practically affecting each of their structures. Because of this unique effect of hydrostatic pressure on proteins, the application of pressure can easily manipulate the population distribution among different conformational states of a protein to a considerable extent at our will, creating what may be called "the magical world of pressure" or "the wonderland for proteins". In this paper, we have succssfully utilized the magical world of pressure in bringing the amyloid fibrils F of wild-type hen lysozyme into the unfolded monomers U and then, upon returning to the Anfinsen regime, back into its original, natively folded state N.

Abstract: Admitting the "Native", "Unfolded" and "Fibril" states as the three basic generic states of proteins in nature, each of which is characterized with its partial molar volume, here we predict that the interconversion among these generic states N, U, F may be performed simply by making a temporal excursion into the so called "the high-pressure regime", created artificially by putting the system under sufficiently high hydrostatic pressure, where we convert N to U and F to U, and then back to "the low-pressure regime" (the "Anfinsen regime"), where we convert U back to N (U→N). Provided that the solution conditions (temperature, pH, etc.) remain largely the same, the idea provides a general method for choosing N, U, or F of a protein, to a great extent at will, assisted by the proper use of the external perturbation pressure. A successful experiment is demonstrated for the case of hen lysozyme, for which the amyloid fibril state F prepared at 1 bar is turned almost fully back into its original native state N at 1 bar by going through the "the high-pressure regime". The outstanding simplicity and effectiveness of pressure in controlling the conformational state of a protein are expected to have a wide variety of applications both in basic and applied bioscience in the future.

Keywords: Anfinsen's dogma; native state N; unfolded state U; fibril state F; protofibrils; hydrostatic pressure; hen lysozyme; circular dichroism; ^{1}H NMR spectroscopy; atomic force microscopy

Citation: Akasaka, K.; Maeno, A. Proteins in Wonderland: The Magical World of Pressure. *Biology* **2022**, *11*, 6. https://doi.org/10.3390/biology11010006

Academic Editors: Dmitri Davydov, Christiane Jung and Martin Schröder

Received: 18 October 2021
Accepted: 16 December 2021
Published: 21 December 2021

1. Introduction

Thermodynamics is a fundamental branch of physics that all creatures on earth must obey to live. The well-known Anfinsen's dogma [1], governing the fate of a newborn polypeptide chain "U" to fold into a unique conformation "N" in an aqueous environment under physiological conditions, is a type of this example. Although certain proteins may need some help from other proteins called chaperones for folding, this process is not considered to alter the essence of Anfinsen's dogma. As such, the "Anfinsen's dogma" may possibly have prevailed on the earthy atmosphere for billions of years of evolution to bring up all (~10 million) archaea, prokaryote and eukaryote species considered to be living presently on earth [2]. On the other hand, by taking Anfinsen's dogma more generally from the thermodynamic and statistical mechanical viewpoint, we can view the unfolding and refolding process of protein as a shift of the conformational distribution induced by thermodynamic perturbation in an aqueous environment [3]. Here, pressure is a particularly important thermodynamic variable besides temperature and solution conditions in controlling the conformational state of a protein in an aqueous environment.

Experimental studies on the conformational state of proteins under pressure perturbation started early in the 1980s when Hui Bon Hoa contributed greatly to advancing various spectroscopic techniques under pressure and promoted their applications [4–6]. Protein high-pressure NMR spectroscopy, re-initiated by Jonas in the 1990s [7], was expanded into a crucial methodology to probe the fluctuating nature of protein structure in later years [8–12]. The method disclosed the notion that, in most globular proteins, the unfolded conformer U is always present in equilibrium with the folded conformer N, even under physiological conditions at 1 bar [8,9].

In accordance with this, an additional state of a protein sometimes called the "misfolded state" [13] has come to gain attention in a wide range of protein systems. It turns out that many of them grow into misfolded oligomers [14], which then turn into a fibrillar state commonly called "protofibrils", which consist of single or a few lines of a linear array of "unfolded" protein monomers forming "the cross β-structure", detailed features of which may vary from protein to protein [15,16]. Importantly, they are known to be the primary cause of a variety of human diseases known as "amyloidosis disease" including Alzheimer disease [17], familial amyloidotic polyneuropathy [18], transthyretin amyloidosis [19], prion disease [20], dialysis-related amyloidosis [21], alpha-synuclein amyloidosis [22] and senile systemic amyloidosis [23] and so on. Furthermore, as it is becoming increasingly clear that the propensity to form amyloid fibrils is a generic property for all proteins including food proteins, protein fibrillization is progressively recognized in food science as a strategy to broaden and improve food protein functionality [24].

Many of the amyloid diseases above arise from single mutations in their wild-type proteins, which often destabilize the N state and increase the equilibrium population of the U state; for example, we previously found in the V30M mutant of transthyretin, that the population of the U conformer increased by as much as 1000-fold, causing fatal amyloidosis [25]. The important point here is that, despite the fact that the protein obeys Anfinsen's dogma to fold, an equilibrium fraction of the protein may always remain unfolded in the cell environment. Then, a crucial question may remain as to how the unfolded state U may turn into the fibrillar state F when there is no substance to catalyze the reaction.

To answer this question, a model study was carried out previously [26], by using an authentic, fully (~100%) unfolded conformer of a protein, prepared from ^{15}N-labeled wild-type hen lysozyme with its four disulfide bonds removed (0SS mutant), to see if they would turn into a protofibril at all and if so, how would it proceed? We found that the protofibrils are formed simply by a prolonged incubation of its aqueous solution over several days at 25 °C at 1 bar [26]. We also found that the protofibrils so formed can then be dissociated back into the monomeric state U (U→F→U) nearly completely simply by applying pressure at 2 kbar for ~50 h [27]. Detailed analysis indicates that the reaction proceeds by a simple reaction, with monomers attached and/or detached at its growing end of the fibril [28]. We believe that the basic mechanisms disclosed here for the simplest system will form the basis for understanding the reality of the protofibril formation and dissociation U→F→U in most amyloidotic proteins.

Under the condition, the concept of the protein conformational regime under physiological conditions at low pressure ("Anfinsen regime") may be extended to include the amyloid fibril state "F" as another generic state of a globular protein in the low-pressure regime (or the Anfinsen regime), basically in dynamic equilibrium with the U and N states as schematically shown in Figure 1a. Here we define state F to be represented by "protofibrils", rather than the "matured amyloid fibrils" which may contain the insoluble entity.

An important property of F as well as of N is that they both are in a high-volume state [29], as they generally have extra space or "vacancy" (called void, cavity, or defects) within their basic architecture, while the state U exists in a low-volume state with most of the extra "vacancies" gone, leaving the polypeptide chain in direct contact with the bulk water. Because of these contrasting properties between U and N–F, their relative thermodynamic stabilities are anticipated to be reversed rather easily by applying a sufficiently high pressure (a few to several kbar).

Indeed, under a high hydrostatic pressure far exceeding 1 kbar (>1 kbar), both the folded conformation N and the fibril state F become less stable than U, fully reversing the order of thermodynamic stability predicted from Anfinsen's dogma in the low-pressure regime, namely U is more stable than N and F at elevated pressures, thereby forming what we call here "the high-pressure regime" (See Figure 1b). Note that "the high-pressure regime" is realizable relatively easily nowadays in high-pressure vessels in scientific laboratories and possibly in food industries where pressures up to several kbar are regularly used.

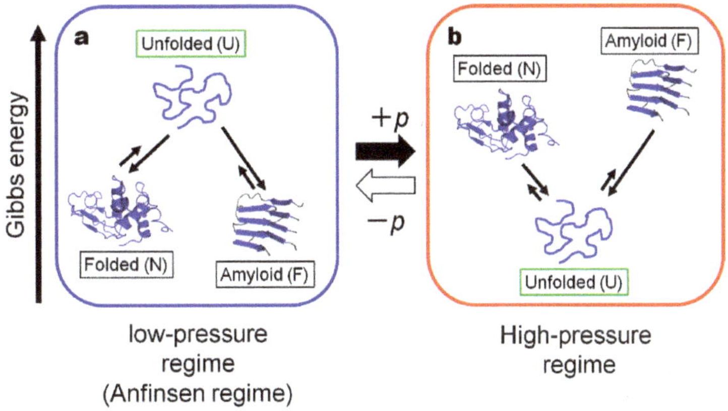

Figure 1. The schematic Gibbs energy diagrams for the proposed three generic forms of a protein; Folded (N), Unfolded (U) and Amyloid fibril (F): (**a**) in the "Anfinsen regime" or the low-pressure regime and (**b**) in the high-pressure regime. The "Anfinsen regime" is the regime realized in nature, while the high-pressure regime is the regime artificially realized in high-pressure vessels. Note that the thermodynamic stabilities of N, U and F are reversed in the two regimes, because of the large $p\Delta V$ contribution. Here the relative Gibbs energy levels for U, N and F are drawn arbitrarily.

2. Thermodynamic Consideration

2.1. In the "Anfinsen Regime" or the Low-Pressure Regime

The well-known Anfinsen's dogma [1], governing the fate of a newly born polypeptide chain U to fold into a unique conformation N, states in essence that, for most proteins in nature under physiological conditions (~at 1 bar), the Gibbs energy $G_U{}^0$ for the unfolded state U is higher than the Gibbs energy $G_N{}^0$ for the folded state N, namely, $\Delta G_{1bar} = \Delta G^0 = G_U{}^0 - G_N{}^0 > 0$, pushing the unfolded polypeptide chain "U" toward the folded state "N". Here for most globular proteins in nature, $\Delta G_{1bar} = \Delta G^0$ takes a small, but the positive value at 1 bar, often within a few tens of kJ/mol, leaving the state N marginally stable against the state U. Here we postulate "amyloid fibril state F" represented by protofibrils to be another generic state of a protein stable at low pressure, giving another minimum in free energy besides the native state N in the "Anfinsen regime".

2.2. In the "High-Pressure Regime"

At high pressure p, the thermodynamic stability of N against U, $\Delta G(p)$, is given approximately to the first order in p by Equation (1),

$$\Delta G(p) = G_U(p) - G_N(p) = \Delta G^0 + \Delta V\,(p - p^0) \quad (1)$$

Here the volume difference ΔV between U and N ($\Delta V = V_U - V_N$) is always negative under or below physiological temperatures [8], making the term $\Delta V\ (p - p^0)$ take a large negative value for large p. The high-volume nature of N against U has been well documented in many proteins. Then at high pressure, the negative $\Delta V\ (p - p^0)$ term (<0) exceeds in magnitude the positive ΔG^0 term (>0), resulting in a negative $\Delta G = G_U - G_N$ (<0), meaning that N turns into U causing "pressure-denaturation" of a protein.

In the case of a typical globular protein of a few kDa in size, the ΔV could be ~−100 mL/mol, making $p\Delta V$ to be ~−20 kJ/mol at 2 kbar and ~−30 kJ/mol at 3 kbar. If ΔG^0, the excess stability of N over U at 1 bar, is typically ~15 kJ/mol, $\Delta G(p)$ in Equation 1 would become ~−5 kJ/mol at 2 kbar and ~−15 kJ/mol at 3 kbar, replacing conformer N (~99.9%) at 1 bar by conformer U (>90%) at 2 kbar, (>99%) at 3 kbar, namely the relative stability of N and U in the Anfinsen regime is likely to be almost fully reversed in the "high-pressure regime" (Figure 1b). When pressure is removed (back to the Anfinsen regime), the state N will recover quickly and reversibly to the original population close to ~99%. Basically, such reversibility has been recognized in most globular proteins including RNase A, hen lysozyme, Staphylococcal nuclease, Apo myoglobin, β-lactoglobulin, P13MTCP1, transthyretin, prion proteins, and ubiquitin, at physiological temperatures or lower [9].

In the case of an amyloid fibril, its high-volume nature was revealed by the results of direct time-dependent densitometry measurement of protofibrils (F) upon its formation from (U) in the intrinsically denatured disulfide-deficient hen lysozyme, which showed a large volume increase by as much as $\Delta V \sim 570$ mL/mol monomer U [29]. The result suggests that the formation of F from U involves a formation of large voids or cavities and/or ionic bonds, in analogy to, or even more than the case for, the formation of N from U. Granting that a high volume is a general property of any amyloid fibrils, pressure is expected to destabilize F significantly against U ($\Delta G = G_U - G_F < 0$), because of the large negative $p\Delta V$ term in Equation (1). Now we can depict a schematic free energy diagram for F, N and U at high pressure in Figure 1b, where the relative stability of F, N and U is reversed from that in the Anfinsen regime at low pressure, the relative stability of N and F depends on the protein concentration among other factors. We may call the regime represented by the scheme in Figure 1b the "high-pressure-regime", which is a fully artificial regime of protein thermodynamics that apparently has not been experienced by most living creatures in their history on earth.

Thus, by switching between the "high-pressure-regime" and the "Anfinsen" regime simply by turning the pressure on and off, we would get a magical power for selecting the conformational state of a protein among N, F and U to a great extent at will. A successful experiment in freely controlling the conformational state among N, F and U will be demonstrated below in the experiment with wild-type hen lysozyme as representative. Here we will demonstrate the nearly full conversion (>90%) of the fibrils (F) back into the folded state (N), simply by temporarily visiting "the magical world of pressure" (the high-pressure regime) and back to the Anfinsen regime (the low-pressure regime).

3. Materials and Methods

Preparation of amyloid fibrils: Lyophilized hen egg white lysozyme (crystallized six-times) was purchased from Seikagaku Kogyo (Tokyo, Japan) and used without further purification. To prepare the amyloid fibrils consisting largely of intact (i.e., non-degraded) hen lysozyme, we used the "seeding method" reported previously in the literature [30]. This seeding method is briefly mentioned as follows. As the first step, the powder of wild type hen lysozyme was dissolved to a final concentration of 8.0 mg/mL in distilled water containing 80 mM NaCl with pH adjusted to 2.2 by HCl, and the solution was incubated at 57 °C, which is close to the transition temperature of hen lysozyme. In the association process to amyloid fibrils of hen lysozyme, the exponential increase in thioflavin T (Th T) fluorescence intensity with increasing incubation time was observed (Figure S1a). After ~11 days, the resultant amyloid fibrils as the first generation was subjected to extensive sonication to produce oligomers, an aliquot of which (10 *w*/*w* %) was mixed into a fresh solution of 90 *w/w* % of intact hen lysozyme (8.0 mg/mL in 80 mM NaCl at pH 2.2) and incubated for 4.5 h at 57 °C. The second-generation fibrils produced in this way were subjected to extensive sonication to produce seeds. Then, an aliquot of these seeds (4 *w/w* %) was mixed with a fresh solution of 96 *w/w* % of intact hen lysozyme (8.0 mg/mL in 80 mM NaCl at pH 2.2) and incubated for 4.5 h at 57 °C to produce the third-generation fibrils consisting almost entirely of intact hen lysozyme molecules, supported by the analysis of SDS-PAGE showing the non-degradation of intact hen lysozyme in the period of fibrillation process (Figure S1b).

Dissociation of amyloid fibrils with pressure: The fibril solution of the third-generation was diluted by 20-fold to produce a fibril solution, containing 0.40 mg/mL fibrils in 80 mM NaCl, pH adjusted to 2.2. This fibril solution was then placed in a homemade Teflon inner vessel (volume~100 μL) and was pressurized at 4 kbar in a pressuring machine Dr. CHEF (KOBELCO, Kobe, Japan) for a varied reaction time between 0.5 and 24 h at 25 °C. After each reaction time, the fibril solution was subjected to the circular dichroism (CD) and ^{1}H NMR measurements without further dilution, while AFM measurements were made after dilution and drying by air on a silica surface. The ^{1}H NMR spectra were measured at 25 °C at 600 MHz on an AVANCE 600 NMR spectrometer (Bruker Biospin, Switzerland) using a standard 5 mm outer diameter tube (Shigemi, Tokyo, Japan). The CD spectra in the far UV region were measured at 25 °C on a J-820 spectropolarimeter (JASCO Co., Tokyo, Japan) using a sample cell of 0.1 cm light path after 1 h of pressure-treatment. The AFM images were obtained at 1 bar at 25 °C with the cyclic contact mode at a frequency of 119 kHz on an SPI-3800 (Seiko Instruments Inc., Tokyo, Japan).

4. Results

4.1. Experimental Demonstration: Turning Amyloid Fibrils "F" Back into the Folded State "N" in Hen Lysozyme

Then, by taking a well-known globular protein hen lysozyme as an example, we will present an actual experimental demonstrating the full conversion of hen lysozyme amyloid fibrils F into the original folded native conformation N by going through the "high-pressure regime"—the magical world of pressure.

The experimental procedure:

(1) N→U→F conversion in the Anfinsen regime: First, in the Anfinsen regime (at 1 bar), we convert the folded conformer N into the unfolded conformer U by heating hen lysozyme solution (8.0 mg/mL, pH 2.2) close to its transition temperature 57 °C at pH 2.2, and then convert U into amyloid fibrils F by seeding with lysozyme oligomers (see Materials and methods). The seeding procedure is repeated to prepare the final fibrils consisting almost exclusively of intact (non-degraded) hen lysozyme molecules.

(2) F→U conversion in the "high-pressure regime": Then, after diluting the fibril solution by 20-fold, we switch to the "high-pressure regime" by applying pressure at 4 kbar at 25 °C and turn the fibrils F into U (actually a mixture of a one-to-one ratio of N and U at 4 kbar) at 25 °C. The process of dissociation of the fibrils with a time of exposure to 4 kbar was step-wise monitored at 1 bar with AFM and ^{1}H NMR.

(3) U→N conversion in the Anfinsen regime: Then by lowering pressure to 1 bar, we switch back to the Anfinsen regime and complete the folding of U back to the original native conformer N at 25 °C (U→N conversion in the Anfinsen regime). The 20-fold dilution assures the pathway U to N rather than the pathway U to F, depending on the protein concentration, in the Anfinsen regime. Thus the entire conformational cycle of hen lysozyme, N→(U)→F→(U)→N, is to be completed.

4.2. The Experimental Result

Figure 2 summarizes the result of the experiment, which starts from N, goes into F, and then returns back to N, along the arrows N→(U)→F→(U)→N* (the asterisk * is to indicate a refolded N, through N and N* should be identical).

Here Figure 2a demonstrates the result with CD as a monitor for both fibrils and monomers, Figure 2b demonstrates the result with AFM as a monitor for fibrils, and Figure 2c demonstrates the result with ^{1}H NMR as a monitor for dissociated monomers from fibrils, all measured at 1 bar at 25 °C.

The far-UV CD spectra (Figure 2a) show that N, showing a characteristic α-rich structure (~30% of α-helix and ~20% of β-sheet) with a minimum at ~208 nm, is converted with an iso-dichroic point at ~211 nm to F, showing a characteristic β-rich structure with a minimum at ~218 nm, and back to the original N nearly completely with an iso-dichroic point at ~211 nm. The AFM figures (only detectable of fibrils) (Figure 2b) start from N with no images, then to F showing typical amyloid fibrils, and then back to N with all fibril images gone, consistent with the observation with CD. The ^{1}H NMR spectra (only detectable of monomers) start from the well-known N signals of hen lysozyme (~100%) (Figure 2c), and is converted to "F signals", actually a trace of the N signals that remain in equilibrium with F, and back to the N* signals showing nearly a full refolding into N (>90%). The time-dependent ^{1}H NMR signals (Figure 2d), monitored intermittently at 1 bar, after exposure of the fibril solution to 4 kbar for a certain period of time, show that the dissociation of the fibrils starts rapidly and is nearly complete within 1 h.

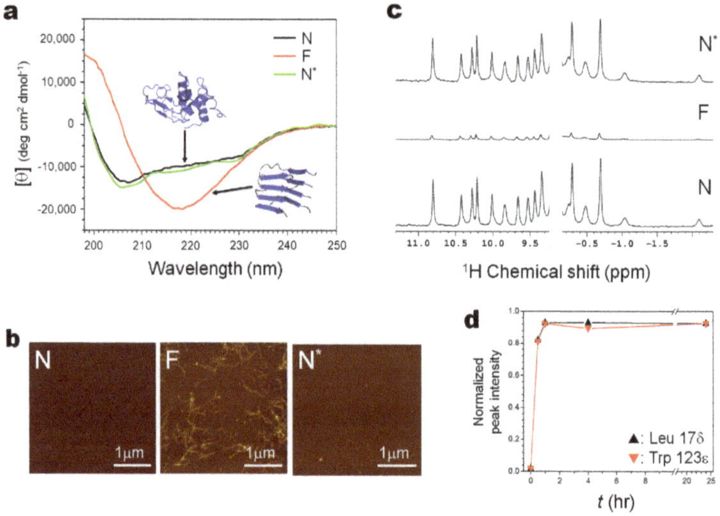

Figure 2. The conversion of the folded form (N) of wild-type hen lysozyme into the amyloid fibril form (F) and then refolding back to the folded form (N), by following the process N→(U)→F→(U)→N*. The experiments are monitored by CD (**a**), AFM (**b**) and ^{1}H NMR (**c**,**d**), all at 1 bar at 25 °C. (The refolded N is designated as N*, showing that it is a refolded N, although their conformations are identical). See Methods for detailed experimental procedures.

(Figure 2a) N→(U)→F→(U)→N* with CD as a monitor for both fibrils (F) and folded monomers (N). The far-UV CD spectra show that N, showing a characteristic β-rich structure with a minimum at ~208 nm (black), is converted with an iso-dichroic point at ~211 nm to F by seeding at 57 °C, showing a characteristic β-rich structure with a minimum at ~218 nm (red), and back to the original N nearly completely with an iso-dichroic point at ~211 nm (green).

(Figure 2b) N→(U)→F→(U)→N* with AFM as a monitor for fibrils (F). The AFM figures (only detectable of fibrils) start from N with no images, then to F showing typical amyloid fibrils, and then back to N with all fibril images gone, consistent with the observation with CD.

(Figure 2c) N→(U)→F→(U)→N* with ^{1}H NMR as a monitor for dissociated monomers. The ^{1}H NMR spectrum (only detectable of monomers) with all NMR peaks characteristic for N of hen lysozyme (~ 100% of an intact protein), is converted to "F" showing only a trace of signals of N (in equilibrium with N) and back to N* (after treatment for 24 h at 4 kbar at 25 °C) showing nearly full refolding into N (>90%).

(Figure 2d) F→(U)→N*, monitoring the dissociation of fibrils with the time-dependent ^{1}H NMR signals of the dissociated monomers, as the fibril solution is treated at 4 kbar at 25 °C for respective time intervals. The result shows that the dissociation is completed within 2 h.

5. Discussion

The example above demonstrates that we can, in fact, choose the conformational state of a protein among N, U and F in a simple and logical way, by temporarily visiting the "high-pressure regime", or "the magical world of pressure", which is surely realizable in high-pressure vessels, and by coming back to the Anfinsen regime to finish the dream. The high-pressure regime is an artificially created "WONDERLAND for protein" in which the relative conformational stability among N, F and U is largely reversed from that in the Anfinsen regime. Choice of the regime between the so-called "Anfinsen" and the "high-pressure" regime can be made simply by "switching pressure off or on" at an appropriate level of pressure.

An increasing number of proteins of physiological relevance have now been recognized as causing amyloidosis, a major hazard to human health in recent years. The formation of amyloidosis fibrils in vivo occurs as an irreversible process in a long time-range and is thought to be the cause of many hitherto incurable human diseases. However, as we have seen here, in a shorter time range, the amyloid fibril formation starts with the formation of protofibrils, which are in equilibrium with their monomeric counterpart and are dissociable under pressure. Thus, the combined use of the low pressure "Anfinsen" and the "high-pressure" regime as shown here, in the early phase of the disease, should have a potential utility in preventing and/or curing amyloid diseases. For the case of food-based amyloidosis, one promising example has been carried out for the fibrils of a prion disease, which are not only dissociated but efficiently degraded by proteinase K under pressure [31]. The result may promise some industrial and biomedical applications in the future. For the case of amyloidosis in human tissues, we might need to invent some new technologies for pressurizing a selective portion of the tissue or the fluid directly. Otherwise, the target tissue or fluid could be temporarily removed from the patient's body and returned after treatment with pressure, as partly realized for the eradication of malignant melanoma [32].

6. Conclusions

The "Anfinsen regime" where the "Anfinsen's dogma" operates has been a reality dominating the current biological world, assuring the prosperity and versatility for all lives on earth including humans, though with a constant danger of the proteins going into stable aggregates with no function. In contrast, the "high-pressure regime" proposed here as a counter regime is also a reality only realized at present in high-pressure vessels in scientific laboratories, in which proteins could temporarily escape from the burden of the Anfinsen's dogma. Through this regime, however, one can have a magical power of freeing the protein from forming amyloid fibrils and then back to the "Anfinsen regime" to promote folding back into the N state. The entire process from N to U to F and back from F to U to N has been successfully demonstrated here in the experiment with wild-type hen lysozyme as a model protein. To realize our dreams further into bio-scientific reality, our traveling into the wonderland of pressure will continue.

Supplementary Materials: The following is available online at: https://www.mdpi.com/article/10.3390/biology11010006/s1. Figure S1: (a) The NaCl concentration-dependent fibrillation process of 4.0 mg/mL hen lysozyme with 4%(w/w) seeds at pH 2.2 at 57 °C, monitored by thioflavin T fluorescence at 482 nm for the varied NaCl concentration of 4, 10, 20, 40 and 80 mM. (b) The SDS-

PAGE analysis of the products produced in the fibrillation reaction of wild-type hen lysozyme (4.0 mg/mL) in the presence of 4% (*w*/*w*) seeds in 80 mM NaCl, at pH 2.2 at 57 °C (cf. (a)) for the incubation times 0–10 h. Lane M is for molecular weight markers and Lane C is for authentic hen lysozyme (14.4 kDa).

Author Contributions: Conceptualization, K.A.; methodology, K.A. and A.M.; software, A.M.; validation, K.A. and A.M.; formal analysis, A.M.; investigation, A.M.; resources, K.A.; data curation, K.A. and A.M.; writing—original draft preparation, K.A. and A.M.; writing—review and editing, K.A.; visualization, K.A. and A.M.; supervision, K.A.; project administration, K.A.; funding acquisition, K.A. All authors have read and agreed to the published version of the manuscript.

Funding: This work was supported by Academic Frontier Program 07F010 of the Ministry of Education, Culture, Sports, Science and Technology of Japan, and the Japan Society for the Promotion of Science (KAKENHI, 22570164).

Institutional Review Board Statement: Not applicable.

Informed Consent Statement: Not applicable.

Data Availability Statement: Not applicable.

Acknowledgments: We thank B. R. Shah for his assistance in the NMR and AFM experiments.

Conflicts of Interest: The authors declare no conflict of interest. The funder had no role in the design of the study; in the collection, analyses, or interpretation of data; in the writing of the manuscript, or in the decision to publish the results.

References

1. Anfinsen, C.B. Principles that govern the folding of protein chains. *Science* **1973**, *181*, 223–230. [CrossRef]
2. Camilo, M.; Derek, P.T.; Sina, A.; Alastair, G.B.S.; Boris, W. How many species are there on earth and in the ocean? *PLoS Biol.* **2011**, *9*, e1001127. [CrossRef]
3. Hirata, F.; Sugita, M.; Yoshida, M.; Akasaka, K. Perspective: Structural fluctuation of protein and Anfinsen's thermodynamic hypothesis. *J. Chem. Phys.* **2018**, *14*, 020901. [CrossRef]
4. Hui Bon Hoa, G.; Douzou, P.; Dahan, N.; Balny, C. High-pressure spectrometry at sub-zero temperatures. *Anal. Biochem.* **1982**, *120*, 125–135. [CrossRef]
5. Hui Bon Hoa, G.; McLean, M.A.; Sligar, S.G. High pressure, a tool for exploring heme protein active sites. *Biochim. Biophys. Acta* **2002**, *1595*, 297–308. [CrossRef]
6. Davydov, D.R.; Hui Bon Hoa, G.; Peterson, J.A. Dynamics of protein-bound water in the heme domain of P450BM3 studied by high-pressure spectroscopy: Cobarrison with P450cam and P450 2B4. *Biochemistry* **1999**, *38*, 751–761. [CrossRef] [PubMed]
7. Jonas, J.; Jonas, A. High pressure NMR spectroscopy of proteins and membranes. *Ann. Rev. Biophys. Biomol. Struct.* **1994**, *23*, 287–318. [CrossRef]
8. Akasaka, K. Exploring the entire conformational space of proteins by high-pressure NMR. *Pure Appl. Chem.* **2003**, *75*, 927–936. [CrossRef]
9. Akasaka, K. Probing conformational fluctuation of proteins by pressure perturbation. *Chem Rev.* **2006**, *106*, 1814–1835. [CrossRef]
10. Kalbitzer, H.R. High pressure NMR methods for characterizing functional sub-states of proteins. *Subcell. Biochem.* **2015**, *72*, 179–197.
11. Akasaka, K. Protein Studies by High Pressure NMR. In *Experimental Approaches of NMR Spectroscopy;* The Nuclear Magnetic Resonance Society of Japan; Springer: Singapore, 2018; pp. 3–36.
12. Dubois, C.; Herrada, I.; Barthe, P.; Roumestand, C. Combining High-Pressure Perturbation with NMR Spectroscopy for a Structural and Dynamical Characterization of Protein Folding Pathways. *Molecules* **2020**, *25*, 5551. [CrossRef] [PubMed]
13. Dobson, C.M. Protein folding and misfolding. *Nature* **2003**, *426*, 884–890. [CrossRef]
14. Bemporad, F.; Chiti, F. Misfolded Oligomers: Experimental Approaches, Mechanism of Formation, and Structure-Toxicity Relationships. *Chem. Biol.* **2012**, *19*, 315–327. [CrossRef]
15. Fitzpatrick, A.W.P.; Debelouchina, G.T.; Bayro, M.J.; Clare, D.K.; Caporini, M.A.; Bajaj, V.S.; Jaroniec, C.P.; Wang, L.; Ladizhansky, V.; Müller, S.A.; et al. Atomic structure and hierarchical assembly of a cross-β amyloid fibril. *Proc. Natl. Acad. Sci. USA* **2013**, *110*, 5468–5473. [CrossRef] [PubMed]
16. Chiti, F.; Dobson, C.M. Protein misfolding, amyloid formation, and human disease: A summary of progress over the last decade. *Annu. Rev. Biochem.* **2017**, *86*, 27–68. [CrossRef]
17. Burns, A.; Iliffe, S. Alzheimer's disease. *BMJ* **2009**, *338*, b158. [CrossRef] [PubMed]
18. Araki, S.; Ando, Y. Transthyretin-related familial amyloidotic poly-neuropathy—Progress in Kumamoto, Japan (1967–2010). *Proc. Jpn. Acad. Ser. B* **2010**, *86*, 694–706. [CrossRef] [PubMed]

19. Yee, A.W.; Aldeghi, M.; Blakeley, M.P.; Ostermann, A.; Mas, P.J.; Moulin, M.; Sanctis, D.; Bowler, M.W.; Dieckmann, C.M.; Mitchell, E.P.; et al. A molecular mechanism for transthyretin amyloidogenesis. *Nat. Commun.* **2019**, *10*, 925. [CrossRef]
20. Prusiner, S.B. Prions. *Proc. Natl. Acad. Sci. USA* **1998**, *95*, 13363–13383. [CrossRef]
21. Portales-Castillo, I.; Yee, J.; Tanaka, H.; Fenves, A.Z. Beta-2 Microglobulin Amyloidosis: Past, Present, and Future. *Kidney360* **2020**, *1*, 1447–1455. [CrossRef]
22. Foguel, D.B.; Suarez, M.C.; Ferrão-Gonzales, A.D.; Porto, T.C.R.; Palmieri, L.; Einsiedler, C.M.; Andrade, L.R.; Lashuel, H.A.; Lansbury, P.T.; Kelly, J.W.; et al. Dissocia-tion of amyloid fibrils of alpha-synuclein and transthyretin by pressure reveals their reversible nature and the formation of water-excluded cavities. *Proc. Natl. Acad. Sci. USA* **2003**, *100*, 9831–9836. [CrossRef]
23. Westermark, P.; Sletten, K.; Johansson, B.; Cornwell, G.G. Fibril in senile systemic amyloidosis is derived from normal transthyretin. *Proc. Natl. Acad. Sci. USA* **1990**, *87*, 2843–2845. [CrossRef]
24. Jansens, K.J.A.; Rombouts, I.; Grootaert, C.; Brijs, K.; Camp, J.V.; Meeren, P.V.; Rousseau, F.; Schymkowitz, J.; Delcour, J.A. Rational design of amyloid-like fibrillary structures for tailoring food protein techno-functionality and their potential health implications. *Compr. Rev. Food Sci. Food Saf.* **2019**, *18*, 84–105. [CrossRef]
25. Niraula, T.N.; Haraoka, K.; Ando, Y.; Li, H.; Yamada, H.; Akasaka, K. Decreased Thermodynamic Stability as a Crucial Factor for Familial Amyloidotic Polyneuropathy. *J. Mol. Biol.* **2002**, *320*, 333–342. [CrossRef]
26. Niraula, T.N.; Konno, T.; Li, H.; Yamada, H.; Akasaka, K.; Tachibana, H. Pressure-dissociable reversible assembly of naturally denatured lysozyme is a precursor for amyloid fibrils. *Proc. Natl. Acad. Sci. USA* **2004**, *101*, 4089–4093. [CrossRef]
27. Kamatari, Y.O.; Yokoyama, S.; Tachibana, H.; Akasaka, K. Pressure-jump NMR study of dissociation and association of amyloid protofibrils. *J. Mol. Biol.* **2005**, *349*, 916–921. [CrossRef] [PubMed]
28. Tachibana, H. Basic equation in statics and kinetics of protein polymerization and the mechanism of the formation and dissociation of amyloid fibrils revealed by pressure perturbation. *Subcell. Biochem.* **2015**, *72*, 279–299.
29. Akasaka, K.; Abdul Latif, A.R.; Nakamura, A.; Matsuo, K.; Tachibana, H.; Gekko, K. Amyloid protofibril is highly voluminous and compressible. *Biochemistry* **2007**, *46*, 10444–10450. [CrossRef]
30. Sasaki, K.; Nakatsuka, K.; Hayashi, I.; Akasaka, K. Efficient conversion of intact hen lysozyme into amyloid fibrils by seeding. *J. Biol. Macromol.* **2008**, *8*, 11–18.
31. Akasaka, K.; Maeno, A.; Murayama, T.; Tachibana, H.; Fujita, Y.; Yamanaka, H.; Nishida, N.; Atarashi, R. Pressure-assisted dissociation and degradation of "proteinase K-resistant" fibrils prepared by seeding with scrapie infected hamster prion protein. *Prion* **2014**, *8*, 314–318. [CrossRef]
32. Morimoto, N.; Mitsui, T.; Sakamoto, M.; Mahara, A.; Yoshimura, K.; Arata, J.; Jinno, C.; Kakudo, N.; Kusumoto, K.; Yamaoka, T. A novel treatment for giant congenital melanocytic nevi combining inactivated autologous nevus tissue by high hydrostatic pressure and a cultured epidermal autograft: First-in-human, open, prospective clinical trial. *Plast. Reconstr. Surg.* **2021**, *9*, 71e–76e. [CrossRef] [PubMed]

biology MDPI

Article

Comparative Assessment of NMR Probes for the Experimental Description of Protein Folding Pathways with High-Pressure NMR

Vincent Van Deuren [1], Yin-Shan Yang [1], Karine de Guillen [1], Cécile Dubois [1], Catherine Anne Royer [2], Christian Roumestand [1,*] and Philippe Barthe [1,*]

1 Centre de Biologie Structurale, CNRS, INSERM, Université de Montpellier, 34090 Montpellier, France; vincent.vandeuren@kuleuven.be (V.V.D.); yang@cbs.cnrs.fr (Y.-S.Y.); karine@cbs.cnrs.fr (K.d.G.); cecile.dubois@cbs.cnrs.fr (C.D.)
2 Department of Biological Sciences, Rensselaer Polytechnic Institute, Troy, NY 12180, USA; royerc@rpi.edu
* Correspondence: christian.roumestand@cbs.cnrs.fr (C.R.); philippe.barthe@cbs.cnrs.fr (P.B.)

Simple Summary: During the last decade, high-pressure multidimensional NMR has emerged as a very powerful tool to describe the folding landscapes of proteins. This is (i) because pressure is a gentle perturbation, the effects of which originate from local properties of the folded state, contrary to chemical or thermal denaturation, and (ii) because multidimensional NMR intrinsically provides multiple probes strategically scattered on the three-dimensional structure of the protein, allowing a quasi-atomic resolution to describe the folding pathway. Residue-specific information obtained from these probes can be used to describe protein folding pathways through the calculation of NMR-derived fractional probabilities of contact at increasing pressure. Here, we used this strategy to evaluate and compare the results obtained from NH amide, CαHα, and CH_3 groups when used as NMR probes to explore the folding pathway of the model protein Δ+PHS Staphylococcal Nuclease.

Abstract: Multidimensional NMR intrinsically provides multiple probes that can be used for deciphering the folding pathways of proteins: NH amide and CαHα groups are strategically located on the backbone of the protein, while CH_3 groups, on the side-chain of methylated residues, are involved in important stabilizing interactions in the hydrophobic core. Combined with high hydrostatic pressure, these observables provide a powerful tool to explore the conformational landscapes of proteins. In the present study, we made a comparative assessment of the NH, CαHα, and CH_3 groups for analyzing the unfolding pathway of Δ+PHS Staphylococcal Nuclease. These probes yield a similar description of the folding pathway, with virtually identical thermodynamic parameters for the unfolding reaction, despite some notable differences. Thus, if partial unfolding begins at identical pressure for these observables (especially in the case of backbone probes) and concerns similar regions of the molecule, the residues involved in contact losses are not necessarily the same. In addition, an unexpected slight shift toward higher pressure was observed in the sequence of the scenario of unfolding with CαHα when compared to amide groups.

Keywords: protein folding; NMR; high hydrostatic pressure; thermodynamic stability

Citation: Van Deuren, V.; Yang, Y.-S.; de Guillen, K.; Dubois, C.; Royer, C.A.; Roumestand, C.; Barthe, P. Comparative Assessment of NMR Probes for the Experimental Description of Protein Folding Pathways with High-Pressure NMR. *Biology* **2021**, *10*, 656. https://doi.org/10.3390/biology10070656

Academic Editors: Dmitri Davydov and Christiane Jung

Received: 9 June 2021
Accepted: 9 July 2021
Published: 12 July 2021

1. Introduction

Hydrostatic pressure is a method of choice in studies of protein folding. This "relatively gentle" perturbation is generally reversible and provides access to thermodynamic parameters at atmospheric pressure, characteristic of the folding/unfolding reaction [1–4]. Contrary to chemical denaturation, it does not modify the composition of the system. Additionally, it does not modify the charges of the molecule, contrary to pH denaturation. Finally, the ΔC_p of the system remains constant over the full reaction, contrary to thermal denaturation. Following the Le Châtelier principle, pressure leads to the unfolding of protein because the molar volume of the unfolded state is smaller than that of the folded state, i.e., the volume change upon unfolding ΔV_u^0 is negative [5,6]. It is now largely admitted that the elimination of the solvent-excluded internal voids due to imperfect protein packing likely represents the largest contribution to the magnitude of ΔV_u^0 [7–11]. Because the distribution of solvent-excluded cavities is specific to each protein's structure, pressure-induced unfolding originates from local properties of the folded state, contrary to unfolding by temperature or chemical denaturants, the effects of which depend on the amount of exposed surface area in the unfolded state.

Due to recent methodological and technical advances, high-pressure NMR (HP-NMR) spectroscopy has emerged as a particularly powerful tool to obtain high-resolution structural description of the protein folding landscape (for reviews [12–18]). This is primarily because an abundance of site-specific probes can be studied simultaneously in a multidimensional NMR spectrum. Strategically located on the protein backbone, amide group resonances (^{1}H,^{15}N) are currently used to monitor the unfolding reaction: each amino acid bears a HN group, with the exception of proline, and is well resolved in the proton and nitrogen-15 spectral dimensions of heteronuclear 2D [^{1}H-^{15}N]-HSQC experiments. Hence, they represent good observables to describe the protein folding pathway at a residue-level resolution. On the other hand, amide protons are acidic and prone to exchange with water at a rate that depends on pressure, thus introducing possible bias in the measurement of thermodynamics parameters ΔV_u^0, ΔG_u^0). CαHα group resonances (^{1}H,^{13}C) could represent an alternative to probe protein unfolding with variable-pressure 2D [^{1}H-^{13}C]-HSQC experiments. They are also ideally distributed along the protein backbone, but Hα protons are not exchangeable, contrary to amide protons. Finally, CH_3 group NMR resonances can also serve probe protein unfolding. Residues bearing methylated side-chains (A, T, M, V, I, L) are usually well distributed in the structure of globular soluble proteins and provide decisive stabilizing hydrophobic interactions in the core of the molecule. Far fewer than amide or CαHα groups, the strategic location of CH_3 groups can nevertheless yield important information on the loss of tertiary contacts during protein unfolding. In the present study, we have used HP-NMR spectroscopy to explore the folding pathway of Staphylococcal Nuclease (SNase) and compare the description given by different NMR probes: amide groups, CαHα groups, and CH_3 groups.

The model protein used in this study (SNase) is a small extracellular enzyme (149 residues) produced by *Staphylococcus aureus* that degrades both DNA and RNA to short oligonucleotides in the presence of Ca^{2+}. It belongs to the OB-fold (Oligonucleotide/oligosaccharide-Binding) superfamily, a widely represented architecture characterized by a 5-stranded β-barrel, capped by an α-helix found between strands 3 and 4 [19,20]. It has long served as model system for protein folding studies [21,22]. In spite of its moderate complexity, SNase displays three structural subdomains (Figure 1) [23–25]. The major N-terminal subdomain (SubD1) consists of the OB-fold itself, encompassing the first 96 residues. The C-terminal helix (residues 122–134) forms the second subdomain (SubD2), linked to SubD1 by an interfacial domain (IntD), essentially formed by a short helix (residues 99–105), a mini-ß-sheet (residues 39–40 and 110–111), and loops. The C-terminal end of the molecule forms a turn (residues 137–141), bearing the sole tryptophan residue (W140), which stabilizes the protein via multiple contacts [26,27]. This organization has been confirmed for a SNase mutant by H/D exchange experiments that reveal three foldons, which correspond more or less to the subdomain description [28].

As in previous published studies, we used a hyper-stable variant of SNase known as Δ+PHS SNase ($\Delta\Delta G \approx 7$ kcal/mol when compared to the wild-type protein) [9,10,29]. This variant bears stabilizing substitutions (G50F, V51N, P117G, H124L, and S128A) and a deletion of the mobile Ω loop (residues 44–49), which is part of the active site of the enzyme.

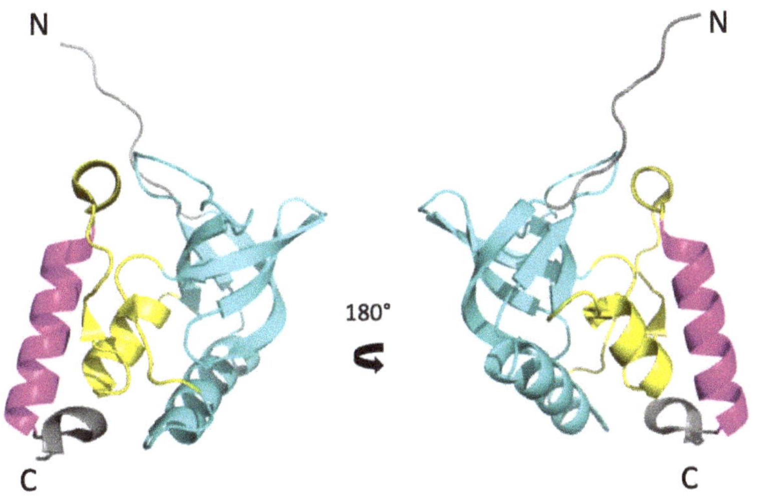

Figure 1. The subdomain organization of the structure of Staphylococcal Nuclease (PDB ID: 3LX0). Two views (180° rotation along the vertical axis) of a cartoon representation of the 3D structure of Δ+PHS Staphylococcal Nuclease. SubD1, IntD, and SubD2 subdomains are colored in cyan, yellow, and magenta, respectively.

2. Materials and Methods

2.1. Protein Expression and Purification

The highly stable Δ+PHS form of SNase was expressed and purified, as described in detail by Shortle and Meeker [30]. The construct Δ+PHS SNase was sub-cloned in pET24a plasmids with kanamycin resistance and introduced in BL21(DE3) bacteria using the heat-shock method. Uniform $^{15}N/^{13}C$ labeling was obtained by growing cells in minimal M9 medium containing $^{15}NH4Cl/^{13}C$-u-labeled glucose as the sole nitrogen and carbon sources. Protein was expressed overnight at 20 °C after induction with 0.2 mM IPTG. The cells were then centrifuged at 5000 rpm for 10 min, and the bacterial pellet was resuspended in an ice-cold buffer containing 25 mM Tris pH8 buffer 2.5 mM EDTA and 6 M Urea (buffer#1). This suspension was kept at 4 °C for 20 min under shaking condition and then centrifugated at 8000 rpm for 15 min. The pellet was resuspended in the same cold buffer but containing 400 mM NaCl (buffer#2). This new suspension was kept at 4 °C for 30 min under gentle shaking condition and then centrifugated at 8000 rpm for 15 min. An equal volume of ice-cold 100% ethanol was added to the supernatant, and precipitation was promoted for 3h at −20 °C. The precipitate was discarded after centrifugation (20 min at 8000 rpm), and an additional two-volumes of ice-cold ethanol was added to the supernatant, and the solution was kept overnight at −20 °C. After the last centrifugation (20 min at 8000 rpm), the precipitate was solubilized in 30 mL of buffer#1 and injected in a Sephadex (Merck-Sigma-Aldrich, France) cationic resin column. Elution was done with a linear gradient of buffer#2. The fractions containing the pure protein were pooled, and the sample was first dialyzed in Tris buffer (10 mM, pH 7) containing 1 M KCl overnight, with stirring under refrigeration, and subsequently in Tris 10 mM pH 7 for 2 h. For NMR studies, the solution was concentrated to about 1 mM (protein concentration), aliquoted to 0.3 mL samples, and freeze-dried. Yields of purified protein were on the order of 60 mg/L. Protein concentration was determined at 280 nm using an extinction coefficient of 0.93.

2.2. Protein NMR Resonance Assignment

The assignment of the amide group ^1H and ^{15}N resonances have been reported in previous works [6,7,21]. The assignment of the CαHα group and CH_3 group ^1H and ^{13}C

resonances were achieved through a 3D [^{1}H,^{13}C] TOCSY-HSQC (isotropic mixing: 60 ms) NMR experiment performed on a 1 mM ^{15}N,^{13}C-labeled Δ+PHS sample (0.2 mL in a conventional 3 mm glass tube), dissolved in Tris 10 mM deuterated buffer at pH 7 (uncorrected from isotopic effects). Additionally, a [^{1}H,^{13}C] NOESY-HSQC (mixing time: 200 ms) was recorded, which helped us solve some ambiguities. Experiments were recorded at 20 °C on a Bruker AVANCE III (Bruker Biospin, Wissenbourg, France) 700 MHz equipped with a 5 mm Z-gradient TCI cryogenic probe head. ^{1}H chemical shifts were directly referenced to the methyl resonance of DSS, while ^{13}C and ^{15}N chemical shifts were referenced indirectly to the ^{13}C/^{1}H and ^{15}N/^{1}H absolute frequency ratios. All NMR experiments were processed with Gifa [31].

2.3. Protein Unfolding

[^{1}H,^{15}N] and [^{1}H,^{13}C] HSQC experiments were recorded at 20 °C on a Bruker AVANCE III 600 MHz spectrometer, equipped with a TXI probe operating at ambient, and at 15 different hydrostatic pressures (1, 30, 200, 400, 600, 800, 1000, 1200, 1400, 1600, 1800, 2000, 2200, 2400, and 2500 bar). The doubly-labeled ^{15}N,^{13}C protein sample was dissolved at a concentration of 1 mM in a Tris 10 mM pH 7 aqueous buffer (+10% D_2O for the lock) and used with a 5 mm o.d. ceramic tube (0.33 mL of sample volume) from Daedalus Innovations (Aston, PA, USA). Guanidinium chloride was added to the sample (1.8 M) in order to drag the protein stability into the pressure range allowed by the experimental set-up (1–2500 bar). Hydrostatic pressure was applied to the sample directly within the magnet using the Xtreme Syringe Pump, also from Daedalus Innovations. Pressure was transmitted by mineral oil, so that no physical separation was needed between the aqueous buffer containing the protein and the transmitting fluid. Each pressure jump was followed by a 12-h relaxation time to allow the protein to reach a steady-state equilibrium before running the 2D experiments. 2D [^{1}H,^{15}N] and [^{1}H,^{13}C] HSQC were recorded sequentially, hence on the same sample and strictly in the same experimental conditions. These experiments were recorded using gradient coherence selection through pulsed field gradients, yielding an excellent suppression of the water resonance in the proton dimension.

The intensities of cross peaks corresponding to NH, CαHα, or CH_3 groups were measured for the folded species at each pressure, and their decrease in pressure was then fitted with a two-state model:

$$I = \frac{I_f + I_u e^{-(\Delta G_u^0 + p\Delta V_u^0)/RT}}{1 + e^{-(\Delta G_u^0 + p\Delta V_u^0)/RT}} \tag{1}$$

where I is the intensity of a native state cross peak measured at a given pressure and I_f and I_u correspond to the cross peak intensities in the folded state (1 bar, $I_f = I_{max}$) and in the unfolded state (2500 bar, $I_u = I_{min}$), respectively. ΔG_u^0 stands for the residue specific apparent free energy of unfolding at atmospheric pressure. ΔV_u^0 corresponds to the residue specific apparent volume of unfolding for pressure denaturation.

Native contact maps were obtained by using software CMView [http://www.bioinformatics.org/cmview/] (accessed on 25 March 2020) with a threshold of 8.5 Å around the Cα of each residue, using the crystal structure of Δ+PHS SNase (PDB ID: 3LX0).

3. Results

3.1. NMR Resonance Assignment

Amide resonances (^{1}H and ^{15}N) were assigned for all amide groups in previous work [9,10,30], and those of CαHα and CH_3 groups (^{1}H and ^{13}C) were assigned through 3D ^{13}C-edited TOCSY and NOESY experiments recorded on a ^{15}N,^{13}C-uniformly enriched Δ+PHS SNase sample dissolved in a deuterated buffer (see Materials and Methods). The assigned HSQC 2D spectra corresponding to these sets of resonances are given as Supplementary Materials (Figures S1–S3). A total of 100 amide cross peaks (73% of the residues) and 81 CαHα cross peaks (59% of the residues) gave neither overlapping cross peaks in the folded state nor in between the folded and unfolded states at 20 °C. Nevertheless, for the accuracy of the comparison, we considered only residues where both NH and CαHα groups were resolvable for further analysis (61 residues, 45% of the sequence). Our construct contains 51 methylated residues (37% of the sequence): 14 alanine, 8 threonine, 4 methionine, 8 valine, 12 leucine, and 5 isoleucine residues. While all CH_3 groups can be assigned unambiguously, only 33 (24% of the sequence) gave cross peaks (at least one cross peak for residues I, L, V, bearing two methyl groups), which showed no overlap in both the folded state or between the folded and unfolded states at 20 °C, and were considered for further analysis. The distribution of the selected residues on the 3D structure of SNase is displayed in Figure 2.

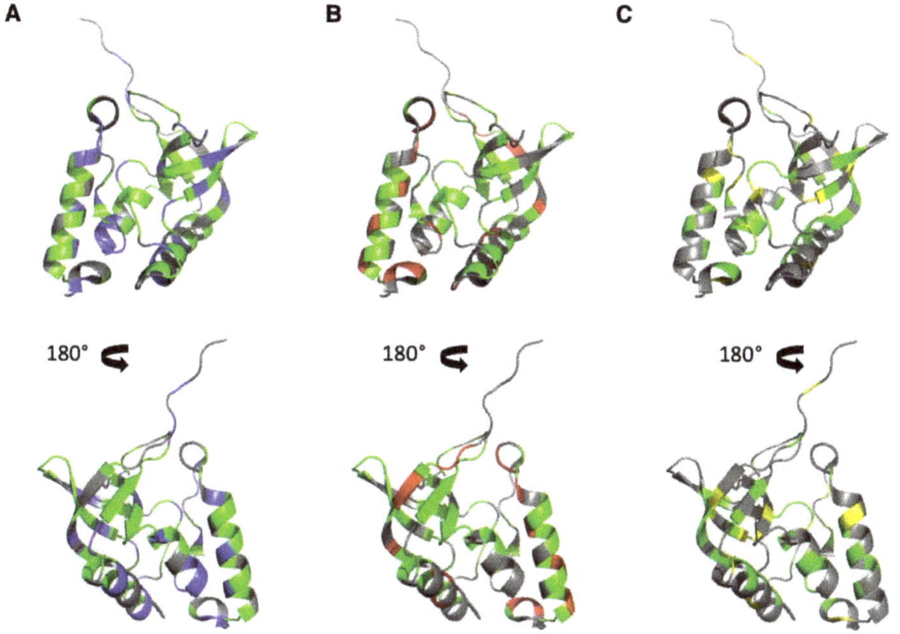

Figure 2. Distribution of the NMR probes used for the HP-NMR denaturation study on the 3D structure of Δ+PHS SNase (PDB ID: 3LX0). (**A–C**): Two views (180° rotation along the vertical axis) of a cartoon representation of the 3D structure of Δ+PHS Staphylococcal Nuclease. In (**A**,**B**), the colored residues correspond to the NH (**A**) (in blue and green) and CαHα (**B**) (in red and green) groups, which were assigned and gave neither overlapping cross peaks in the folded state nor in between the folded and unfolded states at 20 °C in the corresponding HSQC spectra. The residues colored in green correspond to residues where both the NH and the CαHα groups gave no overlapping cross peaks. In (**C**), the colored residues (in yellow and green) correspond to all methylated residues. Those colored in green correspond to residues that gave no overlapping in the 2D [^{1}H,^{13}C] HSQC spectra (folded and unfolded states). In this figure, all residues colored in green were used for the HP NMR study.

3.2. HP-NMR Denaturation Study: Measuring the Thermodynamic Parameters for the Unfolding Reaction

2D [^{1}H,^{15}N] and [^{1}H,^{13}C] HSQC experiments were recorded at variable pressure within the 1–2500 bar pressure range and at 20 °C. In all these spectra, the intensity of each native state cross peak decreases as a function of pressure, while the intensity of peaks corresponding to the unfolded state increases concomitantly (Figure 3). This supports a slow equilibrium on the NMR timescale for each residue between the native and unfolded state and a two-state transition for each residue between their native/unfolded states during the unfolding process. Thus, this simple model can be used to interpret the loss of intensity for each native state cross peak, even though the global protein unfolding does not likely conform to a two-state transition, locally [18].

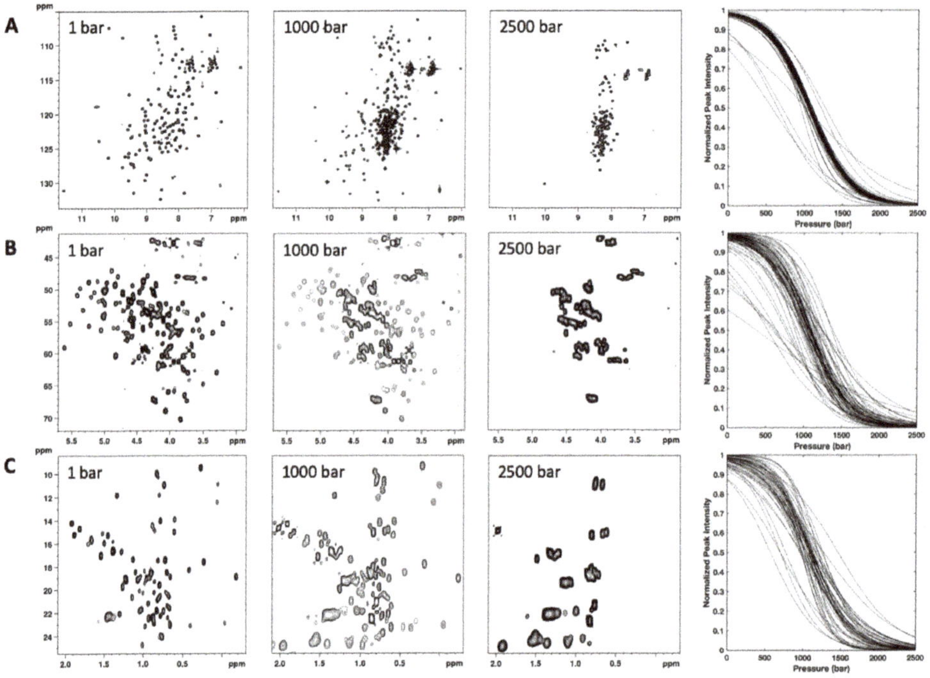

Figure 3. NMR detected high-pressure unfolding of Δ+PHS SNase. From left to right, examples of 2D [^{1}H,^{15}N] (**A**) and [^{1}H,^{13}C] (**B**,**C**) HSQC spectra recorded at 1, 1000, and 2500 bar are displayed. In (**B**,**C**), only a zoom on the CαHα or on the CH_3 cross peak region, respectively, is displayed. The rightmost panels report overlays of the normalized residue-specific denaturation curves obtained from the fits of the pressure-dependent sigmoidal decrease of (**A**) NH amide, (**B**) CαHα, and **C**) CH_3 cross peak intensities in the corresponding HSQC spectra with Equation [1]. Representative examples of experimental fits are given in Supplementary Materials (Figure S4).

A substantial number of local NMR probes (61 NH and CαHα cross peaks, 33 CH_3 cross peaks) can be accurately fitted to the two-state pressure-induced unfolding model described in the Materials and Methods (Equation (1)), yielding local apparent values for ΔG_u^0 and ΔV_u^0 (Figure 4). Although the two-state model was adequate to fit all individual unfolding curves at a residue level, significantly different residue-specific values for apparent free energy ΔG_u^0 and apparent volume change ΔV_u^0 of unfolding were observed, suggesting a deviation from a two-state behavior for the global unfolding of the protein for all probes used for the study.

Interestingly, although values obtained from CαHα groups and CH_3 groups show a broader distribution than those obtained from NH groups, virtually identical average values (within the experimental errors) were obtained for the three probes used. Amide groups yield an average ΔG_u^0 value of 2282 ± 275 cal/mol and a ΔV_u^0 of −91 ± 10 mL/mol, CαHα groups yield an average ΔG_u^0 value of 2245 ± 763 cal/mol and a ΔV_u^0 of −92 ± 22 mL/mol, and CH_3 groups yield an average ΔG_u^0 value of 2252 ± 597 cal/mol and a ΔV_u^0 of −91 ± 21 mL/mol (Figure 4). Note that, for NH and CαHα probes, these values were not biased by the residue selection that we made, keeping only those for which residue-specific curves could be obtained for both atom groups. When considering the 100 amide cross peaks and the 81 CαHα groups that can be fitted accurately with Equation (1) (Supplementary Materials, Figure S5), similar values were obtained: ΔG_u^0 value of 2221 ± 391 cal/mol and a ΔV_u^0 of -90 ± 13 mL/mol for amide cross peaks; ΔG_u^0 value of 2224 ± 721 cal/mol and a ΔV_u^0 of -91 ± 22 mL/mol for CαHα cross peaks. It should be noticed that the apparent global values obtained for ΔG_u^0 and ΔV_u^0 (2394 ± 82 cal/mol and -87 ± 3 mL/mol, respectively) were also in good agreement with the average values of the corresponding apparent residue-specific values extracted from NH, CαHα, or CH_3 denaturation curves, supporting the two-state equilibrium regime for folding or unfolding. These global values were obtained by fitting the increase of the resonance at 0.8 ppm (which corresponds roughly to the resonance of the methyl groups in the unfolded state) on a series of 1D spectra recorded at increasing pressure [18] (Supplementary Materials, Figure S6). This constitutes reassuring results, since the global (or averaged) thermodynamic parameters measured by the different NMR probes are supposed to reflect a similar global behavior of the same system under the same perturbation, even though differences can be expected at a local, residue-specific level.

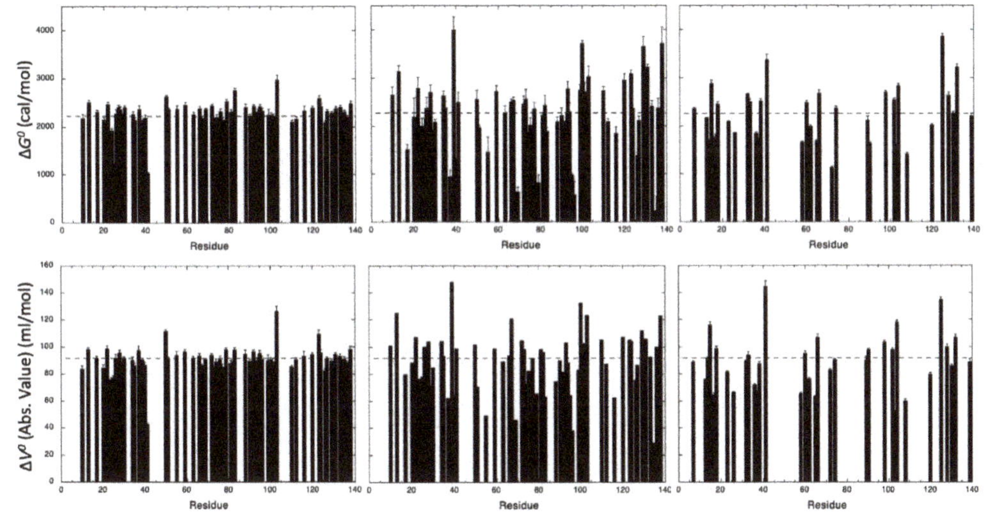

Figure 4. Thermodynamic parameters measured for the unfolding reaction of Δ+PHS SNase. ΔG^0 (upper panels) and ΔV^0 (absolute value, lower panels) obtained from the fit with Equation (1) of the pressure-dependent sigmoidal decrease of the residue cross peak intensities of (from left to right) NH amide groups, CαHα groups, and CH_3 groups. For I, L and V residues, when denaturation curves have been obtained for each of the two cross peaks (corresponding to the two methyl groups), averaged values of ΔG^0 and ΔV^0 are displayed. The dashed lines represent the mean values of the measured thermodynamic parameters. The values of ΔG^0, ΔV^0 and also $P_{1/2}$ (the half-denaturation pressure) are gathered in Table S1 (Supplementary Materials).

3.3. HP-NMR Denaturation Study: Exploring the Folding Pathways of Δ+PHS SNase

In the case of NH and CαHα groups, we used the now classical strategy to track possible intermediates in the folding pathway of Δ+PHS SNase [10,18]. This strategy is based on exploiting the information brought by normalized residue-specific denaturation curves: for a given residue "*i*", the value of 1 at a given pressure ($I = I_f = 1$; Equation (1)) can be associated with a probability P_i of 1 (100%) to find this residue "*i*" in the native state, while for a residue "*j*", the value of 0 at the same pressure, ($I = I_U = 0$) can be associated with a probability P_j equal to zero to find this residue "*j*" in a native state. These probabilities are called fractional probabilities because they are related to the "native fraction" for a given residue. If these two residues *i* and *j* are in an intermediate situation ($0 < P_i$ and $P_j < 1$) at a given pressure, and if they are in contact in the native 3D structure (at atmospheric pressure), their fractional probability P_{ij}, in contact at this pressure, is given by the geometric mean of the two individual probabilities: $P_{ij} = \sqrt{P_i \times P_j}$ [12] (Figure 5) [18,32].

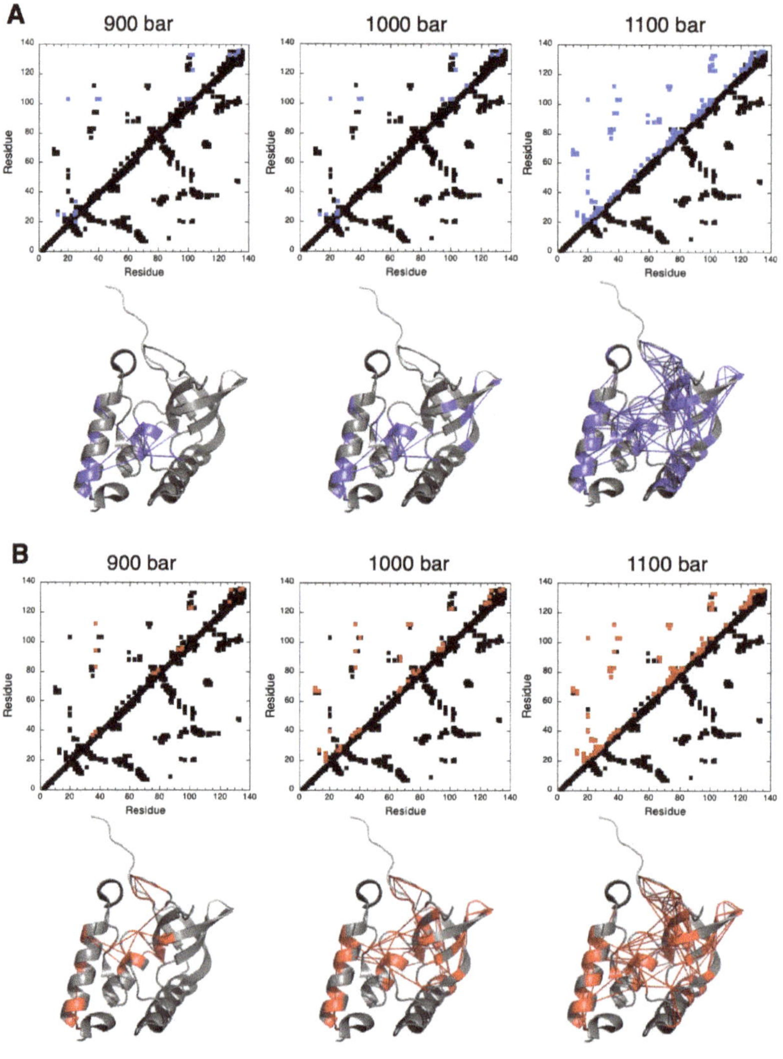

Figure 5. Pressure denaturation of Δ+PHS SNase probed by NH and CαHα backbone atoms. (**A**) Upper panels: contact maps built from the crystal structure of Δ+PHS SNase (PDB ID: 3LX0) at 900, 1000, and 1100 bar, as indicated. Contacts below the diagonal have been calculated with CMview: they correspond to residues where the distance to the corresponding Cα is lower than 8.5 Å. Above the diagonal, the contacts displayed correspond to residues for which fractional probability can be measured from normalized residue-specific denaturation curves obtained from NH cross peaks. In addition, contacts have been colored in blue when contact probabilities P_{ij} lower than 0.5 are observed. Lower panels: visualization of the probabilities of contact on ribbon representations of Δ+PHS SNase at 900, 1000, and 1100 bar, as indicated. The blue lines represent contacts that are significantly weakened ($P_{ij} \leq 0.5$) at the indicated pressure. Residues involved in these contacts are also colored in blue. (**B**) Similar as in (**A**), but the fractional probabilities have been calculated from normalized residue-specific denaturation curves obtained from CαHα cross peaks. In the contact maps, contacts have been colored in red when contact probabilities P_{ij} are lower than 0.5. These weakened contacts are visualized on the 3D structure of Δ+PHS SNase by red lines, and the residues involved in these contacts are also colored in red.

Whichever the probe considered (NH or CαHα groups), unfolding appears to follow a similar scenario. At 900 bar, we observed a partial loss of contacts ($P_{ij} \leq 0.5$) between residues from the interfacial domain (IntD) to residues in SubD1 (the OB-fold domain) and SubD2 (the C-terminal helix) (Figure 5). Although this partial unfolding globally concerns the same area of the 3D structure whatever the probe used, in the details, the residues directly involved are not the same. When using amide groups, fractional contact probabilities below 0.5 were measured essentially for two central residues: L103, located in the short helix of IntD, and K133, located in SubD2. Residue L103 displays weakened contacts with residue G20 in SubD1, with residues V39, D40, T41, A94, V99, N100, and E101 within IntD itself and with residues Q123 and K133, located in SubD2. Residue K133 displays weakened contacts with residues in SubD2 (K127, Q131, E135, and K136) and with residues in IntD (E101 and L103). When considering CαHα groups, weakened contacts essentially concern residue L37 in IntD (with V39 and D83 in subD1 and R35, A94, and A112 within IntD itself), residue G79, located in a loop connecting the β4-strand to the β5-strand from the β-barrel of SubD1 (with F76, D77, and R81 in the same loop), residue Q123 in SubD2 (with N100 and E101 in IntD), and residue E135, also in SubD2 (with K127 and K133 in SubD2) (Figure 5).

At 1000 bar, partial unfolding concerns additional residues in the same areas and the loss of some contacts in the OB-fold itself between residues in the C-terminal turn of the helix and in the first ß-strand of the barrel. Intriguingly, at this pressure, partial unfolding seems to concern more residues when considering fractional probabilities calculated from residue-specific denaturation curves obtained from CαHα probes than from those obtained from NH amide probes. More weakened contacts ($P_{ij} \leq 0.5$) can be detected in the fractional contact maps built from CαHα residue-specific denaturation curves (involving a total of 47 residues) than from those from NH residue-specific denaturation curves (involving only 24 residues). This suggests a sharper unfolding transition when probed by the CαHα groups.

Indeed, at a slightly higher pressure (1050 bar), the number of weakened contacts detected from NH probes becomes closer (38 residues involved) to that detected from CαHα probes at 1000 bar (Supplementary Materials, Figure S7). Moreover, among these 38 residues, 31 (≈82%) also belong to the group of 47 residues involved in weakened contacts ($P_{ij} \leq 0.5$) when probing the unfolding transition with CαHα groups (at 1000 bar). This strongly suggests a similar scenario for the partial unfolding of Δ+PHS SNase, which is slightly shifted to a higher pressure when described by NH probes.

Finally, at 1100 bar, regardless of the probe under consideration, a quasi-global unfolding of the molecule is observed, with the loss ($P_{ij} \leq 0.5$) of most of the contacts in the 3D structure, including those stabilizing the ß-barrel in the OB-fold domain (Figure 5).

When compared to NH or CαHα groups, methyl groups constitute scarce probes for analyzing the folding landscape of the protein (33 selected CH_3 groups against 61 for NH or CαHα, in the results presented here), and contacts between them are few. Thus, we directly used the individual fractional probabilities P_i instead of deriving fractional probabilities of contact P_{ij} between residues. Using this simplified approach, it was not possible to determine which contacts in the 3D structure were lost, but we assessed whether a methylated residue was in a native or unfolded environment at a given pressure. The first methylated residues exhibiting fractional probabilities lower than 0.5 were detected at 1000 bar. When displayed in the 3D structure of Δ+PHS SNase, they were located either in the interfacial domain or in the OB-fold domain and C-terminal helix, with side chains pointing toward the interfacial domain (Figure 6). Also consisted was L14, a residue located on the first ß-strand of the ß-barrel, the side chain of which pointing toward the C-terminal turn of the helix of the OB-fold domain. Fractional probabilities lower than 0.5 concern only residues located in these two areas up to a pressure of 1100 bar. Above (1200 bar), most of the methylated residues report an unfolded environment. Thus, it seems that the folding pathway probed by the methylated side chains is very similar to that probed by the backbone atoms.

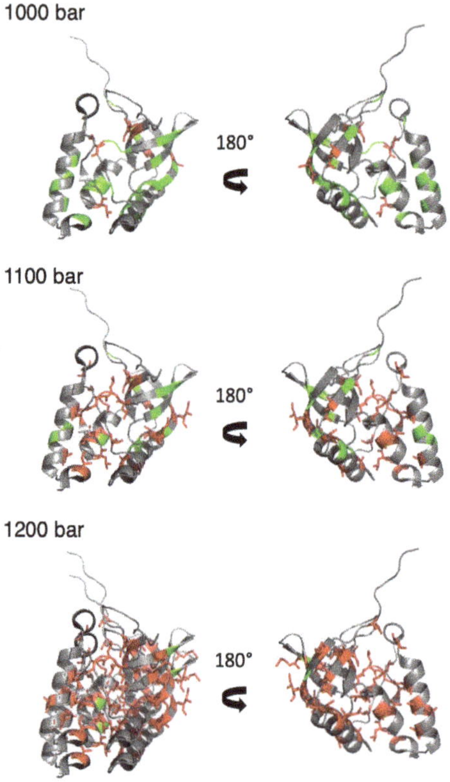

Figure 6. Pressure denaturation of Δ+PHS SNase probed by side chain CH_3 groups. Two views related by a 180° rotation along the vertical axis of a ribbon representation of the 3D structure of Δ+PHS SNase (PDB ID: 3LX0). The green and red color correspond to methylated residues, with fractional probabilities greater or lower than 0.5, respectively. In addition, the side chains of the methylated residues displaying fractional probabilities lower than 0.5 are represented by red sticks. Results obtained at three different pressures (1000, 1100, and 1200 bar) are displayed from top to bottom, as indicated.

4. Discussion

Due to the better resolution of the 2D [^{1}H,^{15}N] HSQC spectrum, NH amide cross peaks provide the most important number of residue-specific NMR probes to explore the folding landscape of Δ+PHS SNase. Indeed, 100 residue-specific denaturation curves can be obtained from non-overlapping cross peaks over 133 non-proline residues. Due to more severe overlapping cross peaks either in the folded state 2D [^{1}H,^{13}C] HSQC spectrum or between the unfolded and unfolded state spectra, a more limited number (81 over 137 residues) can be obtained from CαHα cross peaks, and this number drops to 33 (over 51 methylated residues) when considering the CH_3 cross peaks. In addition, some CαHα cross peaks can be obscured possibly by the water resonance, in the middle of the Hα proton resonances, even if, in the present case, the water suppression scheme (coherence selection through pulsed field gradients) worked well, yielding virtually no artefact, probably due to the rather high protein concentration (1 mM) in the NMR sample.

Whichever the probes used, the fit of cross peak intensity decrease with pressure to a two-state model yields virtually identical average values for the apparent thermodynamic parameters ΔG_u^0 and ΔV_u^0, supporting the theory that NH, CαHα, or CH_3 probes equally sense the denaturation reaction. In the detail, we observed a broader distribution of the residue-specific values of ΔG_u^0 and ΔV_u^0 in the case of CαHα and CH_3 groups than in the case of NH groups. Thus, apparently, the unfolding reaction seems more cooperative when probed with NH amide groups. We do not have a clear explanation for this observation, except maybe the fact that all the amide groups are involved in H-bonds, contrary to CαHα or CH_3 groups. Breaking these H-bonds is mandatory for a NH groups to sense a disordered environment. Since the free-energy associated with H-bonds does not vary significantly within the protein sequence, this probably confers a common and quasi-identical "unfolding contribution" for all amide groups. The differences observed between the apparent thermodynamic parameters ΔG_u^0 and ΔV_u^0, measured for NH groups, should be due to the contribution of the variable distribution of water-excluded voids around them, yielding significant differences in their pressure sensitivity. Since CαHα and CH_3 groups are not involved in H-bonds, they should be sensitive only to this latter contribution.

Fractional probabilities of contact P_{ij}, deduced from either NH or CαHα NMR probes, globally describe a similar folding pathway: the protein denaturation starts at 900 bar with the partial unfolding of IntD and SubD2 sub-domains, whereas SubD1 (the OB-fold domain) remains virtually non-affected until 1100 bar. These results are consistent with those obtained in previous work, demonstrating the existence of a folding intermediate state, where only the OB-fold domain is folded [10]. A similar folding pathway can also be observed when using CH_3 probes. When increasing pressure, the first methylated residues sensing an unfolded environment are located in IntD or in SubD1 and SubD2 but with side chains pointing toward IntD. This supports local unfolding of IntD and SubD2 sub-domains. Nevertheless, since fractional probabilities of contact cannot be calculated from CH_3 probes, a structural description of a possible folding intermediate becomes difficult. Interestingly, the global value for ΔG_u^0 and ΔV_u^0 measured on 1D spectra from the increase with pressure of the resonance corresponding to the unfolded CH_3 groups is similar to the average values of residue-specific ΔG_u^0 and ΔV_u^0 measured on 2D spectra for each individual CH_3 group. This means that the thermodynamic parameters measured at equilibrium for Δ+PHS SNase are similar for the folding and unfolding reaction. This strongly supports a two-state equilibrium between the folded and unfolded states, without the appearance of a pressure-stabilized folding intermediate (or molten-globule), as has been observed for the pp32 L60A variant [33].

Although residue-specific NH or CαHα probes are located in the backbone of the protein and borne by the same residue, even in cases where local unfolding reported by these probes concerns the same area of the protein, the loss of contacts revealed by their fractional probabilities does not necessarily concern the same residues. As mentioned above, this is probably due to the combined effects of H-bonds (for amide protons) and voids distribution around these atom groups.

Interestingly, the sequence of the scenario of the protein unfolding is slightly shifted to higher pressure when probed with CαHα groups, as if the unfolding transition was sharper when compare to results obtained with NH probes. This is an unexpected result since amide protons are exchangeable. Because solvent exchange increase with pressure [34], this effect should contribute to the intensity decrease of NH cross peaks with pressure. We should observe a steeper slope for the residue-specific denaturation curves obtained from NH amides. The reverse result is obtained, and again we do not have a clear explanation for that. Here also, the involvement of amide protons in H-bonds might be responsible of this rather counter-intuitive effect. On the other hand, this result clearly demonstrates that amide proton exchange with water is negligible and probably contributes marginally to the decrease of amide cross peak intensity in the native state spectrum during unfolding.

5. Conclusions

Among the three NMR probes (NH, CαHα, or CH_3 groups) studied here to investigate the protein folding pathways, NH and CαHα groups appear to be the best candidates, even if all three of them describe similar scenarios. Indeed, NH and CαHα groups are shared by all (non-proline) residues, although methylated residues constitute only 37% of the Δ+PHS

SNase sequence. Moreover, they are strategically located on the protein backbone, an ideal situation to probe protein unfolding. Finally, fractional probabilities of contact can be easily calculated from NH and CαHα probes, which is not the case for CH_3 probes, yielding a possible structural description of potential folding intermediates [10].

Unaffected by water suppression and displaying a better spectral resolution, the 2D [^1H,^{15}N] HSQC spectrum gives a larger number of probes when compared to the CαHα region of the 2D [^1H,^{13}C] HSQC spectrum. Moreover, we have shown here that the contribution of solvent exchange to amide cross peak intensity can be safely neglected, since thermodynamic parameters of the unfolding reaction and the folding pathway described both by NH groups and CαHα groups are similar. In addition, the fact that [^1H,^{15}N] HSQC can be recorded in an unexpansive ^{15}N-uniformly-labeled sample (when compared to ^{15}N,^{13}C-, or even the ^{13}C-u-labeled sample) makes NH amide groups very attractive probes for exploring the folding pathway of proteins. On the other hand, due to the more favorable values of natural abundancy and the gyromagnetic ratio of ^{13}C, the use of CαHα groups can constitute an interesting alternative for non-recombinant (and non-isotopically-enriched) proteins. Indeed, the use of cryogenic probes allows to record [^1H,^{13}C] HSQC with a good resolution in about 2 h on protein samples of moderate concentration (1–2 mM). In that case, problems due to water suppression can be circumvented by dissolving the protein sample in deuterated buffers.

Supplementary Materials: The following are available online at https://www.mdpi.com/article/10.3390/biology10070656/s1: Table S1: Thermodynamic parameters values obtained for Δ+PHS; Figure S1: Assignment of Δ+PHS SNase amide groups; Figure S2: Assignment of Δ+PHS SNase CαHα groups; Figure S3: Assignment of Δ+PHS SNase CH_3 groups; Figure S4: Representative examples of experimental fits; Figure S5: Thermodynamic parameters measured for the unfolding reaction of Δ+PHS SNase; Figure S6: Monitoring the unfolding reaction of Δ+PHS SNase with 1D HP-NMR spectroscopy; Figure S7: Fractional contact map obtained at 1050 bar from NH probes.

Author Contributions: V.V.D. carried out HP NMR experiments and analysis. K.d.G. and C.D. prepared the ^{15}N,^{13}C-u-labeled Δ+PHS SNase protein samples. Y.-S.Y. made the NMR resonance assignment. P.B. wrote software for the analysis of the HP data and participated in the coordination of the project with C.A.R. and C.R. and the writing of the manuscript. C.R. supervised the project, conceived experiments, participated in the interpretation, and wrote the article. All authors have read and agreed to the published version of the manuscript.

Funding: This work was supported by French Infrastructure for Integrated Structural Biology (FRISBI) grant No. ANR-10-INSB-05.

Institutional Review Board Statement: Not applicable.

Informed Consent Statement: Informed consent was obtained from all subjects involved in the study.

Data Availability Statement: Data supporting reported results are available upon request to corresponding authors.

Conflicts of Interest: The authors declare no conflict of interest.

References

1. Heremans, K.; Smeller, L. Protein structure and dynamics at high pressure. *Biochim. Biophys. Acta* **1998**, *1386*, 353–370. [CrossRef]
2. Kamatari, Y.O.; Kitahara, R.; Yamada, H.; Yokoyama, S.; Akasaka, K. High-pressure NMR spectroscopy for characterizing folding intermediates and denatured states of proteins. *Methods* **2004**, *34*, 133–143. [CrossRef]
3. Balny, C.; Masson, P.; Heremans, K. High pressure effects on biological macromolecules: From structural changes to alteration of cellular processes. *Biochim. Biophys. Acta* **2002**, *1595*, 3–10. [CrossRef]
4. Akasaka, K.; Kitahara, R.; Kamatari, Y.O. Exploring the folding energy landscape with pressure. *Arch. Biochem. Biophys.* **2013**, *531*, 110–115. [CrossRef]
5. Royer, C.A. Revisiting volume changes in pressure-induced protein unfolding. *Biochim. Biophys. Acta* **2002**, *1595*, 201–209. [CrossRef]
6. Meersman, F.; Dobson, C.M.; Heremans, K. Protein unfolding, amyloid fibril formation and configurational energy landscapes under high pressure conditions. *Chem. Soc. Rev.* **2006**, *35*, 908–917. [CrossRef] [PubMed]
7. Royer, C.A. Why and How Does Pressure Unfold Proteins? *Subcell. Biochem.* **2015**, *72*, 59–71.

8. Rouget, J.; Aksel, T.; Roche, J.; Saldana, J.; Garcia, A.E.; Barrick, D.; Royer, C.A. Size and sequence and the volume change of protein folding. *J. Am. Chem. Soc.* **2011**, *133*, 6020–6027. [CrossRef] [PubMed]
9. Roche, J.; Dellarole, M.J.; Caro, A.; Guca, E.; Norberto, D.R.; Yang, Y.-S.; Garcia, A.E.; Roumestand, C.; García-Moreno, B.; Royer, C.A. Remodeling of the folding free-energy landscape of staphylococcal nuclease by cavity-creating mutations. *Biochemistry* **2012**, *51*, 9535–9546. [CrossRef]
10. Roche, J.; Caro, J.A.; Norberto, D.R.; Barthe, P.; Roumestand, C.; Schlessman, J.L.; Garcia, A.E.; García-Moreno, B.E.; Royer, C.A. Cavities determine the pressure unfolding of proteins. *Proc. Natl. Acad. Sci. USA* **2012**, *109*, 6945–6950. [CrossRef]
11. Xue, M.; Wakamoto, T.; Kejlberg, C.; Yoshimura, Y.; Nielsen, T.A.; Risor, M.W.; Sanggaard, K.W.; Kitahara, R.; Mulder, F.A.A. How internal cavities destabilize a protein. *Proc. Natl. Acad. Sci. USA* **2019**, *116*, 21031–21036. [CrossRef]
12. Jonas, J.; Jonas, A. High-pressure NMR spectroscopy of proteins and membranes. *Annu. Rev. Biophys. Biomol. Struct.* **1994**, *23*, 287–318. [CrossRef]
13. Akasaka, K.; Yamada, H. On-line cell high-pressure nuclear magnetic resonance technique: Application to protein studies. *Methods Enzymol.* **2001**, *338*, 134–158.
14. Kremer, W. High-pressure NMR studies in proteins. *Annu. Rep. NMR Spectrosc.* **2006**, *57*, 177–203.
15. Roche, J.; Royer, C.A.; Roumestand, C. Monitoring protein folding through high pressure NMR spectroscopy. *Prog. Nucl. Magn. Reson. Spectrosc.* **2017**, *102–103*, 15–31. [CrossRef] [PubMed]
16. Caro, J.A.; Wand, A.J. Practical aspects of high-pressure NMR spectroscopy and its applications in protein biophysics and structural biology. *Methods* **2018**, *148*, 67–80. [CrossRef]
17. Roche, J.; Royer, C.A.; Roumestand, C. Exploring Protein Conformational Landscapes Using High-Pressure NMR. *Methods Enzymol.* **2019**, *614*, 293–320.
18. Dubois, C.; Herrada, I.; Barthe, P.; Roumestand, C. Combining High-Pressure Perturbation with NMR Spectroscopy for a Structural and Dynamical Characterization of Protein Folding Pathways. *Molecules* **2020**, *25*, 5551. [CrossRef]
19. Murzin, A.G. OB (oligonucleotide/olisaccharide binding)-fold: Common structural and functional solution for non-homologous sequences. *EMBO J.* **1993**, *12*, 861–867. [CrossRef]
20. Arcus, V. OB-fold domains: A snapshot of the evolution of sequence, structure and function. *Curr. Opin. Struct. Biol.* **2002**, *12*, 794–801. [CrossRef]
21. Taniuchi, H.; Anfinsen, C.B. An experimental approach to the study of the folding of the Staphylococcal nuclease. *J. Biol. Chem.* **1969**, *244*, 3864–3875. [CrossRef]
22. Shortle, D.; Meeker, A.K. Residual structure in large fragments of staphylococcal nuclease: Effects of amino acids substitutions. *Biochemistry* **1998**, *28*, 936–944. [CrossRef]
23. Alexandrescu, A.T.; Gittis, A.G.; Abeygunwardana, C.; Shortle, D. NMR structure of a stable OB-fold sub-domain isolated from staphylococcal nuclease. *J. Mol. Biol.* **1995**, *250*, 134–143. [CrossRef]
24. Ye, K.; Jing, G.; Wang, J. Interactions between subdomains in the partially folded state of staphylococcal nuclease. *Biochim. Biophys. Acta.* **2000**, *1479*, 123–134. [CrossRef]
25. Watson, E.; Matousek, W.M.; Irimies, E.L.; Alexandrescu, A.T. Partially folded states of staphylococcal nuclease highlight the conserved structural hierarchy of OB-fold proteins. *Biochemistry* **2007**, *46*, 9484–9494. [CrossRef]
26. Hu, H.-Y.; Wu, M.-C.; Fang, H.-J.; Forrest, M.D.; Hu, C.-K.; Tsong, T.Y.; Chen, H.M. The role of tryptophan in staphylococcal nuclease stability. *Biophys. Chem.* **2010**, *151*, 170–177. [CrossRef]
27. Wang, M.; Feng, Y.; Yao, H.; Wang, J. Importance of the C-terminal loop L137-S141 for the folding and folding stability of staphylococcal nuclease stability. *Biochemistry* **2010**, *49*, 4318–4326. [CrossRef]
28. Bedard, S.; Mayne, L.C.; Petersen, R.W.; Wand, A.J.; Englander, S.W. The foldon substructure of staphylococcal nuclease. *J. Mol. Biol.* **2008**, *376*, 1142–1154. [CrossRef]
29. Roche, J.; Caro, J.A.; Dellarole, M.; Guca, E.; Royer, C.A.; García-Moreno, B.; Garcia, A.E. Roumestand, C. Structural, energetic and dynamic responses of the native state ensemble of staphylococcal nuclease to cavity-creating mutations. *Proteins* **2013**, *81*, 1069–1080. [CrossRef]
30. Shortle, D.; Meeker, A.K.; Freire, E. Stability mutants of staphylococcal nuclease: Large compensating enthalpy-entropy changes for the reversible denaturation reaction. *Biochemistry* **1988**, *27*, 4761–4768. [CrossRef]
31. Pons, J.L.; Malliavin, T.E.; Delsuc, M.A. Gifa V. 4: A complete package for NMR data set processing. *J. Biomol. NMR* **1996**, *8*, 445–452. [CrossRef]
32. Fossat, M.J.; Dao, T.P.; Jenkins, K.; Dellarole, M.; Yang, Y.-S.; McCallum, S.A.; Garcia, A.E.; Barrick, D.; Roumestand, C.; Royer, C.A. High-Resolution Mapping of a Repeat Protein Folding Free Energy Landscape. *Biophys. J.* **2016**, *111*, 2368–2376. [CrossRef]
33. Jenkins, K.A.; Fossat, M.J.; Zhang, S.; Rai, D.K.; Klein, S.; Gillilan, R.; White, Z.; Gerlich, G.; McCallum, S.A.; Winter, R.; et al. The consequences of cavity creation on the folding landscape of a repeat protein depend upon context. *Proc. Natl. Acad. Sci. USA.* **2018**, *115*, 8153–8161. [CrossRef]
34. Fuentes, E.J.; Wand, A.J. Local stability and dynamics of apocytochrome b562 examined by the dependence of hydrogen exchange on hydrostatic pressure. *Biochemistry* **1998**, *37*, 9877–9883. [CrossRef]

biology

MDPI

Article

Conformational Rearrangements in the Redox Cycling of NADPH-Cytochrome P450 Reductase from *Sorghum bicolor* Explored with FRET and Pressure-Perturbation Spectroscopy

Bixia Zhang, ChulHee Kang * and Dmitri R. Davydov *

Department of Chemistry, Washington State University, Pullman, WA 99164, USA; bixia.zhang@wsu.edu
* Correspondence: chkang@wsu.edu (C.K.); d.davydov@wsu.edu (D.R.D.)

Simple Summary: NADPH-cytochrome P450 reductase (CPR) enzymes are known to undergo an ample conformational transition between the closed and open states in the process of their redox cycling. To explore the conformational landscape of CPR from the potential biofuel crop *Sorghum bicolor* (SbCPR), we incorporated a FRET donor/acceptor pair into the enzyme and employed rapid scanning stop-flow and pressure perturbation spectroscopy to characterize the equilibrium between its open and closed states at different stages of the redox cycle. Our results suggest the presence of several open conformational sub-states differing in the system volume change associated with the opening transition (ΔV^0). Although the closed conformation always predominates in the conformational landscape, the population of the open conformations increases by order of magnitude upon the two-electron reduction and the formation of the disemiquinone state of the enzyme. In addition to elucidating the functional choreography of plant CPRs, our study demonstrates the high exploratory potential of a combination of the pressure-perturbation approach with the FRET-based monitoring of protein conformational transitions.

Citation: Zhang, B.; Kang, C.; Davydov, D.R. Conformational Rearrangements in the Redox Cycling of NADPH-Cytochrome P450 Reductase from *Sorghum bicolor* Explored with FRET and Pressure-Perturbation Spectroscopy. *Biology* **2022**, *11*, 510. https://doi.org/10.3390/biology11040510

Academic Editor: Martin Ronis

Received: 4 March 2022
Accepted: 23 March 2022
Published: 25 March 2022

Abstract: NADPH-cytochrome P450 reductase (CPR) from *Sorghum bicolor* (SbCPR) serves as an electron donor for cytochrome P450 essential for monolignol and lignin production in this biofuel crop. The CPR enzymes undergo an ample conformational transition between the closed and open states in their functioning. This transition is triggered by electron transfer between the FAD and FMN and provides access of the partner protein to the electron-donating FMN domain. To characterize the electron transfer mechanisms in the monolignol biosynthetic pathway better, we explore the conformational transitions in SbCPR with rapid scanning stop-flow and pressure-perturbation spectroscopy. We used FRET between a pair of donor and acceptor probes incorporated into the FAD and FMN domains of SbCPR, respectively, to characterize the equilibrium between the open and closed states and explore its modulation in connection with the redox state of the enzyme. We demonstrate that, although the closed conformation always predominates in the conformational landscape, the population of open state increases by order of magnitude upon the formation of the disemiquinone state. Our results are consistent with several open conformation sub-states differing in the volume change (ΔV^0) of the opening transition. While the ΔV^0 characteristic of the oxidized enzyme is as large as −88 mL/mol, the interaction of the enzyme with the nucleotide cofactor and the formation of the double-semiquinone state of CPR decrease this value to −34 and −18 mL/mol, respectively. This observation suggests that the interdomain electron transfer in CPR increases protein hydration, while promoting more open conformation. In addition to elucidating the functional choreography of plant CPRs, our study demonstrates the high exploratory potential of a combination of the pressure-perturbation approach with the FRET-based monitoring of protein conformational transitions.

Keywords: cytochrome P450 reductase; conformational change; FRET; pressure-perturbation spectroscopy; protein hydration; reduction kinetics; stop-flow spectroscopy; *Sorghum bicolor*

1. Introduction

Cytochromes P450, the heme-thiolate enzymes found in all domains of life, from *Eubacteria* and *Archaea* to *Eukarya*, probably appeared about 3.5 billion years ago [1], when the oxygen content in the atmosphere was negligible. It is suggested that ancient cytochromes P450 acted as reducing enzymes and could play the role of NO reductases [2]. When green plants began to release oxygen into the atmosphere about 2 billion years ago, cytochromes P450 became involved in the synthesis and oxidative metabolism of fatty acids and steroids [3]. Later, the catalytic oxidation of hydrophobic compounds became the primary function of cytochromes P450.

Nowadays, cytochromes P450 act as terminal oxidases in monooxygenase systems, oxidizing various exogenous and endogenous substrates. They are involved in the oxidative metabolism and detoxification of low molecular weight foreign lipophilic compounds (xenobiotics) as well as in the synthesis of pigments, hormones, second messengers, antibiotics, and toxins. To perform these functions better, the eukaryotic P450s became membrane incorporated. In most cases, they are associated with the membranes of the endoplasmic reticulum (ER), where they interact with their partner proteins via lateral diffusion and the formation of dissociative complexes.

All known eukaryotic cytochromes P450 and most bacterial analogs are not self-sufficient in their catalytic function. The monooxygenase reaction requires two electrons, which are usually transferred to cytochrome P450 from a protein partner. For most eukaryotic cytochromes P450, the role of electron donor is played by NADPH-cytochrome P450 reductase (CPR), a flavoprotein that contains two flavin cofactors, FAD and FMN. These flavins are situated in distinct protein domains termed FAD and FMN domains. These two domains are connected with a flexible connecting loop. The reducing equivalents from NADPH are first acquired by FAD and then transferred to FMN, which serves as an ultimate electron donor for P450.

While the majority of animal cytochrome P450 species are involved in xenobiotic metabolism, the predominant part of the plant P450s participates in biosynthetic pathways. They play a critical role in synthesizing lignin, UV protectants, pigments, defense compounds, fatty acids, hormones, and secondary messengers. In particular, cytochrome-P450-dependent cinnamate-4-hydroxylase (C4H), *p*-coumaroyl quinate/shikimate-3′-hydroxylase (C3′H), and ferulate-5-hydroxylase (F5H) are the critical branching points in the phenylpropanoid metabolizing pathway, which is required for the biosynthesis of monolignol and serves as a starting point for the production of flavonoids, coumarins, lignans, and lignin.

This investigation represents a part of our studies aimed at elucidating the mechanisms of function and regulation of phenylpropanoid-metabolizing monooxygenases from *Sorghum bicolor*, a U.S. strategic plant for biofuel production [4–6]. The detailed mechanistic knowledge of these enzymes will enable specific manipulation of lignin composition and content and thus economize the industrial cost of biofuel production. Furthermore, the high flexibility of the hinge region of SbCPR demonstrated in our previous report [7] offers potential for manipulating the functional properties of the enzyme through rational engineering in this region. The present study explores the functional mechanisms of NADPH-cytochrome P450 reductase 2b, one of the three CPR enzymes in *Sorghum bicolor* serving as electron donors for C4H, C3′H, and F5H P450 enzymes. This enzyme is referred to as SbCPR from now on.

In general, the functional redox cycling in SbCPR enzymes follows the scheme common to all known CPRs. Their reduction from the completely oxidized (FAD, FMN) to the four-electron reduced state ($FADH_2$, $FMNH_2$) includes (1) hydride transfer from NADPH to FAD, resulting in a two-electron reduced ($FADH_2$, FMN) state; (2) inter-flavin electron transfer from $FADH_2$ to FMN with the formation of the neutral (blue) disemiquinone ($FADH^{\bullet}$, $FMNH^{\bullet}$); (3) establishing a transient equilibrium between the latter and the other two-electron reduced states (FAD, $FMNH_2$), ($FADH_2$, FMN) and anionic semiquinones ($FAD^{\bullet -}$, $FMN^{\bullet -}$); (4) supply of another pair of electrons from NADPH yielding the four-electron reduced ($FADH_2$, $FMNH_2$) state. This sequence of events is illustrated in Scheme 1.

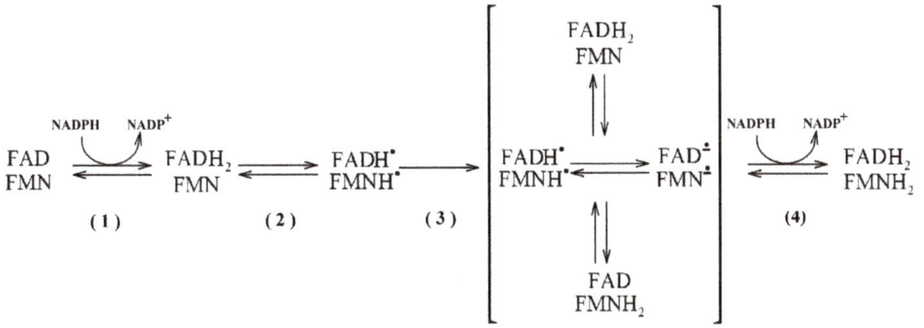

Scheme 1. Scheme of electron transfer events in CPR.

In most eukaryotic monooxygenases, this four-electron reduced state is believed to serve as the P450 electron donor so that FMN cofactor interchanges between the hydroquinone and semiquinone states. By contrast, the FMN moiety in the bacterial CPR-P450 chimera P450BM-3 shuttles between the semiquinone and oxidized states instead [8]. However, in all cases, the transfer of electrons between the FAD and FMN domains remains an obligatory step in the CPR redox cycle.

In this perspective, understanding electron transfer mechanisms and the respective conformational rearrangements has become a challenge for researchers. In the first solved CPR structure [9] and several subsequently published structures of CPR from various species [10–12], the distance between FAD and FMN is around 4 Å, which is considered favorable for the inter-flavin electron transfer. However, this proximity of the two domains does not allow the electron acceptor protein to reach FMN. This circumstance and the largely disordered structure of the connecting loop brought forward a hypothesis of a large-scale opening-and-closing transition involved in the CPR electron transfer mechanism.

In further X-ray crystallographic studies, the CPR variant with a shortened connecting loop was found locked in the open state, which is flawed in terms of inter-flavin electron transfer, but effective in the transfer from FMN to the heme [13]. In contrast, a variant of rat CPR where the two domains are interconnected with a disulfide bond [14] was found locked in the closed conformation. These and other resolved CPR structures [11,12,15,16] demonstrated exceptional conformational flexibility of CPR and emphasized the pivotal functional role of the transitions between the enzyme's closed and open states.

The conformational landscape of CPR and its relevance to the redox cycling of the enzyme was further explored with a wide variety of biophysical techniques ranging from NMR [17] and small-angle neutron and X-ray scattering (SANS and SAX, [18–21]) to ion mobility mass spectrometry [22] and single-molecule fluorescence resonance energy transfer (FRET [23–26]). Despite some contradictory observations in these studies, all of them are consistent in demonstrating a transition of the closed state of the enzyme into an open conformation upon the interdomain electron transfer event and the formation of the disemiquinone state (see [27] for a review). At the same time, these studies also demonstrated that the initial two-state model is insufficient to adequately depict the conformational landscape of CPR.

According to the current concepts, instead of being represented by two discrete states, the enzyme exists in a dynamic equilibrium among multiple conformations differing in the relative positioning of the FMN and FAD domains [27]. Most available data suggest that the closed conformations predominate in the completely oxidized CPR [18–21,24,26]. Some studies also suggest the further displacement of the conformational equilibrium towards the closed state upon the binding of NADPH to the oxidized enzyme [25,27]. There are also strong indications of the predominance of the closed conformations in the four-electron reduced enzyme [20,21,23,26].

Despite a foreseeable similarity of CPR enzymes from different organisms in general mechanisms of electron transport and the related protein choreography, the enzymes from different kingdoms of life may differ considerably in the kinetic and thermodynamic parameters of the individual steps of the redox cycle. Thus, the structure study of *Arabidopsis thaliana* suggests that the oxidized state of plant CPR enzymes may have considerably more open conformation than that characteristic of their mammalian counterparts [11]. Furthermore, the studies of the kinetics of electron transfer in plant CPR demonstrate that the rate of electron transfer from NADPH to FAD in these enzymes is over 50 times faster than in their mammalian counterparts [28].

In the present study, we explore the conformational equilibrium in SbCPR and its modulation during the redox cycle of the enzyme with the use of a combination of the FRET-based detection of protein conformational rearrangements with the rapid scanning absorbance and fluorescence stop-flow technique and the pressure-perturbation approach. While the FRET-based methods and rapid scanning stop-flow techniques have already been applied in both mammalian [24,25,27] and plant [26] CPR studies, the present study represents the first attempt to explore the conformational landscape of CPR with pressure perturbation.

In pressure-perturbation studies, hydrostatic pressure is a variable parameter affecting the protein conformational landscapes. Along with the effects of temperature, varying pressure is indispensable for a detailed understanding of the mechanisms of protein conformational transitions. The basis of pressure effects is the change in system volume that accompanies biochemical processes [29–32]. According to Le Chatelier's principle, increased pressure enhances processes accompanied by a decrease in system volume and, conversely, inhibits processes occurring with a volume increase. A prevalent part of the volume changes in protein transitions stems from the changes in interactions with solvents [33–38]. These include water penetration into the cavities and water constriction around solvent-exposed polar groups of the protein [31,38–43]. Thus, the volume change resulting from the penetration of one water molecule into a protein cavity is equal to -18 mL/mol, while the solvation of a singly charged ion in water is characterized by ΔV values of the order of -10 mL/mol [31]. Generally speaking, pressure increase enhances protein hydration, which therefore constitutes the core of pressure-induced protein transitions [33,34,37,43–46].

Ample conformational transitions necessary for CPR redox cycling are implied to be associated with significant changes in the protein–solvent interactions. The process of protein opening is reported to involve the breaking of several salt bridges [11,12,24] and the subsequent hydration of the newly exposed charges on the protein surface. Therefore, pressure perturbation is the method of choice for exploring the CPR conformational landscape. It allows to judge the changes in protein hydration in the redox cycling of the enzyme and provides a simple means for determining the position of equilibria in the system of open and closed conformation at its different redox states.

To make the studies possible, we incorporate a FRET donor/acceptor pair into the FAD and FMN domains of SbCPR. Our study demonstrates that, although the closed conformation always predominates in the conformational landscape, the population of open state increases by order of magnitude upon the formation of the disemiquinone state. Our results are consistent with several open conformation sub-states differing in the opening transition volume change (ΔV^0). The details of the SbCPR electron transfer mechanism revealed in this study will provide vital information for engineering the monolignol pathway and subsequent lignin polymerization in order to improve the use of *Sorghum bicolor* as a biofuel plant. In addition to elucidating the functional choreography of plant CPRs, our study demonstrates the high exploratory potential of a combination of the pressure-perturbation approach with the FRET-based monitoring of protein conformational dynamics.

2. Materials and Methods

2.1. Materials

DY-520XL and DY-731 were the products of Dyomics GMBH (Jena, Germany). Monobromobimane (MBBr) was obtained from Invitrogen/Molecular Probes (Eugene, OR, USA), now a part of ThermoFisher Scientific. Igepal CO-630, glucose oxidase, catalase, NADPH, glucose-6-phosphate, and glucose-6-phosphate-dehydrogenase were obtained from Sigma-Aldrich (St. Louis, MO, USA). 2′5′-ADP was purchased from Santa Cruz Biotechnology (Dallas, TX, USA). All other chemicals were of the highest grade commercially available and were used without further purification.

2.2. Cloning, Protein Expression, and Purification

The SbCPR cDNA corresponding to the *Sorghum bicolor* gene SORBI_3007G088000 was modified with a truncation of its N-terminal transmembrane sequence (Δ2–50) and the addition of the C-terminal hexahistidine tag. The resulting construct was cloned into a pET-30a (+) vector. For the SbCPR C596S mutant, site-directed mutations were created in the SbCPR coding region by PCR-based amplification using Phusion High-Fidelity DNA polymerase (New England Biolabs, Ipswich, MA, USA). The amplification was performed using the forward primer CTTCGGAAGCAGAAATAGCAAGATGGACT, and the reverse primer TATTTCTGCTTCCGAAGAAGAACACGGATG was followed by *Dpn*I (New England Biolabs, Ipswich, MA, USA) digestion to remove the template strand prior to transformation to XL1-blue competent cell for amplification. C596S mutation was confirmed by DNA sequencing (Fisher Scientific, Waltham, MA, USA). The replacement was performed to limit the possible location of the incorporated fluorescent probes to Cys-235 and Cys-536 (see Section 3.1). The purification methods were the same for the wild-type and C596S mutant. The vectors were transformed into *Escherichia coli* Rosetta 2 (DE3) cells. Three liters of Lysogeny Broth medium complemented with 25 μg mL^{-1} chloramphenicol and 50 μg mL^{-1} kanamycin were inoculated with 20 mL from the culture. The cells were grown at 37 °C until the optical density of the culture at 600 nm reached 0.6~0.8. At this point, the temperature was set at 25 °C and 0.5 mM IPTG was added. After the incubation of the culture for 16 h, the cells were harvested by centrifugation at 5000 rpm for 20 min at 4 °C and resuspended in the Buffer A (50 mM Tris-HCl, 300 mM NaCl, pH 8.0) with 20 mM imidazole. After sonicating on ice for 30 min with a Model 450 sonicator (Branson Ultrasonics, Danbury, CT, USA), the cell debris was removed by ultracentrifugation. The clear lysate was loaded onto the column of Ni-NTA agarose (Qiagen, Germantown, MD, USA) and extensively washed with the same buffer. Modified CPR protein was eluted by Buffer A containing 250 mM imidazole, pH 8.0. After concentrating the protein to 2 mg mL^{-1}, its solution was dialyzed against 5 mM potassium phosphate buffer and applied onto a CHT ceramic hydroxyapatite column (Bio-Rad, Hercules, CA, USA). The fraction containing SbCPR was eluted by a linear phosphate gradient and then concentrated to ~30 mg/mL. Final purity was analyzed by SDS-PAGE, and the concentration was determined by Bradford assay (Bio-Rad).

2.3. Incorporation of Thiol-Reactive Fluorescent Probes

In this study, we used DY-520XL and DY731 fluorescent dyes manufactured by Dyomics GMBH, Jena, Germany) as FRET donor and acceptor fluorophores. Both probes were used as maleimide derivatives (product numbers 520XL-03 and 731-03, respectively). Incorporating these probes into SbCPR involves their attachment to the thiol groups of the cysteine residues of the protein. Prior to modification, SbCPR was stored in 125 mM K-phosphate buffer, pH 7.4, containing 2 mM TCEP (Storage Buffer). TCEP was removed by passing the protein solution through a spin-out column of Bio-Gel P6 desalting resin (Bio-Rad, Hercules, CA, USA) equilibrated with 125 mM K-phosphate buffer, pH 7.4. After diluting the protein with the same buffer to the concentration of 10 μM, a 3 mM solution of DY-520XL maleimide in acetone was added to the final concentration of 10 μM, and the solution was incubated at 4 °C under continuous stirring. The increase in the fluorescence of DY-520XL at 630 nm (excitation at 520 nm) in the process of modification was monitored to ensure reaction completion. After the stabilization of fluorescence in approximately one hour of incubation, an acetone solution of the second probe (DY731 maleimide) was added to the final concentration of 10 μM. The reaction was followed by monitoring a decrease in the fluorescence of DY-520XL. The process of the second modification required 3–4 h for completion. Finally, the reaction was terminated by adding reduced glutathione to the concentration of 1 mM. The protein was concentrated to 100–200 μM and passed through a spin-out column of Bio-Gel P6 equilibrated with 125 mM potassium phosphate buffer, pH 7.4 to remove glutathione adducts unreacted dyes. The stoichiometry of labeling by DY-520XL and DY-731 was determined based on the spectrum of absorbance of the modified protein. This calculation used the extinction coefficients of 0.05 μM^{-1} cm^{-1} at 520 nm and 0.24 μM^{-1} cm^{-1} at 736 nm for DY-520XL and DY-731, respectively, as specified by the manufacturer.

2.4. Rapid Kinetic Studies with Absorbance and Fluorescence Spectroscopy

The kinetics of the NADPH-dependent reduction of SbCPR were studied with rapid-scanning stop-flow spectroscopy. The experiments were performed at 5 °C in 20 mM HEPES buffer, pH 7.4, containing an oxygen-scavenging system consisting of 60 mM glucose, 300 units/mL glucose oxidase, and 2000 units/mL catalase. The concentration of SbCPR and NADPH in the optical cell was equal to 20 μM and 200 μM, respectively. The solution of NADPH also contained 2 mM glucose-6-phosphate and 4 units/mL glucose-6-phosphate dehydrogenase, which were added to keep the concentration of NADPH constant. The stop-flow experiments were performed with the use of RX 2000 Rapid Mixing Stopped-flow Accessory manufactured by Applied Photophysics Ltd. (Leatherhead, Surrey, U.K.) connected to the master channel of an MC2000-2 two-channel CCD spectrometer (Ocean Optics, Inc., Dunedin, FL, USA) equipped with a custom-made thermostated cell holder and a PX-2 pulsed xenon lamp light source (Ocean Optics). The RX 2000 Accessory was custom modified to allow remote control of mixing from the data acquisition software. The absorbance spectra in the range of 320–700 nm were collected with the time intervals changing from 2 ms to 2 s per spectrum using custom data acquisition software.

Rapid kinetics of the changes in SbCPR conformation during the reduction process were studied with FRET-based monitoring in a setup similar to that described above for the absorbance spectroscopy. In these experiments, the concentration of SbCPR-2DY and NADPH in the optical cell was equal to 5 and 100 μM, respectively, and the temperature was maintained at 5 °C. The composition of the other ingredients was the same as indicated above for the absorbance spectroscopy experiments. In these studies, the master channel of the MC2000-2 spectrometer was connected with a Vis-NIR 3 mm liquid light guide (Model 77635, Newport Corporation, Irvine, CA, USA) to the fluorescence window of the cell holder. The excitation light was provided with an M505F1 light-emitting diode (Thorlabs Inc., Newton, NJ, USA) emitting at 505 nm and functioning in a continuous wave mode. We used M617L3 light-emitting diode (Thorlabs Inc.) emitting at 617 nm as a light source in the experiments with direct excitation of the acceptor fluorophore. The fluorescence spectra were recorded in the range of 580–950 nm collected with the time intervals changing from 10 ms to 2 s per spectrum using custom data acquisition software.

2.5. Pressure Perturbation Experiments

Pressure-perturbation experiments were performed using a custom-built high-pressure optical cell [47] connected to a manual pressure generator (High Pressure Equipment, Erie, PA, USA) capable of generating a pressure of up to 6000 bar. The emission spectra were recorded with an MC2000-2 spectrometer (Ocean Optics) connected with a Vis-NIR 3 mm liquid light guide (Model 77635, Newport Corporation, Irvine, CA, USA) to the fluorescence window of the high-pressure cell. The spectra were recorded in the 580–900 nm region with a step of 1 nm. All spectra were corrected for the changes in protein concentration due to pressure-dependent compression of water as described earlier [48]. The excitation light was provided with an M505F1 light-emitting diode (Thorlabs Inc., Newton, NJ, USA) emitting at 505 nm in the continuous wave mode. The experiments were performed with 5 μM SbCPR-2DY at 25 °C in 20 mM Na-Hepes buffer. The experiments with the reduced SbCPR-2DY were carried out in the presence of an oxygen-scavenging system consisting of glucose oxidase (30 units/mL), 60 mM glucose, and 2000 units/mL catalase. The NADPH concentrations used in the experiments with the partially and fully reduced enzyme were equal to 5 and 100 μM, respectively. The experiments in the presence of 2′,5′-ADP were performed at 1 mM concentration of the latter.

2.6. *Data Fitting*

All data treatment and fitting, as well as the data acquisition in the absorbance and fluorescence spectroscopy experiments, were performed using our custom-designed SpectraLab software [48]. The latest version of the software package is freely available on the author's website [49].

2.6.1. Interpretation of the Results of Rapid Scanning Absorbance Spectroscopy

The series of spectra obtained in the rapid scanning absorbance stop-flow experiments were subjected to the Principal Component Analysis (PCA), a linear algebra method commonly used to reduce the dimensionality of large datasets [50]. It analyzes a set of M individual datasets (absorbance or fluorescence spectra in our case) of the dimensionality N (number data points in each spectrum). This dataset is used to construct the N × N covariance matrix, which is then transformed to find M-1 eigenvectors paired with M eigenvalues. The combination of each eigenvector with the corresponding set of eigenvalues is termed the Principal Component. The eigenvectors may be considered unified differences between the basis vector (the first spectrum in the series in our case) and other vectors (spectra) under analysis. The PCs are sorted based on their statistical significance. The first PC represents the most typical difference between the individual datasets (spectra), and the higher-order PCs contain the least significant deviations from the basis. This way, organizing information in PC allows reducing dimensionality without losing much information by discarding the components with low statistical significance. In practice, each dataset may be reconstituted with increasing accuracy by successive summarizing the basis vector and the eigenvectors multiplied by the respective eigenvalues. Thus, the set of eigenvalues deduced from the analysis of a spectral series reflects the changes in the amplitude of spectral alterations represented in the respective eigenvector, which might be considered a unified differential spectrum that characterizes the process under study. PCA is widely used for analyzing the results of rapid scanning kinetic experiments [51–54].

In our experiments, the first Principal Component yielded from this procedure typically covered over 98.5% of the total spectral changes. The time dependence of its eigenvalue was interpreted as reflecting the general kinetics of reduction. Approximation of these kinetics by a three-exponential equation was used to determine the kinetic constants of the individual phases of the reduction process.

2.6.2. Interpretation of the Results of Fluorescence Spectroscopy

The quantitative interpretation of FRET results was based on the application of PCA to a series of emission spectra recorded in rapid kinetics or pressure perturbation experiments. Approximation of the first principal vector (>98% of the observed changes) with a combination of the prototypical spectra of emission of DY-520XL and DY731 normalized proportionally to their quantum yields (see Appendix A) allowed us to resolve the changes in the integral intensities of emission of each of the dyes and interpret them in terms of FRET efficiency. The quantum-yield-normalized intensities of the donor and acceptor fluorescence obtained in this way were used to determine the FRET efficiency according to the following equation:

$$E = (I_a/\Phi_a)/(I_a/\Phi_a + I_d/\Phi_d) \quad (1)$$

where I_a is the emission intensity of the acceptor, I_d is the residual donor emission in the presence of acceptor, and Φ_a and Φ_d are the quantum yields of the fluorescence of the acceptor and the donor, respectively.

Distances between the donor and acceptor fluorophores (R) were calculated using the following equation:

$$R = R_0 \cdot \sqrt[6]{(E^{-1} - 1)} \quad (2)$$

where R_0 is the Förster distance calculated using the absorbance and emission spectra of the protein-bound donor and acceptor fluorophores. These calculations were performed using PhotoChemCad software [55], assuming the values of the orientation factor (κ) and the refractive index (n) to be equal to 0.667 and 1.4, respectively.

2.6.3. Fitting of the Results of Pressure-Perturbation Experiments

The interpretation of the effect of pressure on protein equilibria in this article is based on the equation for the pressure dependence of the equilibrium constant ([56], Equation (1)):

$$\partial(\ln K_{eq})/\partial p = -\left(\Delta V^0\right)/RT \quad (3)$$

or in integral form, [57] (p. 212, Equtation (9)):

$$K_{eq} = K_{eq}^0 \cdot e^{-P\Delta V^0/RT} = e^{(P_{1/2}-P)\Delta V^0/RT} \quad (4)$$

where K_{eq} is the equilibrium constant of the reaction at pressure P, $P_{½}$ is the pressure at which $K_{eq} = 1$ ("half pressure" of the conversion), ΔV^0 is the standard molar reaction volume, and $K^0{}_{eq}$ is the equilibrium constant extrapolated to zero pressure, $K^0{}_{eq} = e^{P_{½}\Delta V^0}/\mathrm{RT}$. For the equilibrium $A \rightleftharpoons B$ and $K_{eq} = [B]/[A]$, Equation (4) may be transformed into the following relationship:

$$\frac{[A]}{C_0} = \frac{1}{1 + K_{eq}^0 \cdot e^{-P\Delta V^0/RT}} = \frac{1}{1 + e^{(P_{1/2}-P)\Delta V^0/RT}} \quad (5)$$

where $C_0 = [A] + [B]$. To determine the ΔV^0 and $P_{½}$ parameters from the experimental datasets describing pressure-induced changes in the amplitude of a signal derived from the fluorescence spectra (A_p), this equation was complemented with the offset (A_0) and scaling factor (A_{max}) parameters and used in the following form:

$$A_p = A_0 + \frac{A_{\max}}{1 + e^{(P_{1/2}-P)\Delta V^0/RT}} \quad (6)$$

Prior to the analysis, all spectra were corrected for the compression of the solvent [48].

2.7. MALDI/TOF Analysis for the Fluorescence Dye Modified Peptides

Prior to MALDI/TOF analysis, the unmodified SbCPR-C596 and its adducts with monobromobimane (MBBr), DY-520XL and DY-731 (see Appendix B) were subjected to SDS-PAGE. After staining the gel slabs, their fragments containing the SbCPR protein band were isolated and subjected to in-gel trypsinolysis, following the established protocol [58]. The digested peptides were analyzed by MALDI/TOF MS. The peptide mass spectra were obtained using procedure and collection programs supplied by the manufacturer (Applied Biosystems, Waltham, MA, USA). The matrix, a-cyano-4-hydroxycinnamic acid, CHCA (Sigma-Aldrich, St. Louis, MO, USA), was prepared as a solution of 10 mg mL^{-1} in 50% water/acetonitrile with 0.1% TFA. The matrix solution was mixed 1:1 with the trypsin digest, applied to the sample plate, and dried. Spectra were collected using a 4800 MALDI TOF/TOF Analyzer (Applied Biosystems, Waltham, MA, USA), using the data collection programs in the positive mode for MS spectra.

3. Results

3.1. Selecting the Attachment Points for the Fluorophores and Construction of the Cysteine-Depleted Variant of SbCPR

To explore the conformational dynamics of SbCPR that accompanies the process of its NADPH-dependent reduction and probe the thermodynamic parameters of the respective conformational transitions with pressure-perturbation spectroscopy, we sought to introduce a FRET donor/acceptor pair into the FAD and FMN domains of the enzyme. The background for selecting DY-520XL and DY-731 maleimides as thiol-reactive fluorophores for these experiments is described in Appendix A. There we also provide characterizations of the photochemical properties of this donor/acceptor pair and its incorporation into SbCPR.

To minimize the perturbations of the protein structure by mutagenesis needed for the site-directed incorporation of the thiol-reactive probes, we elected to employ some of the native cysteine residues of the protein for its modification. SbCPR contains nine cysteine residues—Cys-235, Cys-306, Cys-325, Cys-352, Cys-503, Cys-520, Cys-536, Cys-596 and Cys659. According to the analysis of the structure of the FAD domain [7] and the homology model of the full-length enzyme, the residues Cys-306, Cys-325, Cys-352, Cys-503, Cys-520, and Cys-659 are buried inside the structure and barely accessible. Cys-235, the only cysteine residue located in the FMN domain, and Cys-536, located on the surface of the FAD/NADPH-binding domain, appear to be easily accessible for modification. Another potentially accessible cysteine in the FAD domain is Cys-596, which is more buried than Cys-536. Thus, we expect to encounter two–three modification-accessible cysteine residues in SbCPR, Cys-235, Cys-536, and Cys-596. Of those three residues, the Cys-235 and Cys-536 provide an optimal combination for positioning the donor/acceptor pair. The position of these residues is indicated in Figure 1, where we show a model of SbCPR based on a combination of the resolved X-ray structure of its FAD domain (PDB ID: 7SUX) [7] with the model of the FMN domain and the connecting loop built with AlphaFold, a machine-learning-based protein structure prediction tool [59]. The model was created by replacing the FAD domain in the AlphaFold-generated model of SbCPR with its X-ray-resolved structure starting at Val-310 residue. To this aim, the AlfaFold-built model of SbCPR and the X-ray structure of the FAD domain were aligned upfront using the MatchMaker tool of the UCSF Chimera software [60].

As described in Appendix B, studying the accessibility of SbCPR cysteines for modification with monobromobimane (MBBr), we demonstrated that the enzyme contains three cysteine residues easily accessible for modification with a thiol-reactive probe. Employing MALDI-TOF mass spectroscopy for probing the points of attachment of the fluorophores, we confirmed the above conclusion that Cys-235, Cys-536, and Cys-596 (listed in the order of decreasing accessibility) are the most modification-accessible cysteine residues in the protein.

To limit the SbCPR modification by thiol-reactive probes to a pair of most readily available cysteine residues, Cys-235 and Cys-536, we removed Cys-596 by mutating it into a serine residue. The resulting C596S variant, with only eight cysteine residues per enzyme molecule, can be readily expressed in *E. coli* and purified with a yield similar to that characteristic of the wild-type SbCPR. The rate of its turnover in the reduction of cytochrome c was also nearly identical to that exhibited by the wild-type enzyme. The C596S variant was therefore used in all experiments described in this article. It is from now on referred to as SbCPR to simplify the narrative.

The sequential modification of the C596S variant of SbCPR with DY520-XL and DY-731 (see Section 2.3) resulted in the protein that contains 0.7–1 molar equivalent of each dye per protein molecule and did not result in any considerable protein precipitation. The modified C596S variant enzyme, which we designate hereafter as SbCPR-2DY, was active in the cytochrome c reduction with the turnover number of 2267 min^{-1}, which is comparable with that observed in the wild-type SbCPR. Our MALDI-TOF MS analysis described in Appendix B suggests that the sequential labeling procedure results in the protein where the DY-520-XL probe is prevalently attached to Cys-235, while DY-731 fluorophore is by preference located at Cys-536.

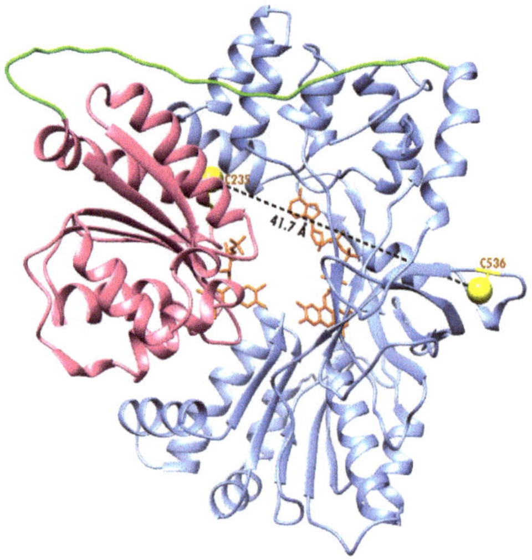

Figure 1. Structural model of SbCPR based on a combination of the resolved X-ray structure of the FAD domain (PDB ID: 7SUX) with the model of FMN domain and the connecting loop built with AlphaFold. The two modification-accessible cysteine residues are shown as yellow spheres. FMN and FAD domains are pink and light blue, respectively, and the connecting loop is green. FAD and FMN molecules are shown as orange stick models. The N-terminal transmembrane helix of the enzyme is not shown.

3.2. Kinetics of the NADPH-Dependent Reduction of SbCPR

In order to explore the time frame of the individual steps of the NADPH-dependent reduction of SbCPR, we examined its kinetics by rapid-scanning stop-flow absorbance spectroscopy. The reduction process was followed by monitoring the changes in absorbance in the 350–700 nm region.

The oxidized state of CPR flavins has two major absorbance bands centered at 380 and 456 nm, respectively. In the neutral (blue) and anionic (red) flavin semiquinones, the amplitude of the band at 456 nm is dramatically decreased. Furthermore, the neutral semiquinone state is distinguished by a broad band centered around 595 nm, which is lacking in the anionic semiquinone. In addition to the complete lack of the 456 and 595 nm bands, the two-electron reduced (hydroquinone) state differs from the semiquinones by decreased absorbance at 380 nm. Therefore, the process of the transition of the enzyme through the stages depicted in Scheme 1 can be followed by analyzing the changes in absorbance at 380, 456, and 595 nm. A decrease in the absorbance at 456 nm reflects the overall reduction process. The changes in the amplitude of the absorbance band at 595 nm reflect the initial appearance and further evanescence of the neutral flavin semiquinones ($FADH^{\bullet}$, $FMNH^{\bullet}$). The formation of the two-electron reduced flavin hydroquinones ($FADH_2$ and $FMNH_2$) can be judged from a decrease in absorbance at 380 nm.

Results of our stop-flow experiments are presented in Table 1 and Figure 2. A series of spectra recorded during the reduction process is exemplified in a 3D plot, shown in Figure 2a. Principal Component Analysis (PCA) of this dataset results in the first and the second principal components (PCs) covering 98.6 and 0.6% of the total changes, respectively. The respective eigenvectors and the sets of eigenvalues are shown in Figure 2b,c. As seen from these plots, the spectra of both PC (their eigenvectors) reveal the features characteristic of the changes in flavins' redox state. The first PC possesses minima at the positions of both absorbance bands of oxidized flavins (380 and 456 nm) and a maximum at 595 nm that corresponds to the absorbance band of the blue semiquinone. While this PC characterizes the overall kinetics of reduction, the second PC, which features the bands at 375 and 595 nm, reflects the difference in the spectral changes between the individual reduction stages (Scheme 1).

Table 1. Parameters of the SbCPR reduction as determined with absorbance and fluorescence stop-flow spectroscopy *.

Phase of the Reduction Process	Apparent End State	Absorbance Spectroscopy	Fluorescence Spectroscopy		
		k_{obs}, s^{-1}	k_{obs}, s^{-1}	FRET Efficiency in the End State	Apparent Inter-Probe Distance in the End State, Å
(initial state)	FAD FMN			0.73 ± 0.03	41.0 ± 1.0
1	$FADH^{\bullet}$ $FMNH^{\bullet}$	168 ± 29	230 ± 71 (0.089)	0.60 ± 0.03	45.1 ± 1.0
2	($FADH_2$ / FMN ↔ $FADH^{\bullet}$ / $FMNH^{\bullet}$ ↔ FAD / $FMNH_2$)	26.9 ± 9.8	17.3 ± 12.7 (0.171)	0.63 ± 0.02	44.2 ± 0.6
3	$FADH^{\bullet}$ / $FMNH_2$ ↔ $FADH_2$ / $FMNH^{\bullet}$	0.021 ± 0.010	0.024 ± 0.012 (0.686)	0.68 ± 0.01	42.7 ± 0.4

* The values given in the table represent the averages of the results of 3–6 individual experiments. The "±" values show the confidence interval calculated for $p = 0.05$. The values given in parentheses represent the results of the Student's t-test for the hypothesis of equality of the k_{obs} values deduced from the absorbance experiments to those obtained in the FRET studies.

For both principal components, the kinetics of the changes in eigenvalues can be adequately approximated with the three-exponential equation (Figure 2c). These approximations yield the sets of kinetic constants that closely match each other. Conversely, an obvious distinction between the two components in the signs and the amplitudes of the individual exponential terms reveals a difference in the spectral signatures of the separate phases of the reduction process. The kinetic constants of the individual phases determined from the fitting of the kinetics of changes in the first eigenvalue to the three-exponential equation and averaged over 12 kinetic runs were found equal to 168 ± 29, 26.9 ± 9.8, and 0.021 ± 0.010 s^{-1}. These values can also be found in Table 1, along with those obtained in the kinetic experiments with FRET-based detection (see below).

Although the use of PCA provides a potent means for global analysis and allows for the accurate determination of the kinetic constants of the individual phases, the identification of the stages of the reduction process that correspond to each of the three exponential terms might be better achieved through the analysis of the absorbance changes at the three representative wavelengths (380, 456 and 595 nm). The respective kinetic curves are exemplified in Figure 3. As seen from this figure, even the first spectrum taken after the mixing is characterized by a substantial increase in absorbance at 595 nm, which is indicative of the formation of the neutral semiquinones. The increase in absorbance at this wavelength continues for approximately 20 ms. It is followed by a partial reversal within the subsequent 200–300 ms. These two initial phases are associated with a profound decrease in the absorbance at 456 nm accompanied by a much less significant attenuation in the optical density at 380 nm.

According to our interpretation, the changes in SbCPR absorbance during the first 500 ms of the reduction process (Figure 3a) suggest that the first resolved kinetic phase corresponds to the inter-flavin electron transfer event (stage (2) in Scheme 1). The subsequent slower phase may be identified to the stage (3), where the transient equilibrium between different two-electron reduced forms of the enzyme is established. These two rapid phases are followed by a very slow further decrease in absorbances at both 456 and 380 nm, accompanied by an increase in the amplitude of the 595 nm band. According to our interpretation, this stage corresponds to the reduction of some part of the enzyme pool to the four-electron reduced state followed by a comproportionation reaction between two- and four-electron reduced SbCPR molecules [61] that leads to the three-electron reduced enzyme ($FADH_2$, $FMNH^{\bullet}$), which appears to be the predominating end-state of the reduction process.

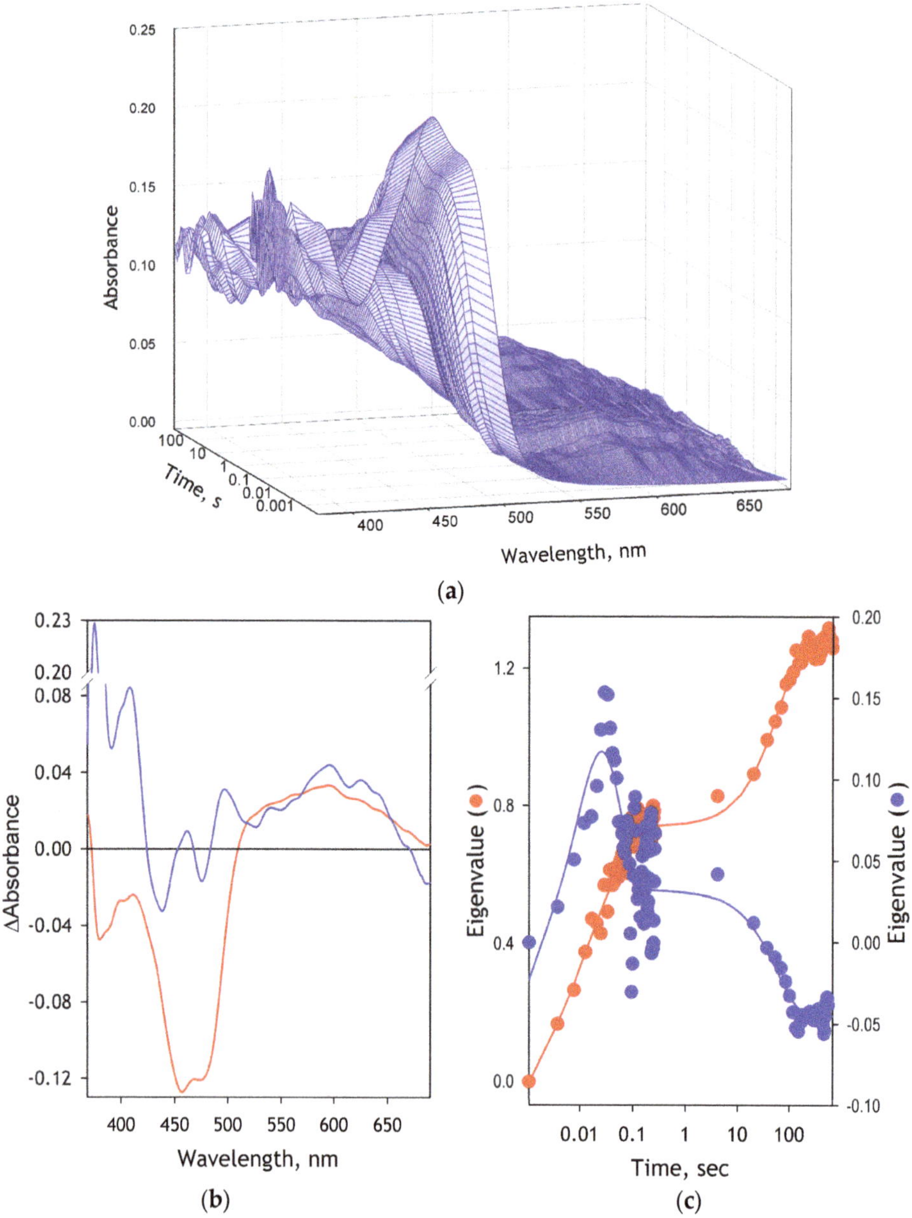

Figure 2. Changes in the spectra of absorbance of SbCPR in the process of its NADPH-dependent reduction. Panel (**a**) exemplifies a series of absorbance spectra recorded in a rapid-scanning stop-flow experiment. Panel (**b**) shows the spectra (eigenvectors) of the first (red) and second (blue) Principal Components obtained with PCA of the above dataset, and panel (**c**) represents the respective sets of eigenvalues plotted against time in semi-logarithmic coordinates. Solid lines in this panel correspond to the approximations of the kinetic curves with the three-exponential equation.

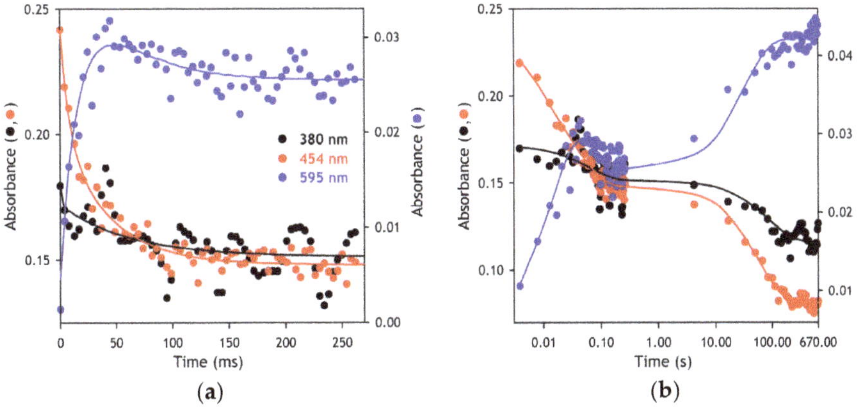

Figure 3. Changes in absorbance of SbCPR at 380, 454, and 595 nm in the process of its NADPH-dependent reduction. Panel (**a**) shows the initial parts of the curves in linear coordinates. In panel (**b**), the same datasets are plotted versus the logarithm of time in the entire time range of the experiment. Solid lines correspond to the approximations of the kinetic curves with the three-exponential equation.

3.3. Conformational Transitions in SbCPR Studied with FRET and Stop-Flow Spectroscopy

To explore the fluctuations of the SbCPR conformational landscape during the redox cycling of the enzyme, we studied the kinetics of changes in FRET in SbCPR-2DY observed in the process of its anaerobic reduction with NADPH with stop-flow technique combined rapid scanning fluorescence spectroscopy. A series of fluorescence spectra taken during the reduction process is exemplified in Figure 4a. As seen from this figure, the addition of NADPH results in a profound drop in the fluorescence of DY731, the FRET acceptor. This extremely rapid decrease is followed by a slow partial reversal associated with a considerable increase in the fluorescence of DY520XL, the FRET donor.

To probe whether the observed changes in the fluorescence of the acceptor reflect the changes in the FRET efficiency and are not associated with the possible alteration of the fluorescence of the acceptor per se, we performed stop-flow experiments with the direct excitation of the acceptor fluorophore at 617 nm. A series of spectra of DY731 fluorescence monitored during the reduction process in this setup is exemplified in Figure 4b. As seen from this plot, the intensity of DY731 fluorescence exhibits no noticeable changes during the reduction. Therefore, the spectral changes observed in the experiments with excitation at 505 nm may be unequivocally attributed to the changes in FRET efficiency.

To assess the FRET efficiency in these experiments and estimate its changes during the reduction, we normalized the series of spectra recorded in the stop-flow experiments on the total intensity of fluorescence of both fluorophores corrected according to their quantum yields (see Appendix A). A series of spectra normalized in this way is shown as a 3D plot in Figure 4c. As described in Materials and Methods, the efficiency of FRET may be directly assessed by calculating the relative intensity of fluorescence of the acceptor normalized in this way (see Equation (1) in Section 2.6.2).

Figure 4d exemplifies a kinetic curve of the changes in FRET efficiency during SbCPR reduction. As seen from this figure, the addition of NADPH to the enzyme results in a very rapid drop in FRET efficiency, followed by a slow two-exponential increase. At the end of this process, the FRET efficiency returns to a level close to that characteristic of the oxidized enzyme. Similar to the kinetics of reduction per se, these kinetic curves may be approximated with a three-exponential equation. The kinetic constants and the phase amplitudes derived from these approximations are found in Table 1.

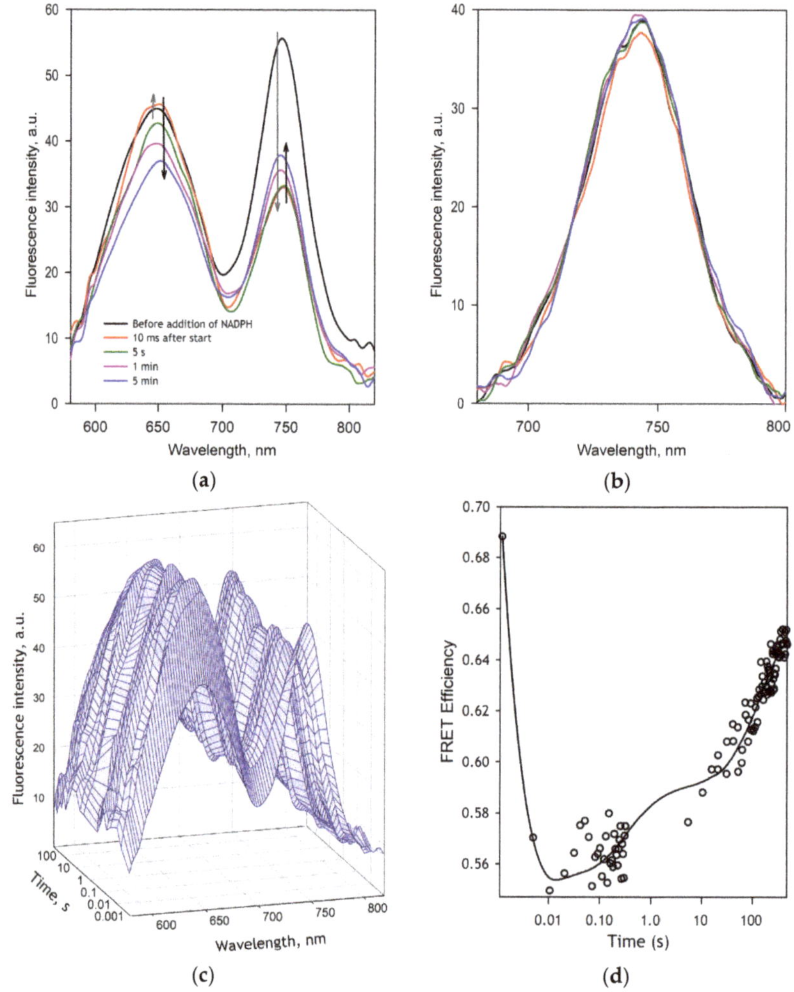

Figure 4. Changes in the fluorescence of SbCPR-2DY in the process of its NADPH-dependent reduction studied by rapid-scanning stop-flow spectroscopy. Panel (**a**) shows a representative set of spectra of fluorescence with excitation at 505 nm registered at different time points. Here, the gray arrows indicate the direction of the changes during the initial 100 ms of the process. Black arrows indicate the direction of the changes during the latter phase of reduction. A series of spectra of fluorescence recorded at the same time points with the direct excitation of the acceptor at 617 nm is shown in panel (**b**). Panel (**c**) illustrates the spectral changes during the reduction as a 3D plot of fluorescence spectra (excitation at 505 nm) normalized on the integral fluorescence intensity. A kinetic curve of the changes in FRET efficiency during the reduction is shown in panel (**d**) in semi-logarithmic coordinates. The solid line shown in this plot corresponds to the approximation of this data set by a three-exponential equation.

As seen from Table 1, where we compare the kinetic parameters of the SbCPR reduction with those characterizing the kinetics of changes in FRET, the two processes exhibit similar values of the rate constants of all three phases. Thus, the rapid initial decrease in FRET intensity may be identified as reflecting the sequence of events resulting in the conversion of the oxidized enzyme (FAD, FMN), first to ($FADH_2$, FMN) then to the double-semiquinone state ($FADH^•$, $FMNH^•$) (stages 1–2 in Scheme 1). A decrease in FRET efficiency in this phase suggests an increase in the average inter-probe distance by ~4 Å. This increase indicates that the formation of the disemiquinone state of the enzyme prompts it to acquire a more open conformation. However, this opening is reversed in the following stages of reduction so that the inner-probe distance in the final, apparent three-electron reduced state approaches that characteristic to the oxidized enzyme.

3.4. Pressure-Perturbation Studies of the Equilibrium between Open and Closed States in SbCPR

The FRET-based detection of the conformational rearrangements in SbCPR established in the above-described experiments opens a gate to apply pressure-perturbation spectroscopy for exploring the conformational landscape of the enzyme and its alterations in redox cycling. The pressure perturbation approach offers unique means for probing the changes in protein–solvent interactions and determining the position of conformational equilibria in different states of the enzyme. Thus, we subjected SbCPR-2DY to a cycle of studies of the effect of pressure on the fluorescence of the donor–acceptor pair. These experiments were performed with the oxidized enzyme, its complex with 2′,5′-ADP (as an NADPH analog), the two-electron reduced enzyme in the presence of equimolar NADPH, and its final, apparently three-electron reduced state at a 20-fold excess of NADPH.

The results of our pressure-perturbation experiments are illustrated in Figure 5, where panels (a,b) exemplify the series of spectra recorded versus increasing pressure with the oxidized and reduced enzyme, respectively. As seen from these plots, rising pressure results in a remarkable increase in the emission band of the acceptor accompanied by a decrease in the donor fluorescence. A similar behavior was also observed with ADP-bound SbCPR and its two-electron reduced state.

Notably, the changes observed with either the completely or partially reduced enzyme were entirely reversible at decompression (see Figure 5b). In contrast, in the oxidized state of either the ligand-free or ADP-bound enzyme, full reversibility was observed only when the enzyme was decompressed from pressures below 1.5 kbar. At higher pressures, the reversibility was only partial (see Figure 5a). Furthermore, the prolonged incubation of the oxidized SbCPR at pressures above 2.5 kbar resulted in an ample time-dependent irreversible decrease in the fluorescence of the acceptor along with increased emission from the donor (data not shown). This observation suggests the slow pressure-induced denaturation of the oxidized enzyme at pressures >2.5 kbar. In contrast, no pressure-induced denaturation was observed with either partially or completely reduced enzymes at pressures as high as 4.2 kbar.

To probe if the pressure effects on the fluorescence of the donor–acceptor pair may be, at least in part, caused by pressure dependence of the quantum yield of each of the probes taken alone, we studied the effect of pressure on the fluorescence of DY-520XL in the single-labeled SbCPR-DY520XL and the fluorescence of DY-731 in SbCPR-2DY subjected to direct excitation at 617 nm. The obtained pressure dependencies are shown in the inset to Figure 5c. This plot shows that both dyes exhibit pressure-dependent quenching of fluorescence, which is better pronounced with DY-731. Thus, the opposite directions of the changes in the intensity of fluorescence of the donor and acceptor fluorophores in the double-labeled enzyme with excitation at the donor band (at 505 nm) suggest a pressure-induced decrease in FRET efficiency, and, therefore, an increase in the distance between the probes at increasing pressure.

The effect of pressure on the intensity of donor fluorescence must equally influence the amplitudes of the bands of both donor and acceptor fluorophores and, therefore, do not affect the calculations of FRET efficiency according to Equation (1). In contrast, the changes in the quantum yield of DY-731 with pressure have to be taken into account in our calculations. To this end, we fitted the pressure dependence of the relative intensity of fluorescence of DY-731 by Equation (6) (Figure 5c, inset) and used this fitting curve to normalize the amplitude of the fluorescence band of the acceptor. The resulting pressure dependencies of FRET efficiency for the four enzyme states are shown in Figure 5c main panel. The respective parameters of pressure-induced transitions are summarized in Table 2.

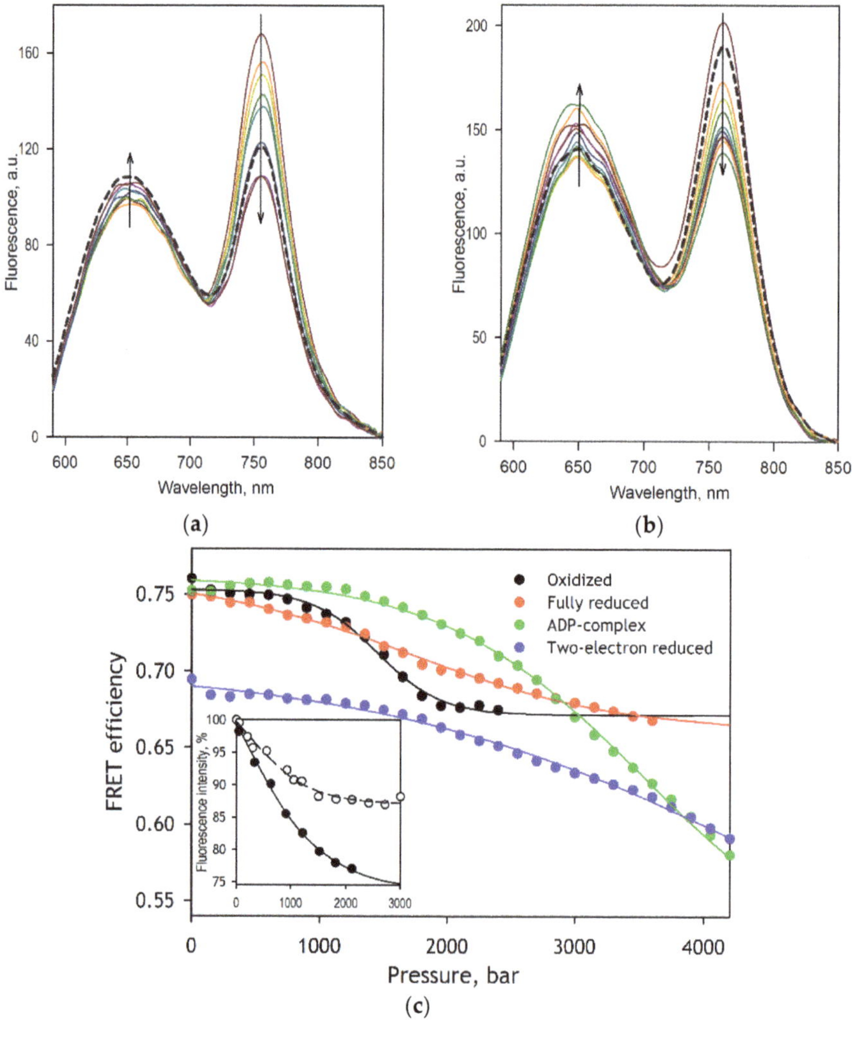

Figure 5. Pressure-induced changes in the spectra of fluorescence of SbCPR-2DY. Panels (**a**,**b**) show the series of spectra recorded at increasing pressure with the oxidized (**a**) and reduced (**b**) enzyme. The spectra shown in solid lines were recorded at 1, 300, 600, 900, 1200, 1500, 1800, 2100, and 2400 bar. In the case of the reduced enzyme, this set is complemented with the spectra recorded at 3000, 3600, and 4200 bar. The spectra shown in thick gray dashed lines were recorded after decompression to the ambient pressure. The pressure dependencies of FRET efficiency obtained with four different enzyme states are exemplified in the main plot of the panel (**c**). Here, the solid lines show the approximations of the datasets with Equation (6). The inset in this panel exemplifies the pressure dependencies of the relative fluorescence intensity of the double-labeled enzyme with excitation at 617 nm (filled circles, solid line) and single-labeled SbCPR-DY520XL with excitation at 505 nm (open circles, dashed line). Lines show the approximations of the datasets with Equation (6).

Table 2. Parameters of the pressure-induced transition in SbCPR-2DY monitored by changes in FRET efficiency *.

State of the Enzyme	$P_{½}$, bar	ΔV^0, mL/mol	K_{eq}	ΔG°, kJ/mol	Low-Pressure End State (Closed)		High-Pressure End State (Open)	
					FRET Efficiency	Distance, Å	FRET Efficiency	Distance, Å
Oxidized	1719 ± 235	−87.8 ± 20.8	0.004 ± 0.004	6.47 ± 1.26	0.76 ± 0.01	38.1 ± 0.3	0.71 ± 0.04	40.1 ± 0.6
ADP-bound	3431 ± 221	−33.7 ± 3.9	0.010 ± 0.002	4.96 ± 0.26	0.77 ± 0.01	37.9 ± 0.3	0.51 ± 0.03	45.8 ± 0.9
Two-electron reduced	4323 ± 32	−17.8 ± 0.6	0.045 ± 0.003	3.34 ± 0.08	0.70 ± 0.001	40.2 ± 0.003	0.39 ± 0.17	50.1 ± 5.9
Fully reduced	2113 ± 578	−27.1 ± 3.6	0.126 ± 0.074	2.49 ± 0.80	0.74 ± 0.03	38.7 ± 0.9	0.59 ± 0.05	43.4 ± 1.6

* The values given in the table represent the averages of the results of 2–6 individual experiments. The individual estimates of ΔV^0 and $P_{½}$ were obtained from fitting the pressure dependencies of the apparent efficiency of FRET (Equation (1)) with Equation (6). These estimates were used to calculate the values of K°_{eq} and ΔG° given in the table. The FRET efficiencies in the end states and the respective inter-probe distances were calculated from parameters A_0 and A_{max} in Equation (6). The "±" values correspond to the confidence interval calculated for $p = 0.05$.

Although pressure increase elicited a decrease in FRET efficiency in all four cases, both the parameters of the pressure-induced transitions and the estimated changes in the inter-probe distance reveal a dramatic difference between the four states of the enzyme. While the distance between the probes in the low-pressure end state (the closed conformation) did not differ considerably between the four states, the inter-probe distances in the high-pressure end state (the open conformation) of the ADP-bound enzyme and its two-electron reduced form were significantly longer than those characteristic to the oxidized and completely reduced forms. While in the latter two cases, the change in the distance upon the transition from more closed to more open conformation was estimated to be 2–4 Å, the opening of the ADP-bound and two-electron reduced enzyme increases the inter-probe difference by 8–10 Å.

A contrasting difference between the oxidized enzyme and its other three states was also observed in the ΔV^0 of the opening transition. If the decrease in the system volume upon its pressure-induced transition was as large as 88 mL/mol for the oxidized enzyme, the binding of 2′,5′-ADP and the reduction of the flavins decreased this change to −33 and −18 mL/mol, respectively. This observation suggests that the conformational change in SbCPR resulting from its interaction with the nucleotide cofactor and further reduction promotes additional protein solvation that minimizes the changes in protein interactions with solvent necessary for acquiring its open conformation.

Importantly, our analysis of the K_{eq} of the pressure-dependent conformational equilibrium suggests that, although the closed conformation predominates in all four enzyme states at ambient pressure, the formation of the disemiquinone state results in a ~10-fold increase in the population of the open state. Interestingly, the further reduction of the enzyme shifts the equilibrium towards the open state even more. However, the "degree of opening" observed in the final, the apparent three-electron reduced state is much lower than in the ADP-bound and two-electron reduced states.

4. Discussion

Incorporating DY520-XL and DY731 fluorescence dyes into the FAD and FMN domains of CPR from *Sorghum bicolor* provided means for the direct observation of conformational rearrangements during the redox cycling of the enzyme. A close match of the kinetic constant derived from the absorbance and fluorescence spectroscopy assays in rapid scanning stop-flow experiments allowed us to track the changes in the average inter-probe distance during the flavoprotein reduction process. Furthermore, applying pressure-perturbation spectroscopy for portraying the conformational landscape of the enzyme, we were able to determine the positions of equilibrium between its open and closed conformations at different points of the electron-transfer pathway. These studies revealed the presence of several open protein sub-states that differ in the protein solvation pattern. Through unveiling the functional choreography of plant CPRs, our study provides the essential information for rational engineering these pivotal enzymes of the monolignol biosynthetic pathway.

The results of our rapid kinetics experiments suggest that the binding of NADPH to the enzyme is exceptionally fast and takes place during the dead time of the stop-flow device (~2 ms). Similar to that reported for human CPR [62], the reduction of SbCPR by NADPH occurs without the intermittent occurrence of the detectable charge-transfer species. The first resolved kinetic phase is the formation of the blue (neutral) disemiquinone resulting from the interdomain electron transfer between $FADH_2$ and FMN immediately coupled to the charge-transfer step. However, the rate constant of this process (around 200 s^{-1} at 5 °C, see Table 1) is an order of magnitude higher than the values reported by Gutierez et al. for human CPR (20 s^{-1} at 25 °C) [62] and by Oprian and Coon for rabbit CPR (28 s^{-1} at unspecified temperature) [63]. Thus, the interdomain electron transfer in SbCPR occurs much faster than in the mammalian enzymes. This observation is consistent with the higher flexibility of the interdomain loop in plant CPRs as compared to the mammalian orthologs, which is suggested by their X-ray structures [7,11].

The second kinetic step presumably corresponds to establishing a transient equilibrium of the red and blue disemiquinones with the other two-electron reduced states, (FAD, $FMNH_2$) and ($FADH_2$, FMN). It has a rate constant of around 20 s^{-1} (Table 1), which is also much higher than those reported for the human (3.7 s^{-1} [62]) and the rabbit (5.4 s^{-1} [63]) enzymes. Notably, the amplitude of the 595 nm band and, respectively, the fractional content of the blue semiquinone species at the end of this phase is considerably higher in SbCPR than that observed with the mammalian reductases.

Interestingly, the kinetics of the reduction of SbCPR reveals a noticeable difference with that reported for another plant CPR, ATR2 enzyme from *Arabidopsis thaliana*. Studying this enzyme, Whitelaw and co-authors reported a resolution of the hydride transfer step (425 s^{-1} at 6 °C) from the interdomain electron transfer stage (49 s^{-1}) [28]. Thus, according to our results, both of these electron transfer events appear to be considerably faster in SbCPR than in ATR2. Furthermore, the fractional content of the blue semiquinone state in the transient equilibrium mixture established after the second phase of reduction is markedly higher in SbCPR than in ATR2, similar to what is observed in the comparison of SbCPR with the mammalian reductases.

The third, extremely slow, kinetic phase of the reduction corresponds to a partial transition of the enzyme to the four-electron reduced state followed by a comproportionation between the two- and four-electron reduced molecules leading to the three-electron reduced enzyme (($FADH_2$, $FADH^\bullet$) $\rightleftharpoons$ ($FMNH^\bullet$, $FMNH_2$)), the apparent final state. This incomplete reducibility of CPR and the formation of a three-electron reduced state through a comproportionation reaction has already been reported for mammalian reductases [64] and the flavoprotein domain of the bacterial P450BM-3 [61].

The changes in FRET efficiency in SbCPR-2DY during its NADPH-dependent reduction are in good agreement with the kinetics of changes in the redox state of the enzyme. The kinetic curves registered in our fluorescence stop-flow experiments obey three-exponential kinetics with the rate constants closely similar to those obtained with absorbance spectroscopy. According to our results, the first resolved phase of reduction that leads to the disemiquinone state is associated with an increase in the averaged inter-probe distance by 4.1 Å. However, the subsequent equilibration between several two-electron reduced states and the further reduction of the enzyme results in the opposite direction of the changes so that the averaged distance observed in the three-electron reduced enzyme is only 1.7 Å larger than in the oxidized enzyme (Table 1).

These results agree with multiple previous reports that demonstrated a transition from the closed conformation to a more open state upon the interdomain electron transfer event and the formation of the disemiquinone state (see [27] for a review). Furthermore, there are strong indications of the predominance of the closed conformations in the three- and four-electron reduced enzyme [20,21,23,26], which is also consistent with our results.

It must be noted that the inter-probe distances estimated in our FRET kinetics experiments do not reflect the distances characteristic of any discrete protein conformations. They rather represent the averages over multiple conformational states, and their changes reflect the redox-state-dependent displacement of equilibrium between these various conformations. To explore better the conformational landscape of SbCPR and characterize its changes in the redox cycling of the enzyme, we used hydrostatic pressure as a tool for displacing the protein equilibria. When combined with such tools for detecting protein structural rearrangements as FRET, the pressure perturbation strategy allows determining the positions of its conformational equilibria in different redox states, assessing the changes in the protein interactions with solvent in its redox cycling, and estimating the inter-probe distances characteristic to the end-states of its conformational breathing.

According to our results, in all four studied states of the enzyme—oxidized ligand-free, oxidized ADP-bound, two-electron, and four-electron reduced—the enzyme exists in the equilibrium between its more closed and more open states. The inter-probe distance in the closed state is not affected by either reduction or the interactions with 2′,5′-ADP (the analog of the nucleotide cofactor). It is estimated to be around 38–40 Å in all four states of the enzyme (Table 2). In contrast, the preferential conformation of the open state exhibits a pronounced change during the redox cycling. While the changes in the inter-probe distance associated with the conformational breathing of the oxidized enzyme are as small as 2 Å, the binding of ADP to SbCPR and its subsequent two-electron reduction increases the distance between the probes in the open conformation to 46–50 Å (Table 2). In agreement with the previous observations [20,21,23,26], the further reduction of the enzyme partially reverts this change and decreases the amplitude of the conformational motion to 4 Å.

A unique feature of the pressure-perturbation approach is its ability to reveal conformational equilibria's endpoints. Suppose that the inter-probe distances observed at any particular pressure represent weighted averages over a population of molecules existing in equilibrium between the low-pressure and pressure-promoted conformational states. Hence, the inter-probe distances estimated by extrapolating pressure dependencies to infinitely high and infinitely low pressures correspond to those characterizing the definite states (or ensembles of states with pressure-insensitive interconversion) representing the endpoints of conformational equilibrium. Therefore, comparing the end states of pressure-dependent transitions of SbCPR at different points of its redox cycle allows probing if the interactions of the enzyme with the nucleotide cofactor or reduction of its flavins results in an emergence of a new conformational state not present in the oxidized enzyme. The remarkable difference of the inter-probe-distance in the pressure-promoted end-state of the oxidized enzyme with those observed in SbCPR-ADP complex and two-electron reduced enzyme suggests that the binding of the nucleotide cofactor is a necessary prerequisite for the wide opening of the enzyme. This inference is consistent with a dramatic difference of the ΔV^0 characteristic to the oxidized enzyme (89 mL/mol) with the ΔV^0 values exhibited by SbCPR in all other probed states. According to this analysis, the nature of the low-amplitude conformational breathing observed in oxidized SbCPR is entirely different from the transitions between the closed and widely open conformations, which become possible only after binding the nucleotide cofactor.

However, it should be taken into account that the changes in the distance between the two protein-incorporated probes monitored in our experiments do not reflect the complete picture of the structural rearrangements, which may involve complex rotational and translational motions of different parts of the protein molecule. Therefore, the inter-probe distance may not be considered a full-fledged measure of the "degree of openness" of the enzyme molecule. Consequently, the actual variations in the accessibility of the FMN domain for interactions with the heme protein acceptor may not be exactly proportional to the variations in the inter-probe distances detected in our experiments.

The most notable and nontrivial conclusion derived from the fitting of the pressure dependencies of the FRET efficiency to Equation (6) is that the closed conformation of the enzyme heavily predominates in all four studied states of the enzyme at ambient pressure. According to the constant of equilibrium determined for the oxidized enzyme, the fraction of the closed form accounts for 99.6% of its total content. Despite a significant increase in the amplitude of the conformational breathing upon the binding of the nucleotide cofactor, its effect on the position of the conformation equilibrium is insignificant (99% of the closed state at 1 bar). However, the reduction of the enzyme with the formation of the disemiquinone displaces the equilibrium appreciably, and the fraction of the closed state decreases to 96%. Surprisingly, despite decreasing the amplitude of motions, the further reduction of SbCPR provokes the further opening of the enzyme so that the fraction of its closed form decreases to 89%.

It has to be noted that the high abundance of the closed conformation of the enzyme in our experiments is furthered by the low ionic strength of the buffer used in our studies (20 mM Na-HEPES, I = 11.6 mM). The conformational equilibrium in CPR enzymes is known to be critically affected by ionic strength, and the abundance of open conformation is considerably increased at high salt concentrations [19,24,25]. This strong ionic strength dependence is caused by the predominant role of charge pairing contacts in the inter-domain interactions [12,65]. The use of the low-ionic-strength media in our experiments was dictated by an objective to accurately determine FRET efficiency in the low-pressure (closed) end-state by displacing the $P_{\frac{1}{2}}$ of the opening transition to higher pressures. It is worth noting that the cytoplasmic ionic strength in cells of plants grown at normal soil salinity varies within 100–200 mM limits [66], which is much higher than the ionic strength of our buffer (11.6 mM). Therefore, the actual position of the SbCPR conformational equilibrium in vivo must be more shifted towards the open state than observed in our experiments.

Another remarkable observation is a dramatic change in the ΔV^0 of the opening transition upon the binding of 2′,5′-ADP and the enzyme reduction. If in the oxidized SbCPR the volume change is as large as −88 mL/mol, the binding of the nucleotide cofactor decreases it (by absolute value) to −33 mL/mol. The subsequent electron transfer to the flavins and formation of the disemiquinone state further decreases ΔV^0 to −18 mL/mol. This observation suggests that the binding of the nucleotide cofactor and two-electron reduction results in some additional hydration of the enzyme, which decreases the changes in protein interactions with solvent necessary for the transition to the open conformation. Suppose we hypothesize that the predominant part of the volume change is originated from the electrostriction of water on the newly opened charges after breaking salt bridges. In that case, we can assume that the opening of the oxidized enzyme involves the dissociation of four salt links. That is calculated from the assumption that the solvation of a single-charged ion incurs the volume change of −10 mL/mol [31]. In contrast, there is only one salt bridge to break for the opening transition of the two-electron reduced enzyme (ΔV^0 = −18 mL/mol).

The analysis of the recently resolved X-ray structure of CPR from the *Candida tropicalis* yeast identified four salt-bridges connecting the FAD and FMN domains in the closed conformation of the enzyme [12]. Comparing this structure with our structural model of SbCPR, we found that three of these charge pairs—D125/R515, E157/K669, and E193/R367—are retained in the sorghum enzyme, where they correspond to the pairs D168/R544, E203/K693, and D238/K414. The fourth one (K57/D338) has no analog in SbCPR despite the conservation of K57 residue, which corresponds to K96 in SbCPR. However, instead, this residue may be a part of a switching salt-link fork between D260 in the connecting loop and K96 and K126 in the FMN domain. Dissociation or switching these salt links may affect the flexibility of the connecting loop and thus modulate the interdomain interactions. Hypothetically, the dissociation of these salt bridges may be involved in the pressure-induced opening of the ligand-free oxidized enzyme. A decrease in the ΔV^0 of the opening transition upon the binding of the nucleotide cofactor and NADPH-dependent reduction may indicate that the interactions of the enzyme with 2′5′-ADP or NADPH promote the dissociation of some of these salt links. Further investigation of this system of molecular tethering and its linkage to the enzyme redox-state by a combination of site-directed mutagenesis and pressure-perturbation FRET spectroscopy may give more insight into the mechanisms controlling the inter-domain interactions in SbCPR.

5. Conclusions

Combining FRET-based detections of conformational motions with pressure-perturbation and rapid scanning stop-flow spectroscopy, we were able to portray the conformational landscape of the enzyme and characterize its changes in the process of enzyme redox cycling. Our results suggest the presence of several open conformational sub-states differing in the opening transition volume change (ΔV^0). Although the closed conformation always predominates in the conformational landscape, the population of the open conformations increases by order of magnitude upon the two-electron reduction and the formation of the disemiquinone state of the enzyme. In addition to elucidating the functional choreography of plant CPRs, our study demonstrates the high exploratory potential of a combination of the pressure-perturbation approach with the FRET-based monitoring of protein conformational rearrangements.

Author Contributions: Conceptualization, D.R.D. and C.K.; methodology, D.R.D. and C.K.; software, D.R.D.; formal analysis, D.R.D. and B.Z.; investigation, B.Z. and D.R.D.; writing—original draft preparation, B.Z.; writing—review and editing, D.R.D. and C.K. All authors have read and agreed to the published version of the manuscript.

Funding: This research was funded by the grants CHE-1804699 and MCB-2043248 from the National Science Foundation (NSF).

Institutional Review Board Statement: Not applicable.

Informed Consent Statement: Not applicable.

Data Availability Statement: Raw experimental datasets may be obtained from the authors upon a reasonable request.

Acknowledgments: We acknowledge Scott E. Sattler at the USDA-ARS, Lincoln, NE 68583, for providing the original clone and Gerhard R. Munske at the Washington State University (LBB1) for conducting MALDI/TOF experiments for determining the modified peptides.

Conflicts of Interest: The authors declare no conflict of interest.

Appendix A. Design and Characterization of the Donor–Acceptor Pair for Intramolecular FRET Experiments in SbCPR

Appendix A.1. Selection of Fluorescent Probes

To explore the conformational landscape of SbCPR and investigate the relationship between the position of the equilibrium between the open and the closed states, we used a FRET-based technique. To avoid any considerable overlap of the excitation and emission spectra of the probes with the bands of absorbance and fluorescence of CPR flavins, we employed a pair of far-red- and infrared-emitting fluorophores. As a fluorescence donor, we chose DY-520XL. This extra-large Stokes shift fluorophore exhibits a broad emission band centered around 640 nm and has its excitation maximum at 525 nm (both positions were determined in aqueous solutions). The acceptor fluorophore was represented by DY-731 dye, which has its excitation and emission maxima around 730 and 750–770 nm, depending on the environment. A vast overlap of the emission band of DY520XL with the spectrum of excitation of DY731 (Figure A1) provides for efficient FRET in this donor–acceptor pair.

Appendix A.2. Determination of Quantum Yield of DY520-XL and the Förster Distance of Its FRET Pair with DY731

To determine the SbCPR Förster distance characteristic to our donor/acceptor pair and quantitatively interpret the results of FRET experiments, we had to estimate the quantum yields of the donor fluorophore first. To this aim, we employed the relative technique of Parker and Rees [67] using Rhodamine 101 as a quantum yield reference [68]. To determine the quantum yield of DY-520XL in its SbCPR-attached state, we measured the spectra of absorbance and fluorescence of diluted solutions of Rhodamine 101 in ethanol and SbCPR C596S variant modified with DY-520XL at 1:1 molar ratio in 20 mM Na-Hepes buffer, pH

7.4. The concentrations were adjusted to the optical density at the wavelength of excitation (520 nm) around 0.08. Two separate sets of measurements were made at 5 and 25 °C, the temperatures used in our kinetic and pressure-perturbation experiments, respectively. According to these measurements, the yield of DY520-XL attached to SbCPR at 25 °C is equal to 0.053. At 5 °C, its value increases to 0.0689.

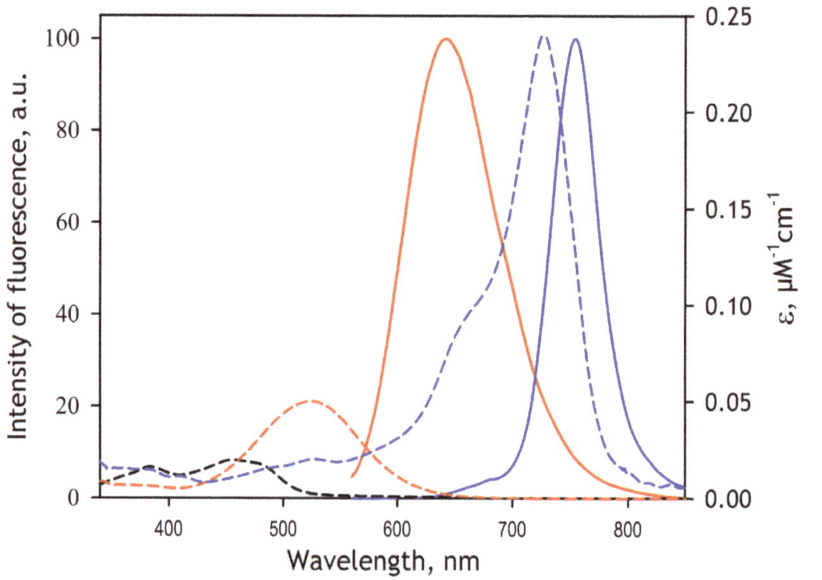

Figure A1. Spectra of absorbance (dashed lines) and fluorescence (solid lines) of DY520-XL (red) and DY731 (blue). The absorbance spectrum of SbCPR is shown in a black dashed line.

To determine the Förster distance characteristic of the donor–acceptor pair, we recorded the fluorescence spectrum of the SbCPR C596S variant modified with DY-520XL (excitation at 505 nm) the spectrum of absorbance of the same protein modified with monobromobimane (MBBr) and DY-731. Here, MBBr, a thiol-reactive probe that does not absorb in the region of interest (520–900 nm), was used as a substitute of DY-520XL to modify the most accessible cysteine of SbCPR (Cys235) prior to attaching the DY731 dye. Using these spectra and the quantum yield of the donor determined as above, we calculated the Förster distance of the DY-520XL/DY-731 pair using PhotoChemCAD software [55]. In these calculations, we assumed the orientation factor and the refractivity coefficient to be equal to 0.6667 and 1.4, respectively. According to these calculations, the Förster distances characteristic to our pair at 5 and 25 °C are equal to 48.30 Å and 46.23 Å, respectively.

Appendix A.3. Direct Determination of FRET Efficiency in SbCPR-2DY

To determine the FRET efficiency in the double-labeled SbCPR-2DY, we compared the intensity of fluorescence of the donor fluorophore in SbCPR-2DY with that in the equimolar mixture of SbCPR C596S variant modified with DY-520XL at 1:1 molar ratio (SbCPR-DY520XL) with the same protein modified with monobromobimane (MBBr) and DY-731 (SbCPR(MBBr, DY-731)). Here, again, we used MBBr as a substitute for DY-520XL to modify the most accessible cysteine of SbCPR (Cys235) prior to attaching the DY731 dye. The solutions were adjusted to the same concentrations of both probes. The incorporation of DY-731 into the protein results in a dramatic increase in the relative amplitude of the acceptor fluorescence band (Figure A2, main panel) at the expense of a profound drop in the intensity of the donor fluorescence (Figure A2, insert). These changes are indicative of an extensive FRET between the dies in the double-labeled protein. The ratio of the integral intensity of fluorescence of the donor in SbCPR-2DY (I_{2DY}) to that in the mixture of SbCPR-DY520XL (I_{mix}) with SbCPR(MBBr, DY-731) was used to determine the FRET efficiency (E) according to the following relationship:

$$E = 1 - \frac{I_{2DY}}{I_{mix}}$$

The estimates of the FRET efficiency in SbCPR-2DY at 25 at 5 °C determined in this way are equal to 0.66 and 0.60, respectively.

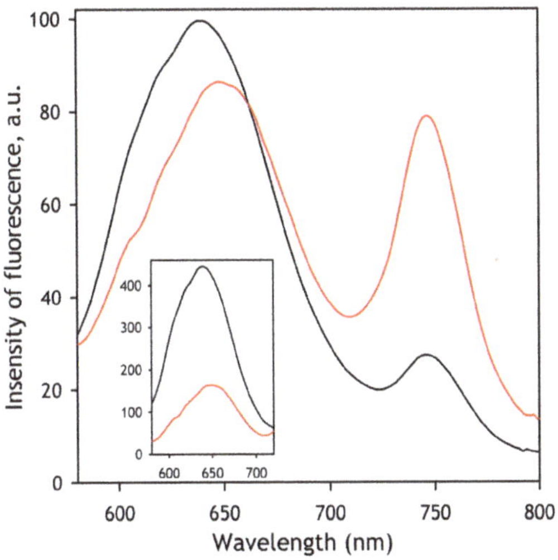

Figure A2. Spectra of fluorescence of SbCPR-2DY (red) and an equimolar mixture of single labeled SbCPR-DY520XL with SbCPR double-labeled with MBBR and DY-731 (black) taken at 5 °C with excitation at 505 nm. The spectra shown in the main panel are normalized to the same integral intensity of fluorescence. The inset shows the donor emission bands unscaled.

These estimates were used to determine the quantum yield of SbCPR-incorporated DY-731, whose knowledge is necessary for estimating the FRET efficiency based on the spectra of fluorescence of SbCPR-2DY. To this aim, we used Equation (1) resolved relative to the quantum yield of the acceptor (Φ_A):

$$\Phi_A = \Phi_D \frac{(1 - E) \cdot I_A}{E \cdot I_D}$$

where Φ_D is the quantum yield of donor fluorescence, E is the FRET efficiency, and I_A and I_D are the integral efficiencies of fluorescence of acceptor and donor, respectively. The values of the quantum yield of DY-731 at 5 and 25 °C calculated in this way are equal to 0.0177 and 0.0158.

The knowledge of the quantum yields of the donor and acceptor allowed for estimating FRET efficiency from the spectra of fluorescence of the double-labeled protein. To this aim, we constructed the sets of the prototypical spectra of SbCPR-incorporated DY-520XL and DY-731 scaled proportionally to their quantum yields. Approximation of the spectra of fluorescence of SbCPR-2DY by a linear combination of these spectral standards was used in this study for estimating the FRET efficiency and studying its changes in rapid kinetics and the pressure-perturbation experiments.

Appendix B. Probing the Accessibility of SbCPR Cysteines and Determining the Position of the Probes in SbCPR-2DY

In our preliminary experiments, we probed the accessibility of SbCPR cysteines for modification with the use of monobromobimane (MBBr) as a thiol-reactive probe. MBBr, which is essentially nonfluorescent until conjugated with thiol groups, readily reacts with low molecular weight thiols (glutathione, N-acetylcysteine, mercaptopurine, etc.), peptides, and proteins. The titration of MBBr-accessible thiol groups in SbCPR was performed by the sequential addition of molar equivalents of MBBr to 10 μM solution SbCPR at 4 °C. After each addition, we recorded the kinetics of the increase in fluorescence at 490 nm (excitation at 395 nm). The first two additions were followed by an increase in MBBr fluorescence, obeying the second-order kinetic equation with the rate constants of 0.008 and 0.028 μM^{-1} s^{-1}, respectively. The increases in fluorescence caused by these two sequential additions were of comparable amplitudes. The addition of the third molar equivalent of MBBr at ~75% completion of the second modification resulted in a more modest and rapid increase in fluorescence, which was associated with the evident precipitation of the protein. The fourth addition did not cause any substantial fluorescence changes. The titration of the remaining unreacted MBBR with reduced glutathione revealed the presence of one unreacted equivalent of the dye. Therefore, according to these results, the protein contains three modification-accessible residues, and the modification of the third one results in protein precipitation.

The results of these preliminary experiments agree with the conclusions driven from the analysis of the SbCPR structural model. Presumably, the residues modified with the first two MBBr equivalents are Cys-235 and Cys-536, while the modification of Cys-596 becomes possible only after incorporating the first two labels and results in the protein precipitation. We validated these conclusions with MALDI-TOF mass spectroscopic analysis of the peptides generated by trypsinolysis of the MBBr-modified enzyme. When adding 3 equivalents of MBBR to the SbCPR, we can see the Cys-235, Cys-536, and Cys-596 with a mass addition of 133 compared to the unlabeled peptides.

To verify the position of the incorporated fluorophores, we subjected the unlabeled protein, its single-labeled adduct with DY520-XL, and the protein sequentially labeled with both probes to MALDI-TOF MS analysis (see Materials and Methods). Unfortunately, our experiments failed to detect the dye-modified peptides, most likely because of the large size and complex ionization modes of the modifying reagents. However, we were able to estimate the positions of the dyes from a comparison of recovery of the cysteine-containing peptides in the unlabeled protein with that in the single- and double-labeled samples. The peptides containing Cys-306, Cys-325, Cys-352, Cys-503, Cys-520, and Cys659, which are thought to be inaccessible for modification, were equally well detected in all three samples. In contrast, the peptide containing Cys-536 was recovered in all samples, but the double-labeled one, while neither of the single- or double-labeled proteins exhibited a detectable Cys-235-containing peptide. These results suggest that our sequential labeling procedure results in the protein where DY-520-XL residue is attached to Cys-235, while DY-731 fluorophore is located at Cys-536 residue.

References

1. Nelson, D.R.; Kamataki, T.; Waxman, D.J.; Guengerich, F.P.; Estabrook, R.W.; Feyereisen, R.; Gonzalez, F.J.; Coon, M.J.; Gunsalus, I.C.; Gotoh, O.; et al. The P450 Superfamily: Update on New Sequences, Gene-Mapping, Accession Numbers, Early Trivial Names of Enzymes, and Nomenclature. *DNA Cell. Biol.* **1993**, *12*, 1–51. [CrossRef] [PubMed]
2. Kahn, R.A.; Durst, F. Function and evolution of plant cytochrome P450. *Evol. Metab. Pathw.* **2000**, *34*, 151–189.
3. Omura, T. Contribution of cytochrome P450 to the diversification of eukaryotic organisms. *Biotechnol. Appl. Biochem.* **2013**, *60*, 4–8. [CrossRef] [PubMed]
4. Sarath, G.; Mitchell, R.B.; Sattler, S.E.; Funnell, D.; Pedersen, J.F.; Graybosch, R.A.; Vogel, K.P. Opportunities and roadblocks in utilizing forages and small grains for liquid fuels. *J. Ind. Microbiol. Biotechnol.* **2008**, *35*, 343–354. [CrossRef] [PubMed]
5. Feltus, F.A.; Vandenbrink, J.P. Bioenergy grass feedstock: Current options and prospects for trait improvement using emerging genetic, genomic, and systems biology toolkits. *Biotechnol. Biofuels.* **2012**, *5*, 80. [CrossRef] [PubMed]
6. Weijde, T.V.D.; Alvim Kamei, C.L.; Torres, A.F.; Vermerris, W.; Dolstra, O.; Visser, R.G.F.; Trindade, L.M. The potential of C4 grasses for cellulosic biofuel production. *Front. Plant. Sci.* **2013**, *4*, 107. [PubMed]

7. Zhang, B.; Munske, G.R.; Timokhin, V.I.; Ralph, J.; Davydov, D.R.; Vermerris, W.; Sattler, S.E.; Kang, C. Functional and structural insight into the flexibility of cytochrome P450 reductases from *Sorghum bicolor* and its implications for lignin composition. *J. Biol. Chem.* **2022**, *298*, 101761. [CrossRef] [PubMed]
8. Sevrioukova, I.F.; Peterson, J.A. NADPH-P-450 Reductase: Structural and Functional Comparisons of the Eukaryotic and Prokaryotic Isoforms. *Biochimie* **1995**, *77*, 562–572. [CrossRef]
9. Wang, M.; Roberts, D.L.; Paschke, R.; Shea, T.M.; Masters, B.S.S.; Kim, J.J.P. Three-dimensional structure of NADPH–cytochrome P450 reductase: Prototype for FMN-and FAD-containing enzymes. *Proc. Natl. Acad. Sci. USA* **1997**, *94*, 8411–8416. [CrossRef] [PubMed]
10. Xia, C.; Panda, S.P.; Marohnic, C.C.; Martásek, P.; Masters, B.S.; Kim, J.J.P. Structural basis for human NADPH-cytochrome P450 oxidoreductase deficiency. *Proc. Natl. Acad. Sci. USA* **2011**, *108*, 13486–13491. [CrossRef] [PubMed]
11. Niu, G.Q.; Zhao, S.; Wang, L.; Dong, W.; Liu, L.; He, Y.K. Structure of the *Arabidopsis thaliana* NADPH-cytochrome P450 reductase 2 (ATR2) provides insight into its function. *FEBS J.* **2017**, *284*, 754–765. [CrossRef]
12. Ebrecht, A.C.; van der Bergh, N.; Harrison, S.T.; Smit, M.S.; Sewell, B.T.; Opperman, D.J. Biochemical and structural insights into the cytochrome P450 reductase from *Candida tropicalis*. *Sci. Rep.* **2019**, *9*, 20088. [CrossRef] [PubMed]
13. Hamdane, D.; Xia, C.; Im, S.C.; Zhang, H.; Kim, J.J.P.; Waskell, L. Structure and function of an NADPH-cytochrome P450 oxidoreductase in an open conformation capable of reducing cytochrome P450. *J. Biol. Chem.* **2009**, *284*, 11374–11384. [CrossRef] [PubMed]
14. Xia, C.; Hamdane, D.; Shen, A.L.; Choi, V.; Kasper, C.B.; Pearl, N.M.; Zhang, H.; Im, S.C.; Waskell, L.; Kim, J.J.P. Conformational Changes of NADPH-Cytochrome P450 Oxidoreductase Are Essential for Catalysis and Cofactor Binding. *J. Biol. Chem.* **2011**, *286*, 16246–16260. [CrossRef]
15. Aigrain, L.; Pompon, D.; Morera, S.; Truan, G. Structure of the open conformation of a functional chimeric NADPH cytochrome P450 reductase. *EMBO Rep.* **2009**, *10*, 742–747. [CrossRef] [PubMed]
16. Sugishima, M.; Sato, H.; Wada, K.; Yamamoto, K. Crystal structure of a NADPH-cytochrome P450 oxidoreductase (CYPOR) and heme oxygenase 1 fusion protein implies a conformational change in CYPOR upon NADPH/NADP(+) binding. *FEBS Lett.* **2019**, *593*, 868–875. [CrossRef]
17. Vincent, B.; Morellet, N.; Fatemi, F.; Aigrain, L.; Truan, G.; Guittet, E.; Lescop, E. The Closed and Compact Domain Organization of the 70-kDa Human Cytochrome P450 Reductase in Its Oxidized State As Revealed by NMR. *J. Mol. Biol.* **2012**, *420*, 296–309. [CrossRef] [PubMed]
18. Ellis, J.; Gutierrez, A.; Barsukov, I.L.; Huang, W.C.; Grossmann, J.G.; Roberts, G.C. Domain Motion in Cytochrome P450 Reductase Conformational Equilibria Revealed by NMR and Small-Angle X-Ray Scattering. *J. Biol. Chem.* **2009**, *284*, 36628–36637. [CrossRef]
19. Huang, W.C.; Ellis, J.; Moody, P.C.; Raven, E.L.; Roberts, G.C. Redox-Linked Domain Movements in the Catalytic Cycle of Cytochrome P450 Reductase. *Structure* **2013**, *21*, 1581–1589. [CrossRef] [PubMed]
20. Freeman, S.L.; Martel, A.; Raven, E.L.; Roberts, G.C. Orchestrated Domain Movement in Catalysis by Cytochrome P450 Reductase. *Sci. Rep.* **2017**, *7*, 1–11. [CrossRef] [PubMed]
21. Freeman, S.L.; Martel, A.; Devos, J.M.; Basran, J.; Raven, E.L.; Roberts, G.C. Solution structure of the cytochrome P450 reductase-cytochrome c complex determined by neutron scattering. *J. Biol. Chem.* **2018**, *293*, 5210–5219. [CrossRef]
22. Jenner, M.; Ellis, J.; Huang, W.C.; Lloyd Raven, E.; Roberts, G.C.; Oldham, N.J. Detection of a protein conformational equilibrium by electrospray ionisation-ion mobility-mass spectrometry. *Angew. Chem. Int. Ed.* **2011**, *50*, 8291–8294. [CrossRef]
23. Hedison, T.M.; Hay, S.; Scrutton, N.S. Real-time analysis of conformational control in electron transfer reactions of human cytochrome P450 reductase with cytochrome c. *FEBS J.* **2015**, *282*, 4357–4375. [CrossRef]
24. Quast, R.B.; Fatemi, F.; Kranendonk, M.; Margeat, E.; Truan, G. Accurate Determination of Human CPR Conformational Equilibrium by smFRET Using Dual Orthogonal Noncanonical Amino Acid Labeling. *Chembiochem* **2019**, *20*, 659–666. [CrossRef] [PubMed]
25. Bavishi, K.; Li, D.; Eiersholt, S.; Hooley, E.N.; Petersen, T.C.; Moller, B.L.; Hatzakis, N.S.; Laursen, T. Direct observation of multiple conformational states in Cytochrome P450 oxidoreductase and their modulation by membrane environment and ionic strength. *Sci. Rep.* **2018**, *8*, 1–9. [CrossRef] [PubMed]
26. Kovrigina, E.A.; Pattengale, B.; Xia, C.; Galiakhmetov, A.R.; Huang, J.; Kim, J.J.P.; Kovrigin, E.L. Conformational States of Cytochrome P450 Oxidoreductase Evaluated by Forster Resonance Energy Transfer Using Ultrafast Transient Absorption Spectroscopy. *Biochemistry* **2016**, *55*, 5973–5976. [CrossRef]
27. Hedison, T.M.; Scrutton, N.S. Tripping the light fantastic in membrane redox biology: Linking dynamic structures to function in ER electron transfer chains. *FEBS J.* **2019**, *286*, 2004–2017. [CrossRef]
28. Whitelaw, D.A.; Tonkin, R.; Meints, C.E.; Wolthers, K.R. Kinetic analysis of electron flux in cytochrome P450 reductases reveals differences in rate-determining steps in plant and mammalian enzymes. *Arch. Biochem. Biophys.* **2015**, *584*, 107–115. [CrossRef]
29. Heremans, K. High-pressure effects on proteins and other biomolecules. *Annu. Rev. Biophys. Bioeng.* **1982**, *11*, 1–21. [CrossRef] [PubMed]
30. Somero, G.N. Adaptations to high hydrostatic pressure. *Ann. Rev. Physiol.* **1992**, *54*, 557–577. [CrossRef] [PubMed]
31. Mozhaev, V.V.; Heremans, K.; Frank, J.; Masson, P.; Balny, C. High pressure effects on protein structure and function. *Proteins: Struct. Funct. Genet.* **1996**, *24*, 81–91. [CrossRef]

32. Davydov, D.R. Merging Thermodynamics and Evolution: How the Studies of High-Pressure Adaptation may Help to Understand Enzymatic Mechanisms. *J. Thermodynam. Cat.* **2012**, *3*, e110. [CrossRef]
33. Masson, P.; Reybaud, J. Hydrophobic interaction electrophoresis under high hydrostatic pressure: Study of the effects of pressure upon the interaction of serum albumin with a long-chain aliphatic ligand. *Electrophoresis* **1988**, *9*, 157–161. [CrossRef] [PubMed]
34. Low, P.S.; Somero, G.N. Activation volumes in enzymic catalysis: Their sources and modification by low-molecular-weight solutes. *Proc. Natl. Acad. Sci. USA* **1975**, *72*, 3014–3018. [CrossRef] [PubMed]
35. Low, P.S.; Somero, G.N. Protein hydration changes during catalysis: New mechanism of enzymic rate-enchancement and ion activation inhibition of catalysis. *Proc. Natl. Acad. USA* **1975**, *72*, 3305–3309. [CrossRef]
36. Weber, G.; Drickamer, H.G. The effect of high pressure upon proteins and other biomolecules. *Q. Rev. Biophys.* **1983**, *16*, 89–112. [CrossRef]
37. Shimizu, S. Estimating hydration changes upon biomolecular reactions from osmotic stress, high pressure, and preferential hydration experiments. *Proc. Natl. Acad. Sci. USA* **2004**, *101*, 1195–1199. [CrossRef] [PubMed]
38. Boonyaratanakornkit, B.B.; Park, C.B.; Clark, D.S. Pressure effects on intra- and intermolecular interactions within proteins. *Biochim. Biophys. Acta-Protein. Struct. Mol. Enzymol.* **2002**, *1595*, 235–249. [CrossRef]
39. Royer, C.A. Revisiting volume changes in pressure-induced protein unfolding. *Biochim. Biophys. Acta-Protein Struct. Mol. Enzymol.* **2002**, *1595*, 201–209. [CrossRef]
40. Imai, T.; Hirata, F. Hydrophobic effects on partial molar volume. *J. Chem. Phys.* **2005**, *122*, 094509. [CrossRef] [PubMed]
41. Mozhaev, V.V.; Heremans, K.; Frank, J.; Masson, P.; Balny, C. Exploiting the effects of high hydrostatic pressure in biotechnological applications. *Trends. Biotechnol.* **1994**, *12*, 493–501. [CrossRef]
42. Chalikian, T.V.; Filfil, R. How large are the volume changes accompanying protein transitions and binding? *Biophys. Chem.* **2003**, *104*, 489–499. [CrossRef]
43. Helms, V. Protein dynamics tightly connected to the dynamics of surrounding and internal water molecules. *ChemPhysChem* **2007**, *8*, 23–33. [CrossRef] [PubMed]
44. Mentre, P.; Hui Bon Hoa, G. Effects of high hydrostatic pressures on living cells: A consequence of the properties of macromolecules and macromolecule-associated water. *Int. Rev. Cell. Mol. Biol.* **2001**, *201*, 1–84.
45. Kharakoz, D.P. Partial volumes and compressibilities of extended polypeptide chains in aqueous solution: Additivity scheme and implication of protein unfolding at normal and high pressure. *Biochemistry* **1997**, *36*, 10276–10285. [CrossRef] [PubMed]
46. Kornblatt, J.A.; Kornblatt, M.J. Water as it applies to the function of enzymes. *Int. Rev. Cytol.* **2002**, *215*, 49–73. [PubMed]
47. Hui Bon Hoa, G.; Douzou, P.; Dahan, N.; Balny, C. High pressure spectrometry at subzero temperatures. *Anal. Biochem.* **1982**, *120*, 125–135. [CrossRef]
48. Davydov, D.R.; Deprez, E.; Hui Bon Hoa, G.; Knyushko, T.V.; Kuznetsova, G.P.; Koen, Y.M.; Archakov, A.I. High-pressure-induced transitions in microsomal cytochrome P450 2B4 in solution: Evidence for conformational inhomogeneity in the oligomers. *Arch. Biochem. Biophys.* **1995**, *320*, 330–344. [CrossRef]
49. Davydov, D.R. SpectraLab Software. Available online: http://cyp3a4.chem.wsu.edu/spectralab.html (accessed on 16 February 2022).
50. Dunteman, G.H. *Principal Component Analysis*; Sage Publications: Newbury Parc, CA, USA, 1989.
51. Cochran, R.N.; Horne, F.H. Strategy for resolving rapid scanning wavelength experiments by principal component analysis. *J. Phys. Chem.* **1980**, *84*, 2561–2567. [CrossRef]
52. Cochran, R.N.; Horne, F.H.; Dye, J.L.; Ceraso, J.; Suelter, C.H. Principal component analysis of rapid scanning wavelength stopped-flow kinetics experiments on the liver alcohol-dehydrogenase catalyzed reduction of para-nitroso-n,n-dimethylaniline by 1,4-dihydronicotinamide adenine-dinucleotide. *J. Phys. Chem.* **1980**, *84*, 2567–2575. [CrossRef]
53. Estela, J.M.; Cladera, A.; Cerda, V. Development and testing of a new computerized method for multicomponent kinetic determinations based on multiwavelength spectrophotometric detection. *Anal. Chim. Acta.* **1995**, *310*, 307–318. [CrossRef]
54. Davydov, D.R.; Sineva, E.V.; Sistla, S.; Davydova, N.Y.; Frank, D.J.; Sligar, S.G.; Halpert, J.R. Electron transfer in the complex of membrane-bound human cytochrome P450 3A4 with the flavin domain of P450BM-3: The effect of oligomerization of the heme protein and intermittent modulation of the spin equilibrium. *Biochim. Biophys. Acta.* **2010**, *1797*, 378–390. [CrossRef] [PubMed]
55. Dixon, J.M.; Taniguchi, M.; Lindsey, J.S. PhotochemCAD 2: A refined program with accompanying spectral databases for photochemical calculations. *Photochem. Photobiol.* **2005**, *81*, 212–213. [CrossRef]
56. Hui Bon Hoa, G.; McLean, M.A.; Sligar, S.G. High pressure, a tool for exploring heme protein active sites. *Biochim. Biophys. Acta.* **2002**, *1595*, 297–308. [CrossRef]
57. Weber, G. *Protein Interactions*; Chapman and Hall: New York, NY, USA, 1991.
58. Shevchenko, A.; Tomas, H.; Havli, J.; Olsen, J.V.; Mann, M. In-gel digestion for mass spectrometric characterization of proteins and proteomes. *Nat. Protoc.* **2006**, *1*, 2856–2860. [CrossRef] [PubMed]
59. Jumper, J.; Evans, R.; Pritzel, A.; Green, T.; Figurnov, M.; Ronneberger, O.; Tunyasuvunakool, K.; Bates, R.; Žídek, A.; Potapenko, A.; et al. Highly accurate protein structure prediction with AlphaFold. *Nature* **2021**, *596*, 583–589. [CrossRef] [PubMed]
60. Pettersen, E.F.; Goddard, T.D.; Huang, C.C.; Couch, G.S.; Greenblatt, D.M.; Meng, E.C.; Ferrin, T.E. UCSF Chimera—A visualization system for exploratory research and analysis. *J. Comput. Chem.* **2004**, *25*, 1605–1612. [CrossRef]

61. Sevrioukova, I.; Truan, G.; Peterson, J.A. The flavoprotein domain of P450BM-3: Expression, purification, and properties of the flavin adenine dinucleotide-and flavin mononucleotide-binding subdomains. *Biochemistry* **1996**, *35*, 7528–7535. [CrossRef] [PubMed]
62. Gutierrez, A.; Lian, L.Y.; Wolf, C.R.; Scrutton, N.S.; Roberts, G.C.K. Stopped-flow kinetic studies of flavin reduction in human cytochrome P450 reductase and its component domains. *Biochemistry* **2001**, *40*, 1964–1975. [CrossRef]
63. Oprian, D.D.; Coon, M.J. Oxidation-reduction states of FMN and FAD in NADPH-cytochrome P-450 reductase during reduction by NADPH. *J. Biol. Chem.* **1982**, *257*, 8935–8944. [CrossRef]
64. Vermilion, J.L.; Coon, M.J. Purified liver microsomal NADPH-cytochrome P-450 reductase. Spectral characterization of oxidation-reduction states. *J. Biol. Chem.* **1978**, *253*, 2694–2704. [CrossRef]
65. Aigrain, L.; Pompon, D.; Truan, G. Role of the interface between the FMN and FAD domains in the control of redox potential and electronic transfer of NADPH-cytochrome P450 reductase. *Biochem. J.* **2011**, *435*, 197–206. [CrossRef] [PubMed]
66. Hariadi, Y.; Marandon, K.; Tian, Y.; Jacobsen, S.E.; Shabala, S. Ionic and osmotic relations in quinoa (Chenopodium quinoa Willd.) plants grown at various salinity levels. *J. Exp. Bot.* **2011**, *62*, 185–193. [CrossRef] [PubMed]
67. Parker, C.A.; Rees, W.T. Correction of fluorescence spectra and measurement of fluorescence quantum efficiency. *Analyst* **1960**, *85*, 587–600. [CrossRef]
68. Rurack, K.; Spieles, M. Fluorescence Quantum Yields of a Series of Red and Near-Infrared Dyes Emitting at 600−1000 nm. *Anal. Chem.* **2011**, *83*, 1232–1242. [CrossRef] [PubMed]

biology MDPI

Article

Pressure Adaptations in Deep-Sea *Moritella* Dihydrofolate Reductases: Compressibility versus Stability

Ryan W. Penhallurick and Toshiko Ichiye *

Department of Chemistry, Georgetown University, Washington, DC 20057, USA; rwp33@georgetown.edu
* Correspondence: ti9@georgetown.edu; Tel.: +1-202-687-3724

Simple Summary: Deep-sea organisms must have proteins that function under high hydrostatic pressure to survive. Adaptations used in proteins from "pressure-loving" piezophiles may include greater compressibility or greater stability against pressure-induced destabilization. However, while greater compressibility can be accomplished by greater void volume, larger cavities in a protein have been associated with greater destabilization and even unfolding as pressure is increased. Here, computer simulations of dihydrofolate reductase from a moderate piezophile and a hyperpiezophile were performed to understand the balance between adaptations for greater compressibility and those against pressure destabilization and unfolding. The results indicate that while compressibility appears to be important for deep-sea microbes, adaptation for the greatest depths may be to prevent water penetration into the interior.

Abstract: Proteins from "pressure-loving" piezophiles appear to adapt by greater compressibility via larger total cavity volume. However, larger cavities in proteins have been associated with lower unfolding pressures. Here, dihydrofolate reductase (DHFR) from a moderate piezophile *Moritella profunda* (Mp) isolated at ~2.9 km in depth and from a hyperpiezophile *Moritella yayanosii* (My) isolated at ~11 km in depth were compared using molecular dynamics simulations. Although previous simulations indicate that MpDHFR is more compressible than a mesophile DHFR, here the average properties and a quasiharmonic analysis indicate that MpDHFR and MyDHFR have similar compressibilities. A cavity analysis also indicates that the three unique mutations in MyDHFR are near cavities, although the cavities are generally similar in size in both. However, while a cleft overlaps an internal cavity, thus forming a pathway from the surface to the interior in MpDHFR, the unique residue Tyr103 found in MyDHFR forms a hydrogen bond with Leu78, and the sidechain separates the cleft from the cavity. Thus, while *Moritella* DHFR may generally be well suited to high-pressure environments because of their greater compressibility, adaptation for greater depths may be to prevent water entry into the interior cavities.

Keywords: deep-sea adaptations; compressibility; cavities; pressure; potential energy landscape

Citation: Penhallurick, R.W.; Ichiye, T. Pressure Adaptations in Deep-Sea *Moritella* Dihydrofolate Reductases: Compressibility versus Stability. *Biology* **2021**, *10*, 1211. https://doi.org/10.3390/biology10111211

Academic Editors: Dmitri Davydov and Christiane Jung

Received: 21 October 2021
Accepted: 17 November 2021
Published: 20 November 2021

1. Introduction

The discovery of life thriving under extreme conditions of temperature, pressure, and composition has led to intriguing questions about the limits at which life can survive. Mechanisms used by "extremophiles" to adapt their biological macromolecules to these extremes could assist in our understanding of these limits of life. Studying the sequence-structure-function relationship of proteins from extremophiles compared to proteins from organisms living under ambient conditions, "mesophiles," is useful in understanding adaptations used to maintain functional enzymes under all conditions [1]. So far, studies of extremophiles have largely focused on temperature adaptation. For instance, the corresponding states hypothesis that enzyme activity is high near the growth conditions (i.e., growth temperature T_G and growth pressure P_G) of the microbe [2] and that maximal activity is achieved by balancing the stability and flexibility of the protein [3] is mainly based on studies of homologous enzymes of temperature-adapted microbes. However, less is understood about adaptations to high hydrostatic pressure largely due to limited access to extreme oceanic depths until recently. Since about 88% of the ocean has biologically high pressures, comprising the largest portion of the biosphere [4,5], and "piezophiles" have now been found in a wide range of environments, including hydrothermal vents, deep-sea trenches, and under the Earth's crust [6,7], studies of adaptation to high pressure are timely.

For proteins, the effects of pressure are compression and denaturation [8]. Below 4 kbar, proteins mostly compress, while generally far above ~4 kbar, single-chain proteins will denature. Although seemingly contrary to volume reduction necessary to lower the free energy, pressure unfolding apparently occurs since water can pack more tightly against polypeptide than polypeptide against polypeptide so that more open solvated states become favorable [9], thus lowering the free energy of the entire system.

Numerous studies of pressure unfolding of proteins have shown that larger cavity size within a protein apparently leads to lower pressure stability [10] because the system volume is lowered when water enters these cavities. Point mutants that increase the cavity volume decrease the stability of the enzyme as pressure increases [11], and even slight, local changes affecting cavity sizes can have profound impacts on destabilization, as well as on the conformational dynamics [12]. Moreover, pressure-induced water penetration into internal cavities of proteins is observed in high-pressure crystallography [13,14] and high-pressure NMR [15].

However, adaptations for smaller cavity volumes in piezophile proteins have not been found. In fact, comparisons of crystal structures of 3-isopropyl malate dehydrogenase (IPMDH) from the obligate piezophile *Shewanella benthica* (Sb) with that from the mesophile *Shewanella oneidensis* (So) find a larger total cavity volume in SbIPMDH, although this was attributed to more numerous small cavities rather than larger cavities [16]. Furthermore, the larger total cavity volume in SbIPMDH was proposed as an adaptation for greater compressibility. In addition, although experimental determination of the compressibilities of proteins is complicated by the need to measure the proteins in solution, studies of the effects of ligand binding [17] and single-point mutations [18] find that relatively small changes to local structure can have large effects on both the compressibility and activity of an enzyme.

Dihydrofolate reductase (DHFR) is an ~160 residue, ~20 kDa enzyme that is a prime target for comparative studies of extremophile proteins because it is ubiquitous. DHFR catalyzes the hydride transfer and protonation of dihydrofolate (DHF) from the coenzyme NADPH to form tetrahydrofolate (THF), an essential precursor in the purine biosynthesis pathway [19,20]. Conformational changes of the loops and subdomains have been found to be important in the catalytic cycle [21–24]. In addition, extensive experimental studies have been compared for DHFR from the mesophile (T_G = 37 °C, P_G = 1 bar) *Escherichia coli* (Ec) with that from the moderate psychropiezophile (T_G = 6 °C, P_G = 220 bar [25]) *Moritella profunda* (Mp) [26–28], as well as other deep-sea piezophiles [29–31]. Although major structural differences are not apparent between crystal structures of MpDHFR and those of EcDHFR [27], MpDHFR has maximum enzyme activity at 500 bar while EcDHFR is monotonically inactivated by pressure above 1 bar. Moreover, MpDHFR appears to have a larger total cavity volume than EcDHFR [27], so it appears to be adapted by having greater compressibility. Another potential adaptation in MpDHFR is the presence of Glu27 rather than Asp27 in EcDHFR. With increasing pressure, the Asp27Glu mutation (D27E) of EcDHFR exhibits increased activity rather than the decreased activity observed in wild-type EcDHFR [28]. However, while Glu27 has been found in all species of *Moritella* DHFR so far, it is not in other piezophile DHFR, indicating it may allow but is not necessary for high-pressure activity [32]. In addition, enzyme activity does not always increase with pressure for DHFR from other deep-sea bacteria from other genera [33]. In addition, the unfolding pressure (P_u) at 25 °C is 2.7 kbar for apo-EcDHFR but only 0.7 kbar for apo-MpDHFR, indicating MpDHFR is actually more sensitive to pressure denaturation than EcDHFR [27].

The marginal stability of DHFR and other enzymes from other deep-sea piezophiles has been noted [33]. Since many of the piezophile proteins studied have been from the cold deep ocean, the marginal stability may be an adaptation for cold temperature rather than for high pressure [34].

Molecular dynamics (MD) simulation can provide an important molecular perspective to experimental studies. Our previous MD simulation studies of EcDHFR and MpDHFR showed that MpDHFR had higher overall atomic fluctuations than EcDHFR, and pressure appeared to increase fluctuations [35,36]. The higher fluctuations in MpDHFR appeared to be due to somewhat fewer hydrogen bonds in MpDHFR compared to EcDHFR. Comparisons of MpDHFR versus EcDHFR [37] and of wild-type versus D27E EcDHFR [38] indicate that strengthening of the strong Thr113 O ... Asp27 O_δ hydrogen bond under pressure leads to the monotonic pressure deactivation in EcDHFR by overcorrelating collective motions while strengthening of the weak Thr113 O ... Glu27 O_ε hydrogen bond to a strength similar to EcDHFR at 1 bar leads the pressure activation in MpDHFR and D27E EcDHFR.

In addition, since the compressibility of a protein is difficult to measure, a quasiharmonic analysis (QHA) is a method based on computer simulations that allows another assessment of compressibility. A QHA probes the local energy landscape through a series of short simulations at a variety of temperatures and pressures around a reference set of conditions [39]. The effective local potential well for a given atom created by its neighbors is assumed to be described by the atomic fluctuations, and the temperature and pressure dependence are defined at a set of reference conditions by the width of the average well $\sigma_0{}^2$, an intrinsic isobaric expansivity α_P, and an intrinsic isothermal compressibility κ_T. At 279 K, 1 bar, the QHA indicates MpDHFR ($\kappa_T = 76 \times 10^{-3}$ / kbar) was more compressible compared to EcDHFR ($\kappa_T = 67 \times 10^{-3}$/kbar) [40], consistent with the crystallographic studies.

Finally, our previous sequence comparison and molecular dynamics studies of DHFR from *Moritella* [41] indicate that in general, *Moritella* DHFR may have been adapted for the cold by having fewer interactions so that they are more flexible, but that this adaptation may also be fortuitously favorable for high pressures by making them more compressible. However, weaker interactions also would lead to lower stability under either or both higher temperatures or higher pressures. DHFR from *Moritella yayanosii* (My), which has an optimum $T_G = 10$ °C and $P_G = 800$ bar [42] but is found at depths of 11 km, was found to remain steadily active up to ~1 kbar, which corresponds to the pressure where it was isolated [30] in contrast to MpDHFR, which begins to lose activity at a much lower pressure, ~500 bar, near its P_u = ~700 bar [27]. Notably, there are only four sequence differences between MpDHFR and MyDHFR. While the absolute activity and catalytic efficiency [27,30] of MyDHFR are greater than that of MpDHFR, how MyDHFR can maintain activity at pressures far beyond the unfolding pressure of MpDHFR is important in understanding pressure adaptations.

All-atom MD simulations at 279 K and 1 and 800 bar of dihydrofolate reductase bound by the cofactor NADPH and substrate DHF, which is the presumed Michaelis complex [21], from the moderate piezophile *M. profunda* and hyperpiezophile *M. yayanosii* were performed to explore adaptations for high pressure, focusing on sequence differences between these homologous enzymes. Note that a consensus sequence numbering of aligned *Moritella* DHFR sequences with *E. coli* DHFR is used in this text (Figure S1), with the original *Moritella* DHFR sequence numbering in parentheses for reference. Of the four sequence differences between the two, the focus is on the residues that are unique to MyDHFR in comparison to all of the *Moritella* DHFR [41]; specifically, the unique residues of MyDHFR, which are Tyr103 (105), Ile119 (121), and His132 (134), while MpDHFR has Cys103, Thr119, and Asn132. General properties such as average mean-square fluctuations, radius of gyration, and hydrogen bonds, as well as QHA, were used to compare compressibilities. In addition, a cavity analysis was used to compare differences in cavity behavior near the unique residues of MyDHFR.

2. Materials and Methods

Methods have been described previously [41], so they are described briefly here and in more detail in Supplemental Material. Coordinate manipulations and analyses were performed using the molecular mechanics package CHARMM [43]. Because of the large amount of literature on *E. coli* DHFR, consensus sequence numbering based on the sequence numbering of *E. coli* DHFR is used (Figure S1). Residues 1 and 67 of the original MpDHFR sequence were renumbered to 0 and 66.5, respectively, to be consistent with gaps in the alignment with *E. coli* DHFR. Coordinates of MpDHFR bound by $NADP^+$ and folate (PDB: 2ZZA), a presumed analog of the Michaelis complex, were obtained from the PDB [27]. The first residue of the structure was incorrectly determined to be Val, so the first residue was corrected to Met, and the C-terminal tail was built (K160), using GalaxyFill [44] in PDB Reader. For MyDHFR, mutations to the MpDHFR template structure (C103Y, T119I, N132H, N150D) were also made using GalaxyFill. Coordinates of $NADP^+$ and folate were modified to the Michaelis complex cofactor NADPH and substrate DHF, respectively, using Ligand Reader and Modeler [45] in CHARMM-GUI. The CHARMM36 all-atom non-polarizable potential energy parameter set was used to model the protein [46,47], water was modeled by TIP4P-Ew [48], the ligand DHF was modeled by CHARMM General Force Field (CGenFF) [49], and cofactor NADPH was modeled by the nucleotide parameter set [50]. MD simulations of *M. profunda* and *M. yayanosii* DHFR at T = 279 K and P = 1, 800 bar were performed using the molecular mechanics package OpenMM [51]. Each system was minimized with 500 iterations of the L-BFGS algorithm [52]. Heating, pressurization, and an initial 5 ns equilibration were performed in the *NPT* ensemble using a leapfrog Verlet integrator with a time step of 0.001 ps, Andersen thermostat [53] and Monte Carlo (MC) barostat [54]. Afterward, a second 5 ns equilibration followed by 50 ns production was performed in the *NVT* ensemble using a velocity Verlet integrator with a timestep of 0.001 ps and a Nosé-Hoover thermostat [55–58].

Average properties were calculated from coordinates written at 1 ps intervals except as noted. Averages and standard deviations were calculated by block averaging over 10 ns blocks. The mean-squared fluctuations of the protein-heavy atoms $\langle \Delta r_{\mathrm{HA}}{}^2 \rangle$ were calculated within 10 ns blocks with respect to the average structure within each block and then averaged over all blocks. The mean-squared fluctuations of C_α atoms, $\langle \Delta r_{C\alpha}{}^2 \rangle$, were calculated from the entire 50 ns production run with respect to the average structure over the entire production run.

Hydrogen bonds were defined as having a distance between the donor hydrogen atom and acceptor atom smaller than 2.40 Å [59] and an angle of D–H . . . A larger than 130°. Chemically equivalent donors or acceptors of the same residue were combined, and bifurcated hydrogen bonds were treated as a single event. Further details on hydrogen bond calculations can be found in Supplemental Material.

Cavities and clefts were calculated using defaults, except, as noted, using McVol [60]. A search grid of 1.0 Å, probe radius of 1.1 Å and a refinement grid of 0.5 Å with 50 Monte Carlo steps per $Å^3$ were used. Volumes were calculated from structures at every 5 ns from the 50 ns simulation. The average volume and root mean square (RMS) fluctuations in volumes for each cavity or cleft were then obtained from volumes over the ten structures, where volumes less than the 1.0 $Å^3$ cutoff were given a volume of 0 $Å^3$. Since many cavities transitioned between cavities and solvent-accessible clefts, they were termed as "cavity" or "cleft" based on the larger population.

A quasiharmonic analysis [39,40] from a *P-T* grid of short, 1 ns simulations in the *NPT* ensemble (with coordinates saved every 0.1 ps) starting from the end of the 5 ns *NVT* equilibration at P = 1 bar, T = 279 K. This *P–T* grid was comprised of all combinations of P = 1, 2500, 5000, 7500, and 10,000 bar and T = 40, 80, 120, 160, 200, 240, 280, 320 K.

The average fluctuations, $\sigma^2(P,T)$, were calculated for each of the 1 ns $P-T$ grid simulations. $\sigma^2(P,T)$ were calculated by averaging fluctuations with respect to the average structure of each 10 ps interval and then performing a second average over the 100 $\times$ 10 ps intervals in the 1 ns simulation. The fits to the quasiharmonic equations were performed in gnuplot. The reference state is P_0 = 1 bar and T_0 = 279 K. First, $\sigma^2(P,T)$, from the MD simulation data at all pressures and $T \geq 200$ K were fit using Equation (1) to $\sigma_0{}^2$, $\alpha_{P,0}$, and $\kappa_{T,0}$.

$$\sigma^2(P,T) = \sigma_0{}^2 \frac{T}{T_0}\left[(1+\kappa_{T,0}\Delta P)\mathrm{e}^{-\alpha_{P,0}\Delta T}\right]^{-2/3} \quad (1)$$

Next, $\sigma^2(P,T)$ from the MD simulation data for all pressures and $T < 200$ K were fit using Equations (2) and (3) to find values for $T_{g,0}$ and c.

$$\sigma_g{}^2(\mathrm{P}) = \sigma_0{}^2\left(\frac{T_g(P)}{T_0}\right)\left[(1+\kappa_{T,0}\Delta P)\mathrm{e}^{-\alpha_{P,0}(T_g(P)-T_0)}\right]^{-2/3} \quad (2)$$

$$T_g(P) = T_{g,0} - c\Delta P \quad (3)$$

3. Results

3.1. Average Properties

The average properties of the *Moritella* DHFRs in the 50 ns MD simulation are similar and do not change much with pressure (Table 1). At 1 bar, there are three fewer hydrogen bonds in MpDHFR compared to that of MyDHFR, while at 800 bar, there is one more hydrogen bond in MpDHFR than MyDHFR, although error bars are large. The radius of gyration, R_g, for MyDHFR appears slightly larger than for MpDHFR (Table 1).

Table 1. Average properties from the 50 ns MD simulation. Average heavy atom mean-square fluctuations, $\langle \Delta r_{HA}{}^2 \rangle$, number of hydrogen bonds, N_{HB}, and radii of gyration, R_g.

Protein	*P* (bar)	$\langle \Delta r_{HA}{}^2 \rangle$ (Å^2)	N_{HB}	$\langle R_g \rangle$ (Å^2)
MpDHFR	1	0.60 ± 0.04	104 ± 1	15.48 ± 0.07
MpDHFR	800	0.61 ± 0.02	106 ± 3	15.50 ± 0.04
MyDHFR	1	0.60 ± 0.06	107 ± 1	15.63 ± 0.03
MyDHFR	800	0.61 ± 0.08	105 ± 1	15.56 ± 0.05

The C_α fluctuations, $\langle \Delta r_{C\alpha}{}^2 \rangle$, as a function of residue number are also quite similar (Figure 1). At 1 bar, MpDHFR appears to have slightly higher fluctuations in the Met20, CD, FG loops, and helix C, while MyDHFR has larger fluctuations in helix F (Figure 1a). At increasing pressure, these fluctuations appear to remain unchanged or decrease for MpDHFR, while fluctuations in the CD loop, helix E, and strand G increase for MyDHFR (Figure 1b).

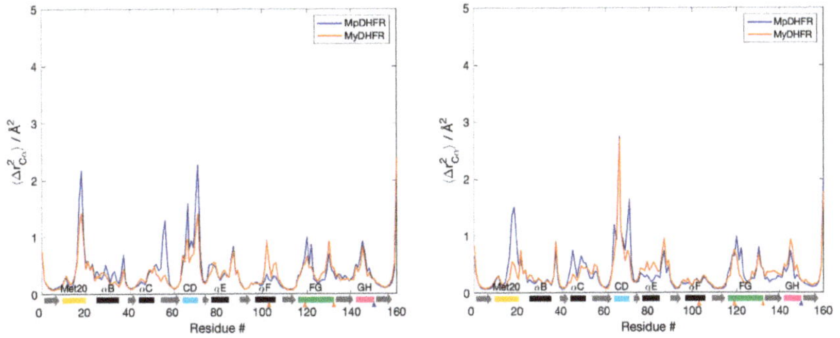

(a) (b)

Figure 1. Backbone fluctuations of *Moritella* DHFRs for the 50 ns simulation at (**a**) 1 and (**b**) 800 bar. α-helices (black rectangles), β-strands (gray arrows), and loops (colored rectangles) are denoted below the axis. Unique residues for MpDHFR (blue) and MyDHFR (orange) are noted with triangles below the axis.

3.2. Hydrogen Bonding

As a whole, the hydrogen bonding in MpDHFR and MyDHFR at 1 bar is also quite similar (Figure 2), as to be expected given the high degree of homology. However, a prominent difference between Mp- and MyDHFRs involves Res103 (105), where the intrahelical Cys103 (105) S_γ ... Ile99 (101) O hydrogen bond within helix F in MpDHFR is replaced by the Tyr103 (105) O_η ... Leu78 (80) O hydrogen bond between helix F and E in MyDHFR, especially at 800 bar (Table S2).

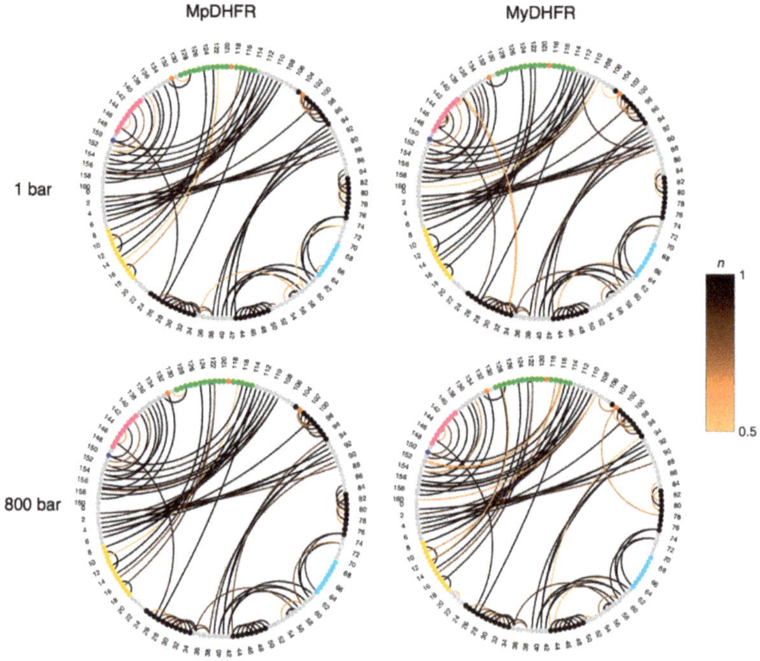

Figure 2. Hydrogen bond occupancy (n) for *Moritella* DHFRs at low and high pressure. Connections between donor/acceptor residues with $n > 0.5$ are shown with the line color proportional to the occupancy of the hydrogen bond. The unique residues for Mp- (dark blue) and MyDHFRs (orange) along with the α-helices (black), and Met20 (yellow), CD (cyan), FG (green), and GH (magenta) loops are identified on the nodes.

3.3. Potential Energy Landscape

The QHA indicates that the potential energy landscapes for MyDHFR and MpDHFR at 279 K and 1 bar are also quite similar (Table 2). However, the wells are somewhat shallower ($\sigma_0{}^2$ is greater) in MyDHFR than MpDHFR. Interestingly, the thermal property $\alpha_{P,0}$ is nearly identical between the two *Moritella* DHFRs, while the compressibility $\kappa_{T,0}$ is slightly greater for MyDHFR than MpDHFR, and barriers between wells $T_{g,0}$ are somewhat lower for MyDHFR than MpDHFR (Table 2).

Table 2. Parameters calculated from QHA. Goodness-of-fit given by reduced χ^2.

DHFR	$\sigma_0{}^2$ (Å^2)	$\alpha_{P,0}$ (10^{-3}/K)	$\kappa_{T,0}$ (10^{-3}/kbar)	χ^2 (10^{-6})	$T_{g,0}$ (K)	$-c$ (K/kbar)	χ^2 (10^{-6})
MpDHFR	0.148 ± 0.001	8.0 ± 0.1	65 ± 2	3.5	191 ± 2	0.5 ± 0.3	0.51
MyDHFR	0.151 ± 0.001	8.1 ± 0.1	70 ± 3	4.0	186 ± 1	1.0 ± 0.2	0.39

3.4. Cavities and Clefts

Five cavities or clefts were found near the unique residues of MyDHFR (Figure 3). The average and root mean square (RMS) fluctuations in the volumes are given in Table 3. Note that the RMS fluctuations are not the error in the average volume but rather the range in values to expect since the volumes are a fluctuating quantity in the simulation. For reference, cavity 1 is found consistently for both DHFR at both pressures. Cavity 1 appears to be relatively independent of species or pressure, with relatively small fluctuations in cavity size. Cleft 2 is found near the unique residue Tyr103 (105) of MyDHFR. Additionally, cavity 2, which can become as large as 9 to 17 Å, appears adjacent to cleft 2, although as a rare event seen in one or at most two of the snapshots and not in MyDHFR at 1 atm. In MpDHFR, both cleft 2 and cavity 2 appear as separate cavities, although they can occasionally merge into a single pathway to the surface (Figure 4) and is also observed in the starting crystal structure (Table S2). However, in MyDHFR, Tyr103 of helix F appears to separate cleft 2 from cavity 2 for much of the simulation while it is hydrogen-bonded to Leu78 (80) of helix E. The Tyr103 ring fills much of the space in which cleft 2 in MpDHFR occupies, shifting and separating cleft 2 from cavity 2. This hydrogen bond becomes stronger at the higher pressure, from an occupancy of ~0.3 at 1 bar to ~0.7 at 800 bar. Furthermore, an inspection of simulations of MyDHFR at 1 bar indicates that when the Tyr103 O_{η} ... Leu78 O hydrogen bond breaks, Tyr103 flips toward the surface of the protein away from helix E, allowing helix E to slip downwards toward the conformation adopted by MpDHFR.

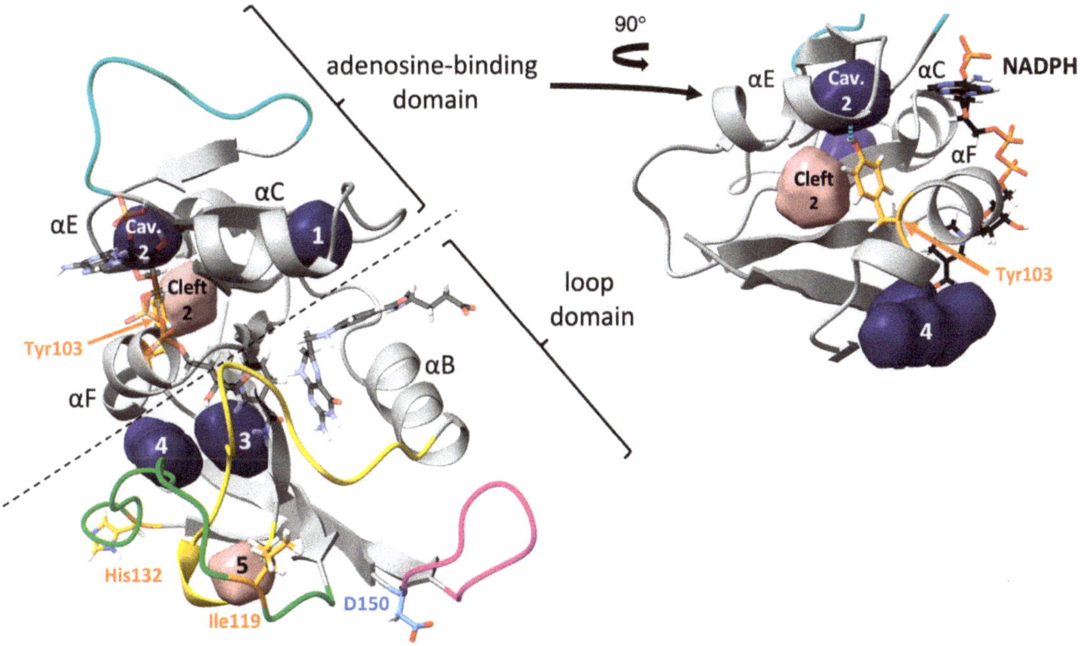

Figure 3. Cavities (dark blue) and clefts (pink) in *Moritella* DHFRs. Ribbon representation of MyDHFR. Unique residues of MyDHFR shown in wire. Cavities discussed in text near-unique residues of MyDHFR identified by arrows. Ligands NADPH and DHF shown in transparent CPK. Met20 (yellow), CD (cyan), FG (green) and GH (magenta) loops are also indicated. Right inset: rotated depiction of adenosine-binding domain with Tyr103 O_{η} ... Leu78 O hydrogen bond (blue dashed line).

Table 3. Average and RMS fluctuations cavity or cleft volumes, V_{cav} (Å^3).

DHFR	P (bar)	Cavity/Cleft					
		1	Cavity 2	Cleft 2	3	4	5
MpDHFR	1	17 ± 8	1 ± 3	5 ± 7	19 ± 5	12 ± 9	4 ± 5
MpDHFR	800	15 ± 5	1 ± 0	3 ± 8	19 ± 3	11 ± 6	2 ± 3
MyDHFR	1	16 ± 6	0 ± 0	10 ± 13	19 ± 5	10 ± 12	8 ± 5
MyDHFR	800	16 ± 3	2 ± 5	8 ± 8	19 ± 5	15 ± 17	2 ± 3

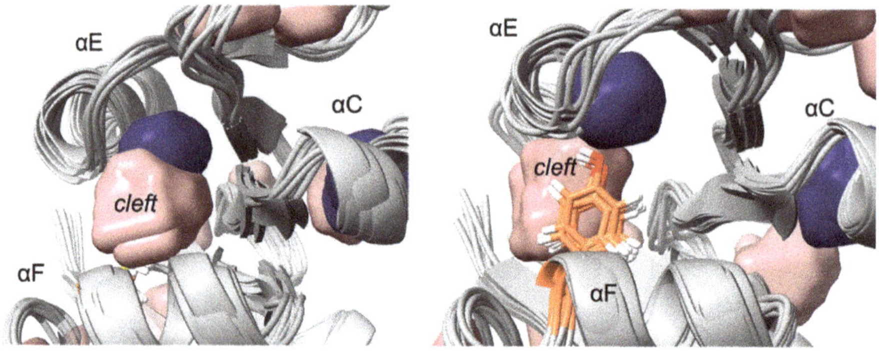

(**a**) (**b**)

Figure 4. Cavity 2 and cleft 2 near Res103. (**a**) Cavity 2 (dark blue) and solvent-accessible cleft 2 (pink) along helix E across from Cys103 in MpDHFR merge at 800 bar, providing solvent access to the internal cavity. (**b**) Cleft 2 remains separated from cavity 2 by Tyr103 (orange) in MyDHFR, possibly preventing solvent penetration into the cavity.

Cavities 3 and 4 are located near the unique residue 132 (134) of MyDHFR, which is at the end of the FG loop, and cleft 5 is embedded within the Met20 and FG loops, adjacent to the unique residue 119 (121) of MyDHFR. Average volumes of cavities 3, 4, and 5 are similar for both proteins and appear to be largely pressure-independent. While cavities 3 and 4 are not observed in the crystal and starting structures (Table S2), this may be accounted for by differences in sidechain conformations due to cryocooling [61] and enhanced solution-state motions at higher temperatures [62]. Crystal structures obtained at various pressures of ternary Michaelis-analog *E. coli* DHFR observed all cavities identified here [63]. MpDHFR has a hydrophilic threonine for Res119, whereas MyDHFR has hydrophobic isoleucine. Inspection of the crystal structure shows a resolved water molecule within cleft 5, while none were resolved within other cavities and clefts.

4. Discussion

Pressure leads to a decreased total volume of the system, which can occur by decreasing the total cavity volume or increasing the hydration of cavities. QHA indicates that the potential energy landscape of MyDHFR may be slightly more compressible than MpDHFR due to slightly shallower potential energy wells (indicated by greater $\sigma_0{}^2$) and lower barriers between wells (indicated by lower $T_{g,0}$) as well as slightly larger R_g. However, the difference in the intrinsic isothermal compressibility between the two of 5×10^{-3}/kbar is much less than between EcDHFR and MpDHFR of 9×10^{-3}/kbar. Note that the previous work comparing compressibilities [40] is for binary THF-bound DHFR while the current work is of ternary NADPH- and DHF-bound DHFR, so the magnitudes are somewhat smaller here, which is expected as there are more bound ligands and cofactors, but not enough to account for the larger differences between EcDHFR and MpDHFR than between MpDHFR and MyDHFR. Thus, while both MpDHFR and MyDHFR are both expected to have larger compressibilities compared to EcDHFR, this is consistent with the idea that this is mainly an adaptation for the cold that is fortuitously favorable for high pressure. However, the compressibility of MpDHFR may be reaching the limit of increased compressibility possible without destabilizing too much for deeper pressures.

Interestingly, the three unique residues of MyDHFR were found near cavities or clefts. Note that the most important factor here is not the average volumes but the fluctuations in the volumes. For instance, while cavity 2 and cleft 2 are generally separate in MpDHFR, occasionally, the two connect and form a pathway from the surface to the interior. In other words, occasional fluctuations could allow water to penetrate the interior, which could lead to distortion of the structure. However, in MyDHFR, Tyr103 of helix F forms a hydrogen bond with Leu78, which separates the two cavities, thus blocking the pathway, especially at the higher pressure, while in MpDHFR, Cys103 forms an intrahelical hydrogen bond so that the open pathway remains accessible to surrounding solvent.

5. Conclusions

Potential adaptations of piezophile proteins appear to have opposite means of being accomplished: greater compressibility by larger total cavity volume versus greater stability against pressure denaturation by smaller cavities. Here, MpDHFR and MyDHFR appear to have similarly large compressibilities, which may be an adaptation for cold (i.e., greater compressibility is also associated with greater flexibility) that fortuitously also makes them function better at high pressure. However, while greater flexibility/compressibility is generally accomplished by fewer or weaker interactions, there may be a limit to how much the flexibility/compressibility can be increased while maintaining the three-dimensional fold so that these two DHFRs may have reached that limit. Moreover, since MpDHFR begins to show deactivation at ~500 bar and unfolding at ~700 bar, the higher pressures that MyDHFR experiences are more likely to result in water penetration. Thus, the evolutionary driver may be preventing water penetration rather than increasing compressibility. Since cleft 2 and cavity 2 can form a pathway from the surface to the interior in MpDHFR, the unique Tyr103 (105) in MyDHFR, which forms a hydrogen bond that prevents the merging of cleft 2 and cavity 2, may be an adaptation to block water from reaching the interior by this pathway.

Supplementary Materials: The following are available online at https://www.mdpi.com/article/10.3390/biology10111211/s1: Detailed methods section, Figure S1: Sequence alignment of MpDHFR and MyDHFR with consensus sequence numbering, Table S1: Starting system information, Table S2: Cavities and clefts for crystal and starting structures, and Table S3: Differences in hydrogen bonding involving residue 103.

Author Contributions: Conceptualization, T.I. and R.W.P.; methodology, T.I. and R.W.P.; validation, T.I. and R.W.P.; formal analysis, T.I.; resources, T.I.; writing, R.W.P.; writing—review and editing, T.I.; visualization, R.W.P.; supervision, T.I.; project administration, T.I.; funding acquisition, T.I. All authors have read and agreed to the published version of the manuscript.

Funding: The authors acknowledge support from the National Institutes of Health through grant number R01-GM122441. T.I. also acknowledges support from the William G. McGowan Charitable Fund.

Institutional Review Board Statement: Not applicable.

Informed Consent Statement: Not applicable.

Data Availability Statement: The data that support the findings of this study are available from the corresponding author upon reasonable request.

Acknowledgments: This work used computer time on the Extreme Science and Engineering Discovery Environment (XSEDE) granted via MCB990010, which is supported by the National Science Foundation grant number OCI-1053575. Additional computational resources were provided by University Information Services at Georgetown University.

Conflicts of Interest: The authors declare no conflict of interest.

References

1. Ichiye, T. What makes proteins work: Exploring life in *P-T-X*. *Phys. Biol.* **2016**, *13*, 063001. [CrossRef] [PubMed]
2. Somero, G.N. Proteins and temperature. *Annu. Rev. Physiol.* **1995**, *57*, 453–468. [CrossRef]
3. Feller, G.; Gerday, C. Psychrophilic enzymes: Hot topics in cold adaptation. *Nat. Rev. Microbiol.* **2003**, *1*, 200–208. [CrossRef] [PubMed]
4. Jebbar, M.; Franzetti, B.; Girard, E.; Oger, P. Microbial diversity and adaptation to high hydrostatic pressure in deep-sea hydrothermal vents prokaryotes. *Extremophiles* **2015**, *19*, 721–740. [CrossRef] [PubMed]
5. Kallmeyer, J.; Pockalny, R.; Adhikari, R.R.; Smith, D.C.; D'Hondt, S. Global distribution of microbial abundance and biomass in subseafloor sediment. *Proc. Natl. Acad. Sci. USA* **2012**, *109*, 16213–16216. [CrossRef]
6. Yayanos, A.A. Deep-sea piezophilic bacteria. *Methods Microbiol.* **2001**, *30*, 615–637.
7. Bartlett, D.; Wright, M.; Yayanos, A.A.; Silverman, M. Isolation of a gene regulated by hydrostatic-pressure in a deep-sea bacterium. *Nature* **1989**, *342*, 572–574. [CrossRef] [PubMed]
8. Gross, M.; Jaenicke, R. Review: Proteins under pressure: The influence of high hydrostatic pressure on structure, function and assembly of proteins and protein complexes. *Eur. J. Biochem.* **1994**, *221*, 617–630. [CrossRef] [PubMed]
9. Silva, J.L.; Weber, G. Pressure stability of proteins. *Annu. Rev. Phys. Chem.* **1993**, *44*, 89–113. [CrossRef]
10. Roche, J.; Caro, J.A.; Norberto, D.R.; Barthe, P.; Roumestand, C.; Schlessman, J.L.; Garcia, A.E.; Garcia-Moreno, B.E.; Royer, C.A. Cavities determine the pressure unfolding of proteins. *Proc. Natl. Acad. Sci. USA* **2012**, *109*, 6945–6950. [CrossRef]
11. Frye, K.J.; Royer, C.A. Probing the contribution of internal cavities to the volume change of protein unfolding under pressure. *Protein Sci.* **1998**, *7*, 2217–2222. [CrossRef] [PubMed]
12. Kitahara, R.; Hata, K.; Maeno, A.; Akasaka, K.; Chimenti, M.S.; Garcia-Moreno, B.; Schroer, M.A.; Jeworrek, C.; Tolan, M.; Winter, R.; et al. Structural plasticity of staphylococcal nuclease probed by perturbation with pressure and pH. *Proteins* **2011**, *79*, 1293–1305. [CrossRef] [PubMed]
13. Collins, M.D.; Quillin, M.L.; Hummer, G.; Matthews, B.W.; Gruner, S.M. Structural rigidity of a large cavity-containing protein revealed by high-pressure crystallography. *J. Mol. Biol.* **2007**, *367*, 752–763. [CrossRef] [PubMed]
14. Nagae, T.; Kawamura, T.; Chavas, L.M.G.; Niwa, K.; Hasegawa, M.; Kato, C.; Watanabe, N. High-pressure-induced water penetration into 3-isopropylmalate dehydrogenase. *Acta Crystallogr. D* **2012**, *68*, 300–309. [CrossRef]
15. Nucci, N.V.; Fuglestad, B.; Athanasoula, E.A.; Wand, A.J. Role of cavities and hydration in the pressure unfolding of T-4 lysozyme. *Proc. Natl. Acad. Sci. USA* **2014**, *111*, 13846–13851. [CrossRef] [PubMed]
16. Nagae, T.; Kato, C.; Watanabe, N. Structural analysis of 3-isopropylmalate dehydrogenase from the obligate piezophile *Shewanella benthica* DB21MT-2 and the nonpiezophile *Shewanella oneidensis* MR-1. *Acta Crystallogr. F* **2012**, *68*, 265–268. [CrossRef] [PubMed]
17. Kamiyama, T.; Gekko, K. Effect of ligand binding on the flexibility of dihydrofolate reductase as revealed by compressibility. *Biochim. Biophys. Acta Protein Struct. Mol. Enzymol.* **2000**, *1478*, 257–266. [CrossRef]
18. Gekko, K.; Kamiyama, T.; Ohmae, E.; Katayanagi, K. Single amino acid substitutions in flexible loops can induce large compressibility changes in dihydrofolate reductase. *J. Biochem.* **2000**, *128*, 21–27. [CrossRef]
19. Wan, Q.; Bennett, B.C.; Wilson, M.A.; Kovalevsky, A.; Langan, P.; Howell, E.E.; Dealwis, C. Toward resolving the catalytic mechanism of dihydrofolate reductase using neutron and ultrahigh-resolution X-ray crystallography. *Proc. Natl. Acad. Sci. USA* **2014**, *111*, 18225–18230. [CrossRef] [PubMed]
20. Liu, C.T.; Francis, K.; Layfield, J.P.; Huang, X.Y.; Hammes-Schiffer, S.; Kohen, A.; Benkovic, S.J. *Escherichia coli* dihydrofolate reductase catalyzed proton and hydride transfers: Temporal order and the roles of Asp27 and Tyr100. *Proc. Natl. Acad. Sci. USA* **2014**, *111*, 18231–18236. [CrossRef] [PubMed]
21. Sawaya, M.R.; Kraut, J. Loop and subdomain movements in the mechanism of *Escherichia coli* dihydrofolate reductase: Crystallographic evidence. *Biochemistry* **1997**, *36*, 586–603. [CrossRef]
22. Epstein, D.M.; Benkovic, S.J.; Wright, P.E. Dynamics of the dihydrofolate reductase-folate complex-catalytic sites and regions known to undergo conformational change exhibit diverse dynamical features. *Biochemistry* **1995**, *34*, 11037–11048. [CrossRef] [PubMed]
23. Boehr, D.D.; McElheny, D.; Dyson, H.J.; Wright, P.E. The dynamic energy landscape of dihydrofolate reductase catalysis. *Science* **2006**, *313*, 1638–1642. [CrossRef]
24. Bhabha, G.; Ekiert, D.C.; Jennewein, M.; Zmasek, C.M.; Tuttle, L.M.; Kroon, G.; Dyson, H.J.; Godzik, A.; Wilson, I.A.; Wright, P.E. Divergent evolution of protein conformational dynamics in dihydrofolate reductase. *Nat. Struct. Mol. Biol.* **2013**, *20*, 1243–1262. [CrossRef]
25. Xu, Y.; Nogi, Y.; Kato, C.; Liang, Z.; Rüger, H.-J.; de Kegel, D.; Glansdorff, N. *Moritella profunda* sp. nov. and *Moritella abyssi* sp. nov., two psychropiezophilic organisms isolated from deep Atlantic sediments. *Int. J. Syst. Evol. Microbiol.* **2003**, *53*, 533–538. [CrossRef]
26. Hata, K.; Kono, R.; Fujisawa, M.; Kitahara, R.; Kamatari, Y.O.; Akasaka, K.; Xu, Y. High pressure NMR study of dihydrofolate reductase from a deep-sea bacterium *Moritella profunda*. *Cell Mol. Biol.* **2004**, *50*, 311–316.
27. Ohmae, E.; Murakami, C.; Tate, S.-I.; Gekko, K.; Hata, K.; Akasaka, K.; Kato, C. Pressure dependence of activity and stability of dihydrofolate reductases of the deep-sea bacterium *Moritella profunda* and *Escherichia coli*. *Biochim. Biophys. Acta* **2012**, *1824*, 511–512. [CrossRef] [PubMed]

28. Ohmae, E.; Miyashita, Y.; Tate, S.; Gekko, K.; Kitazawa, S.; Kitahara, R.; Kuwajima, K. Solvent environments significantly affect the enzymatic function of *Escherichia coli* dihydrofolate reductase: Comparison of wild-type protein and active-site mutant D27E. *Biochim. Biophys. Acta* **2013**, *1834*, 2782–2794. [CrossRef]
29. Ohmae, E.; Kubota, K.; Nakasone, K.; Kato, C.; Gekko, K. Pressure-dependent activity of dihydrofolate reductase from a deep-sea bacterium *Shewanella violacea* strain DSS12. *Chem. Lett.* **2004**, *33*, 798–799. [CrossRef]
30. Murakami, C.; Ohmae, E.; Tate, S.-I.; Gekko, K.; Nakasone, K.; Kato, C. Cloning and characterization of dihydrofolate reductases from deep-sea bacteria. *J. Biochem.* **2010**, *147*, 591–599. [CrossRef] [PubMed]
31. Murakami, C.; Ohmae, E.; Tate, S.-I.; Gekko, K.; Nakasone, K.; Kato, C. Comparative study on dihydrofolate reductases from *Shewanella* species living in deep-sea and ambient atmospheric-pressure environments. *Extremophiles* **2010**, *15*, 165–175. [CrossRef]
32. Ichiye, T. Enzymes from piezophiles. *Semin. Cell Dev. Biol.* **2018**, *84*, 138–146. [CrossRef]
33. Ohmae, E.; Miyashita, Y.; Kato, C. Thermodynamic and functional characteristics of deep-sea enzymes revealed by pressure effects. *Extremophiles* **2013**, *17*, 701–709. [CrossRef]
34. Evans, R.M.; Behiry, E.M.; Tey, L.-H.; Guo, J.; Loveridge, E.J.; Allemann, R.K. Catalysis by dihydrofolate reductase from the psychropiezophile *Moritella profunda*. *ChemBioChem* **2010**, *11*, 2010–2017. [CrossRef]
35. Huang, Q.; Rodgers, J.M.; Hemley, R.J.; Ichiye, T. Extreme biophysics: Enzymes under pressure. *J. Comput. Chem.* **2017**, *38*, 1174–1182. [CrossRef]
36. Huang, Q.; Tran, K.N.; Rodgers, J.M.; Bartlett, D.H.; Hemley, R.J.; Ichiye, T. A molecular perspective on the limits of life: Enzymes under pressure. *Condens. Matter Phys.* **2016**, *19*, 22801–22817. [CrossRef]
37. Huang, Q.; Rodgers, J.M.; Hemley, R.J.; Ichiye, T. Adaptations for pressure and temperature effects on loop motion in *Escherichia coli* and *Moritella profunda* dihydrofolate reductase. *High Press. Res.* **2019**, *39*, 225–237. [CrossRef]
38. Penhallurick, R.W.; Harold, A.; Durnal, M.D.; Ichiye, T. How adding a single methylene to dihydrofolate reductase can change its conformational dynamics. *J. Chem. Phys.* **2021**, *154*, 165103. [CrossRef]
39. Rodgers, J.M.; Hemley, R.J.; Ichiye, T. Quasiharmonic analysis of protein energy landscapes from pressure-temperature molecular dynamics simulations. *J. Chem. Phys.* **2017**, *147*, 125103–125110. [CrossRef]
40. Huang, Q.; Rodgers, J.M.; Hemley, R.J.; Ichiye, T. Quasiharmonic Analysis of the Energy Landscapes of Dihydrofolate Reductase from Piezophiles and Mesophiles. *J. Phys. Chem. B* **2018**, *122*, 5527–5533. [CrossRef]
41. Penhallurick, R.W.; Durnal, M.D.; Harold, A.; Ichiye, T. Adaptations for Pressure and Temperature in Dihydrofolate Reductases. *Microorganisms* **2021**, *9*, 1706. [CrossRef]
42. Nogi, Y.; Kato, C. Taxonomic studies of extremely barophilic bacteria isolated from the Mariana Trench and description of *Moritella yayanosii* sp. nov., a new barophilic bacterial isolate. *Extremophiles* **1999**, *3*, 71–77.
43. Brooks, B.R.; Brooks, C.L., III; MacKerell, A.D., Jr.; Nilsson, L.; Petrella, R.J.; Roux, B.; Won, Y.; Archontis, G.; Bartels, C.; Boresch, S.; et al. CHARMM: The biomolecular simulation program. *J. Comput. Chem.* **2009**, *30*, 1545–1614. [CrossRef]
44. Coutsias, E.A.; Seok, C.; Jacobson, M.P.; Dill, K.A. A kinematic view of loop closure. *J. Comput. Chem.* **2004**, *25*, 510–528. [CrossRef]
45. Kim, S.; Lee, J.; Jo, S.; Brooks, C.L.; Lee, H.S.; Im, W. CHARMM-GUI ligand reader and modeler for CHARMM force field generation of small molecules. *J. Comput. Chem.* **2017**, *38*, 1879–1886. [CrossRef]
46. MacKerell, A.D., Jr.; Bashford, D.; Bellot, M.; Dunbrack, R.L., Jr.; Field, M.J.; Fischer, S.; Gao, J.; Guo, H.; Ha, S.; Joseph, D.; et al. All-atom empirical potential for molecular modeling and dynamics studies of proteins. *J. Phys. Chem. B* **1998**, *102*, 3586–3616. [CrossRef]
47. Best, R.B.; Zhu, X.; Shim, J.; Lopes, P.E.; Mittal, J.; Feig, M.; Mackerell, A.D., Jr. Optimization of the additive CHARMM all-atom protein force field targeting improved sampling of the backbone phi, psi and side-chain chi(1) and chi(2) dihedral angles. *J. Chem. Theory Comput.* **2012**, *8*, 3257–3273. [CrossRef]
48. Horn, H.W.; Swope, W.C.; Pitera, J.W.; Madura, J.D.; Dick, T.J.; Hura, G.L.; Head-Gordon, T. Development of an improved four-site water model for biomolecular simulations: TIP4P-Ew. *J. Chem. Phys.* **2004**, *120*, 9665–9678. [CrossRef]
49. Vanommeslaeghe, K.; Hatcher, E.; Acharya, C.; Kundu, S.; Zhong, S.; Shim, J.; Darian, E.; Guvench, O.; Lopes, P.; Vorobyov, I.; et al. CHARMM general force field: A force field for drug-like molecules compatible with the CHARMM all-atom additive biological force fields. *J. Comput. Chem.* **2010**, *31*, 671–690. [CrossRef]
50. Pavelites, J.J.; Gao, J.L.; Bash, P.A.; Mackerell, A.D. A molecular mechanics force field for NAD(+), NADH; the pyrophosphate groups of nucleotides. *J. Comput. Chem.* **1997**, *18*, 221–239. [CrossRef]
51. Eastman, P.; Swails, J.; Chodera, J.D.; McGibbon, R.T.; Zhao, Y.; Beauchamp, K.A.; Wang, L.P.; Simmonett, A.C.; Harrigan, M.P.; Stern, C.D.; et al. OpenMM 7: Rapid development of high performance algorithms for molecular dynamics. *PLoS Comput. Biol.* **2017**, *13*, e1005659. [CrossRef]
52. Liu, D.C.; Nocedal, J. On the Limited Memory BFGS Method for Large-Scale Optimization. *Math. Program.* **1989**, *45*, 503–528. [CrossRef]
53. Andersen, H.C. Molecular-dynamics simulations at constant pressure and/or temperature. *J. Chem. Phys.* **1980**, *72*, 2384–2393. [CrossRef]
54. Aqvist, J.; Wennerstrom, P.; Nervall, M.; Bjelic, S.; Brandsdal, B.O. Molecular dynamics simulations of water and biomolecules wit a Monte Carlo constant pressure algorithm. *Chem. Phys. Lett.* **2004**, *384*, 288–294. [CrossRef]
55. Nosé, S. A unified formulation of the constant temperature molecular dynamics methods. *J. Chem. Phys.* **1984**, *81*, 511–519. [CrossRef]

56. Hoover, W.G. Canonical dynamics: Equilibrium phase-space distributions. *Phys. Rev. A* **1985**, *31*, 1695–1697. [CrossRef]
57. Martyna, G.J.; Klein, M.L.; Tuckerman, M. Nose-Hoover Chains—The Canonical Ensemble via Continuous Dynamics. *J. Chem. Phys.* **1992**, *97*, 2635–2643. [CrossRef]
58. Martyna, G.J.; Tuckerman, M.E.; Tobias, D.J.; Klein, M.L. Explicit reversible integrators for extended systems dynamics. *Mol. Phys.* **1996**, *87*, 1117–1157. [CrossRef]
59. De Loof, H.; Nilsson, L.; Rigler, R. Molecular dynamics simulation of galanin in aqueous and nonaqueous solution. *J. Am. Chem. Soc.* **1992**, *114*, 4028–4035. [CrossRef]
60. Till, M.S.; Ullmann, G.M. McVol—A program for calculating protein volumes and identifying cavities by a Monte Carlo algorithm. *J. Mol. Model.* **2010**, *16*, 419–429. [CrossRef]
61. Keedy, D.A.; van den Bedem, H.; Sivak, D.A.; Petsko, G.A.; Ringe, D.; Wilson, M.A.; Fraser, J.S. Crystal Cryocooling Distorts Conformational Heterogeneity in a Model Michaelis Complex of DHFR. *Structure* **2014**, *22*, 899–910. [CrossRef]
62. Fenwick, R.B.; van den Bedem, H.; Fraser, J.S.; Wright, P.E. Integrated description of protein dynamics from room-temperature X-ray crystallography and NMR. *Proc. Natl. Acad. Sci. USA* **2014**, *111*, E445–E454. [CrossRef]
63. Nagae, T.; Yamada, H.; Watanabe, N. High-pressure protein crystal structure analysis of *Escherichia coli* dihydrofolate reductase complexed with folate and NADP+. *Acta Crystallogr. D* **2018**, *74*, 895–905. [CrossRef]

biology

MDPI

Article

The Effects of Temperature and Pressure on Protein-Ligand Binding in the Presence of Mars-Relevant Salts †

Nisrine Jahmidi-Azizi [1], Rosario Oliva [1,*], Stewart Gault [2], Charles S. Cockell [2] and Roland Winter [1,*]

[1] Physical Chemistry I—Biophysical Chemistry, Department of Chemistry and Chemical Biology, TU Dortmund University, Otto-Hahn Street 4a, 44227 Dortmund, Germany; nisrine.jahmidi@tu-dortmund.de
[2] UK Centre for Astrobiology, SUPA School of Physics and Astronomy, University of Edinburgh, James Clerk Maxwell Building, Peter Guthrie Tait Road, Edinburgh EH9 3FD, UK; s.a.gault@sms.ed.ac.uk (S.G.); c.s.cockell@ed.ac.uk (C.S.C.)
* Correspondence: rosario.oliva@tu-dortmund.de (R.O.); roland.winter@tu-dortmund.de (R.W.)
† The manuscript is dedicated to Dr. Gaston Hui Bon Hoa.

Simple Summary: Interactions of ligands with proteins are central to all reactions in the biological cell. How such reactions are affected by harsh environmental conditions, such as low temperatures, high pressures, and high concentrations of biologically destructive salts, is still largely unknown. Our work focused on specific salts found on Mars to understand whether the planet's potentially liquid, water-rich subsurface harbors conditions that are theoretically favorable for life. Our data show that, while magnesium chloride and sulfate do not significantly alter protein–ligand interactions, the perchlorate ion strongly affects protein–ligand binding. However, the temperature and pressure conditions encountered on Mars do not necessarily preclude protein–ligand interactions of the type studied here.

Abstract: Protein–ligand interactions are fundamental to all biochemical processes. Generally, these processes are studied at ambient temperature and pressure conditions. We investigated the binding of the small ligand 8-anilinonaphthalene-1-sulfonic acid (ANS) to the multifunctional protein bovine serum albumin (BSA) at ambient and low temperatures and at high pressure conditions, in the presence of ions associated with the surface and subsurface of Mars, including the chaotropic perchlorate ion. We found that salts such as magnesium chloride and sulfate only slightly affect the protein–ligand complex formation. In contrast, magnesium perchlorate strongly affects the interaction between ANS and BSA at the single site level, leading to a change in stoichiometry and strength of ligand binding. Interestingly, both a decrease in temperature and an increase in pressure favor the ligand binding process, resulting in a negative change in protein–ligand binding volume. This suggests that biochemical reactions that are fundamental for the regulation of biological processes are theoretically possible outside standard temperature and pressure conditions, such as in the harsh conditions of the Martian subsurface.

Keywords: protein–ligand binding; high pressure; Martian salts; perchlorate; BSA; ANS

Citation: Jahmidi-Azizi, N.; Oliva, R.; Gault, S.; Cockell, C.S.; Winter, R. The Effects of Temperature and Pressure on Protein-Ligand Binding in the Presence of Mars-Relevant Salts. *Biology* **2021**, *10*, 687. https://doi.org/10.3390/biology10070687

Academic Editors: Dmitri Davydov and Christiane Jung

Received: 25 June 2021
Accepted: 16 July 2021
Published: 20 July 2021

1. Introduction

Protein–ligand recognition and binding are fundamental to all biochemical processes and are essential for all life forms [1–5]. Hence, elucidating the nature and strength of the driving forces involved in the ligand binding processes is of particular interest in the biosciences. In most cases, non-covalent bonds, such as electrostatic and hydrophobic interactions, ensure formation of the protein–ligand complexes [5]. In a molecular picture, protein–ligand interactions may not strictly follow a simple binding process; instead, they may be accompanied by conformational as well as hydration changes of the protein and potentially also the ligand. Owing to the inherent complexity of the process, many aspects of ligand binding have not been fully explored, yet. This is particularly true for complex solution conditions, such as ligand binding in cellulo or in the presence of high concentrations of co-solutes or at extreme environmental conditions, such as at low/high temperatures and high hydrostatic pressures (HHP). HHP environments are, for example, encountered in the deep sea or in subsurface environments where pressures up to the kbar regime are encountered (1 kbar = 100 MPa). Hence, knowledge about high hydrostatic pressure effects on biological systems is also fundamental for our understanding of life being exposed to such harsh conditions and of the physical limits of life in general [6–10].

Of interest is to explore the theoretical capacity of other planetary bodies, such as Mars, to support life. Mars is known to have hosted a vigorous hydrological regime in its early history. Although we do not know if Mars ever hosted life, we could ask the question whether conditions on that planet could theoretically support similar biological processes observed on Earth and therefore whether Mars or Mars-like geological conditions on any planet would act as a barrier to life as we know it. In particular, as water was lost from Mars, brines may have formed. Today, the planet hosts localized high concentrations of salts such as chlorides [11], sulfates [12], and perchlorates [13]. Although the surface of Mars is today at the triple point, the subsurface may still host liquid water as it did in the past [14–16]. These chemical constituents of the planetary environment raise the question of how they, in combination with high pressures associated with the subsurface, would influence the theoretical habitability of that planet.

In this work, we set out to investigate the effect of temperature, pressure, and Mars-relevant salts, including $MgCl_2$, $Mg(ClO_4)_2$, and $MgSO_4$, on the binding characteristics of the small aromatic ligand 8-anilinonaphthalene-1-sulfonic acid (ANS) to the multifunctional protein bovine serum albumin (BSA). To this end, pressure-dependent fluorescence spectroscopy was applied, supplemented by circular dichroism (CD) experiments.

2. Materials and Methods

2.1. Materials

The protein bovine serum albumin (BSA, molecular weight of 66 kDa, 583 residues) in the form of lyophilized powder, the fluorophore 8-anilinonaphthalene-1-sulfonic acid (ANS), the salts $MgCl_2$, $Mg(ClO_4)_2$ and $MgSO_4$ were all purchased from Sigma Aldrich Chemicals (Taufkirchen, Germany). All the sample solutions were prepared in the pressure stable 10 mM Tris-HCl buffer, at the pH of 7.4. Deionized water was used for all buffer and sample preparations.

2.2. Samples Preparation

The stock solution of the protein BSA was prepared by dissolving the lyophilized powder in Tris-HCl buffer. The exact concentration was determined by measuring the absorbance at 280 nm with a UV-1800 spectrometer from Shimadzu Corporation (Kyoto, Japan), using a molar extinction coefficient of 43600 M^{-1} cm^{-1} [17]. A stock solution of the fluorophore ANS was prepared by dissolving it in water. After dilution in buffer, the exact concentration was determined by measuring the absorbance, using a molar extinction coefficient of ε (350 nm) = 4950 M^{-1} cm^{-1} [17]. All the samples were prepared by diluting BSA and ANS in 10 mM Tris-HCl buffer, pH 7.4, in the absence and presence of 250 mM $MgCl_2$, $Mg(ClO_4)_2$ or $MgSO_4$.

2.3. Steady-State Fluorescence Spectroscopy

The extent of complex formation between ANS and BSA was followed by means of steady-state fluorescence spectroscopy using a K2 fluorometer from ISS, Inc. (Champaign, IL, USA). The binding isotherms were obtained by recording ANS emission spectra by exciting the solutions at 350 nm and recording the emission intensities in the range 400–550 nm. The width slits of the excitation and emission monochromators were both set to 8 nm. Briefly, a series of solutions with a fixed concentration of ANS at ~5 μM were prepared, and the concentration of BSA was varied between 0 and ~40 μM. Then estimation of the binding constants (K_b) was performed by using a plot of $\Delta F = F - F_0$ (where F is the fluorescence intensity of ANS at the maximum in the presence of BSA, and F_0 is the intensity of ANS in the absence of BSA) as a function of total BSA concentration and fitting the experimental data according to an equivalent and independent binding sites model or to two classes of non-equivalent and independent binding-site models, as described in detail in Reference [17].

For the pressure dependent measurements, the high-pressure cell system from ISS and quartz cuvettes were used. The pressure was controlled by means of a manual pump, and water was used as pressurizing fluid. A pressure range from 1 to 2000 bar was explored. The ANS and BSA solutions were mixed, vortexed, and then filled into the sample cell, which was sealed with DuraSeal^{TM} laboratory stretch film and placed into the high-pressure vessel. The stretch film allowed for the pressure transmission in the sample cuvette.

2.4. *Circular Dichroism Spectroscopy*

Circular dichroism (CD) spectroscopy experiments were performed in the Far-UV region (190–260 nm) in order to determine the secondary structure of the protein BSA in the presence of 250 mM of $MgCl_2$, $Mg(ClO_4)_2$, or $MgSO_4$ and at the temperatures of 5, 15, and 25 °C. CD spectra of a 14 μM BSA solution were recorded by using a 0.01 cm path-length quartz by means of a Jasco J-715 spectropolarimeter (Jasco Corporation, Tokyo, Japan). The instrument parameters were set as follows: scan rate of 50 nm min^{-1}, response of 2 s, and bandwidth of 4 nm. For each sample, a background blank (neat buffer or salts-containing buffer) was subtracted. The recorded spectra are the results of three accumulations, and they were normalized per mole of residue.

3. Results

In a previous study it was shown that the small aromatic ligand ANS is able to bind to the protein BSA with a binding constant, K_b, of the order of 10^6 M^{-1} in 10 mM Tris-HCl buffer (neat buffer conditions) at ambient temperature, i.e., 25 °C [11]. It was also demonstrated that three ANS molecules are bound on average to one BSA molecule and that the binding process can be well described by assuming that all the three ANS molecules can interact with the same affinity [17]. In order to investigate the impact of the Mars-relevant salts on the complex formation between ANS and BSA, we performed a series of fluorescence spectroscopic experiments. By varying the temperature and pressure, a temperature range from 5 to 25 °C and a pressure range from ambient pressure (1 bar) to 2000 bar was covered.

First, we explored the impact of 250 mM $MgCl_2$, $Mg(ClO_4)_2$, and $MgSO_4$ on the ligand binding process at 25 °C and ambient pressure (1 bar). To be able to determine the binding constant, it is of fundamental importance to exactly know the stoichiometry of the complex formed. In this way, a proper binding model can be applied in the data analysis of the measured binding isotherms, providing the most appropriate value of the binding constant, K_b. We applied the method of continuous variation (or Job's plot) for the estimation of the binding stoichiometry [18–20] by means of steady-state fluorescence spectroscopy. A series of solutions were prepared such that the total concentration (i.e., [ANS] + [BSA]) is constant, while the mole fractions of the interacting partners were varied. Discontinuities in the plot of fluorescence intensity vs. x_{ANS} (where x_{ANS} is the mole fraction of ANS) are indicative of the stoichiometry of the complex formed. Figure 1 shows the Job's plot obtained in the presence of the three salts at T = 25 °C and p = 1 bar.

An inspection of Figure 1A reveals the presence of one inflection point in the presence of $MgCl_2$ which is centered at $x_{ANS} \approx 0.75$, indicating the formation of a 1:3 (BSA:ANS) complex. Qualitatively, the same result was also obtained in the $MgSO_4$ containing solution: the presence of one inflection point at $x_{ANS} \approx 0.75$ suggests that, again, three ANS molecules are bound to one BSA molecule (Figure 1B). The same stoichiometry was previously observed in the same buffer but in the absence of any salt [17], suggesting that both magnesium chloride and sulfate have no significant impact on the stoichiometry of the BSA:ANS complex.

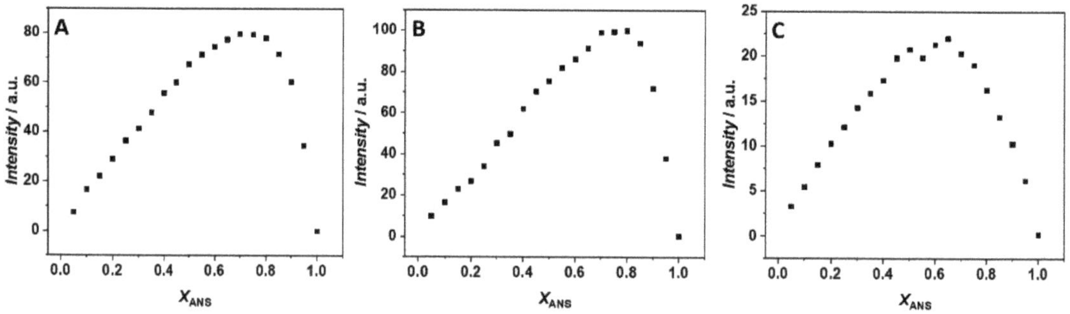

Figure 1. Job's plot for ANS/BSA complex formation obtained at the temperature of 25 °C and pressure of 1 bar in the presence of 250 mM (**A**) $MgCl_2$, (**B**) $MgSO_4$, and (**C**) $Mg(ClO_4)_2$. The total concentration ([ANS] + [BSA]) was 35 µM. The fluorescence intensity is reported in arbitrary units (a.u.).

A completely different scenario was observed in the presence of $Mg(ClO_4)_2$. The Job's plot is characterized by the presence of two distinct inflection points (Figure 1C). One is centered at $x_{ANS} = 0.5$, and the other one at $x_{ANS} \approx 0.65$, suggesting that only two ANS molecules are bound to one BSA molecule. The presence of two distinct inflection points is indicative of a non-equivalence of binding sites; otherwise, only one inflection point should be observed, as in the case of the $MgCl_2$ and $MgSO_4$ solutions. Thus, $Mg(ClO_4)_2$ is able to strongly modulate the formation of the complex at the level of single binding sites, inhibiting the binding to one site and leading to the loss of equivalence of the two remaining sites.

Then, we explored the effect of temperature on the stoichiometry of the ANS:BSA complex. We determined the Job's plots also at 5 and 15 °C. The Job's plot data obtained in the presence of $MgCl_2$, $MgSO_4$, and $Mg(ClO_4)_2$ are reported in Supplementary Materials Figures S1–S3, respectively. An inspection of Supplementary Materials Figures S1–S3 reveals that a decrease in temperature to 5 °C does not alter the stoichiometry of the protein–ligand complex. As in the case at T = 25 °C, stoichiometries of 3:1, 3:1, and 2:1 ANS:BSA were observed for the complex formation in the presence of $MgCl_2$, $MgSO_4$, and $Mg(ClO_4)_2$, respectively (Table 1).

Table 1. Binding constants (K_b) and stoichiometries for the BSA:ANS complex formation in 10 mM Tris-HCl buffer, pH 7.4, in the presence of the indicated salts and at temperatures (T) of 5, 15, and 25 °C.

Solution Conditions	T/°C	K_{b1}/M^{-1} × 10^6	K_{b2}/M^{-1} × 10^6	^1n
250 mM $MgCl_2$	5	1.0 ± 0.1	-	1:3
	15	0.36 ± 0.13	-	1:3
	25	4.9 ± 0.2	-	1:3
250 mM $MgSO_4$	5	0.62 ± 0.15	-	1:3
	15	0.39 ± 0.14	-	1:3
	25	2.9 ± 0.3	-	1:3
250 mM $Mg(ClO_4)_2$	5	0.19± 0.13	0.19 ± 0.13	1:2
	15	0.15 ± 0.04	0.13 ± 0.02	1:2
	25	0.59 ± 0.22	1.2 ± 0.1	1:2

Note: ^1n represents the stoichiometry of binding as BSA:ANS.

Once the stoichiometries of the complex in the presence of the salts and at the three different temperatures are known, it is possible to estimate the binding constants, K_b, performing titration experiments by means of steady-state fluorescence spectroscopy. In these experiments, a solution of ANS was titrated with a BSA solution. The ANS is characterized by a very low quantum yield when it is free in solution [21]. Instead, when the aromatic ligand is bound to the protein's hydrophobic pockets, a strong increase of the fluorescence intensity is observed. Thus, the extent of binding can be readily determined by following the fluorescence increase of ANS. The subsequent data analysis was performed according to the stoichiometries inferred by the Job's plot experiments. In $MgCl_2$ and $MgSO_4$ containing buffer with one class of site only, the experimental points of the titration experiment were fitted according to an equivalent and independent binding sites model. Instead, in the presence of $Mg(ClO_4)_2$, two distinct binding modes were observed; hence, a two-classes-of-independent-binding-sites model was used. Figure 2A–C depict the binding isotherms at ambient pressure, obtained in the presence of 250 mM $MgCl_2$, $MgSO_4$, and $Mg(ClO_4)_2$ at 5, 15, and 25 °C. The values of the binding constants determined are collected in Table 1.

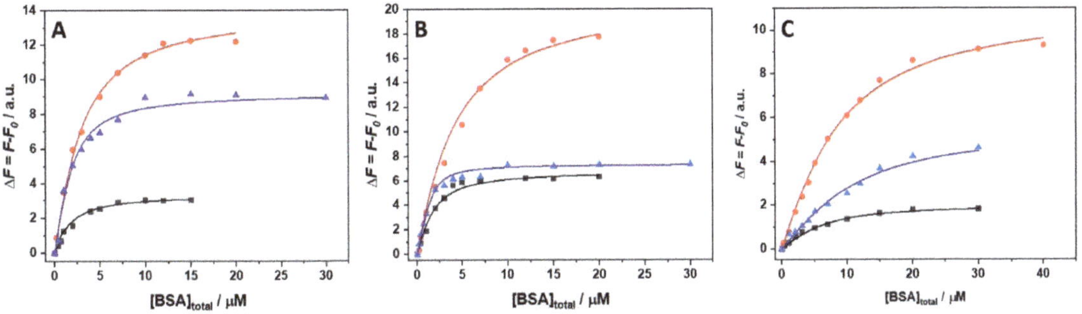

Figure 2. Binding isotherms for complex formation between the bovine serum albumin (BSA) and 8-anilinonaphthalene-1-sulfonic acid (ANS) obtained at the temperatures of 5 °C (black squares), 15 °C (red circles), and 25 °C (blue triangles) at $p = 1$ bar in the presence of 250 mM (**A**) $MgCl_2$, (**B**) $MgSO_4$, and (**C**) $Mg(ClO_4)_2$. The solid lines represent the best fit of experimental data according to an equivalent and independent binding sites model for the experiments performed in the presence of $MgCl_2$ and $MgSO_4$, and to two classes of independent binding-sites models for the experiments carried out in the presence of $Mg(ClO_4)_2$. The binding isotherms were obtained by plotting $\Delta F = F - F_0$ (where F is the fluorescence intensity of ANS at the maximum in the presence of BSA, and F_0 is the intensity of ANS in the absence of BSA) as a function of total BSA concentration.

In the presence of $MgCl_2$, decreasing the temperature from 25 to 15 °C, a prominent decrease of K_b (~90%) was observed. At 5 °C, the K_b-value is only slightly higher compared to the value at 15 °C, however. Thus, the system exhibits a complex non-linear temperature dependence of the overall binding constant measured. A very similar behavior was also observed in the presence of $MgSO_4$, i.e., the decrease of the temperature disfavors formation of the complex, but in a non-linear way. In the presence of $Mg(ClO_4)_2$, the K_b-values decrease as well upon lowering the temperature. The decrease of K_{b1} seems to be less pronounced with respect to the decrease of K_{b2}, indicating that the two different binding sites are characterized by different binding energetics, which is probably due to the differences in the non-covalent interactions established upon binding. It is important to note that decreasing the temperature leads to similar values of the two binding constants.

Principally, the differences observed for the effect of temperature and salt on complex formation could be ascribed to conformational changes of the protein structure. To test this possibility, circular dichroism (CD) spectra of BSA in the far-UV range were recorded. In this spectral region, information about the secondary structure of the protein can be obtained [22,23]. The spectra were acquired at temperatures of 5, 15, and 25 °C, and in the presence of the three different salts. Figure 3 shows the CD spectra of BSA recorded at 25 °C in the presence of 250 mM $MgCl_2$, $Mg(ClO_4)_2$, and $MgSO_4$. For reference, the CD spectrum of BSA in neat buffer (10 mM Tris-HCl, pH 7.4) is also shown.

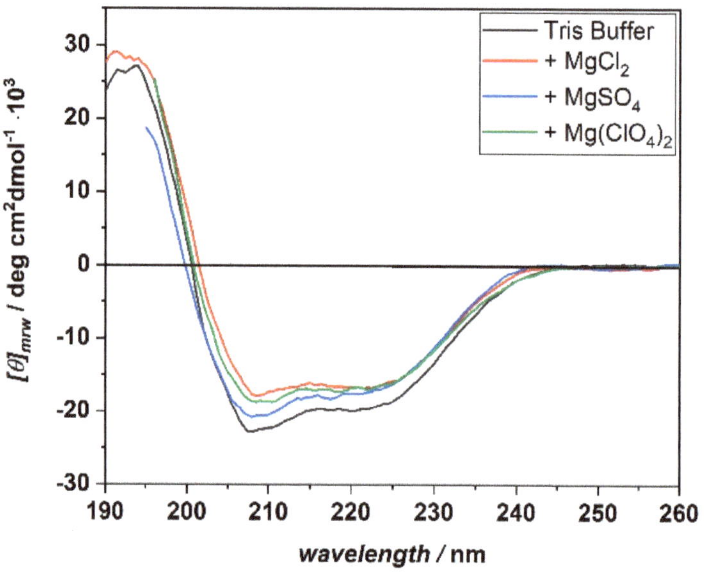

Figure 3. Far-UV CD spectra of BSA in the presence of 250 mM $MgCl_2$ (red spectrum), $MgSO_4$ (blue spectrum), and $Mg(ClO_4)_2$ (green spectrum). For reference, the CD spectrum of BSA in neat buffer condition (black spectrum) is also reported. All the spectra were acquired at the temperature of 25 °C, in 10 mM Tris-HCl buffer, pH 7.4. The CD spectra are reported by plotting the molar ellipticity ($[\theta]_{mrw}$) as a function of the wavelength, in nm.

The CD spectrum of BSA at neat buffer conditions is characterized by the presence of two minima located at about 208 and 222 nm. In addition, a positive band centered at around 195 nm is present. These spectral features are characteristic of a protein which adopts an α-helical conformation, which is in agreement with its reported structure [24]. In the salt-containing media, the CD spectra of BSA show the same general features as in the neat buffer case, signifying that even in the presence of high concentrations of these Mars-relevant salts, the protein's secondary structure seems to be retained. The same result was obtained for the measurements carried out at the temperatures of 5 and 15 °C (Supplementary Materials Figure S4). Thus, the differences observed in the binding affinities and stoichiometries do not seem to be related to a conformational change of the protein structure. However, small and localized changes cannot be excluded a priori.

In the next step, we explored the impact of high hydrostatic pressure (HHP) on the binding of ANS to BSA in the presence of the three salts and in the temperature range between 5 and 25 °C. To this end, we performed the same titration experiments following the complex formation by means of HHP fluorescence spectroscopy. As an example, Figure 4 depicts the binding isotherms obtained for the ANS titration with a solution of BSA in the presence of 250 mM $MgCl_2$ at T = 25 °C and in the pressure range between 1 and 2000 bar. The binding constants determined for all samples are shown in Table 2.

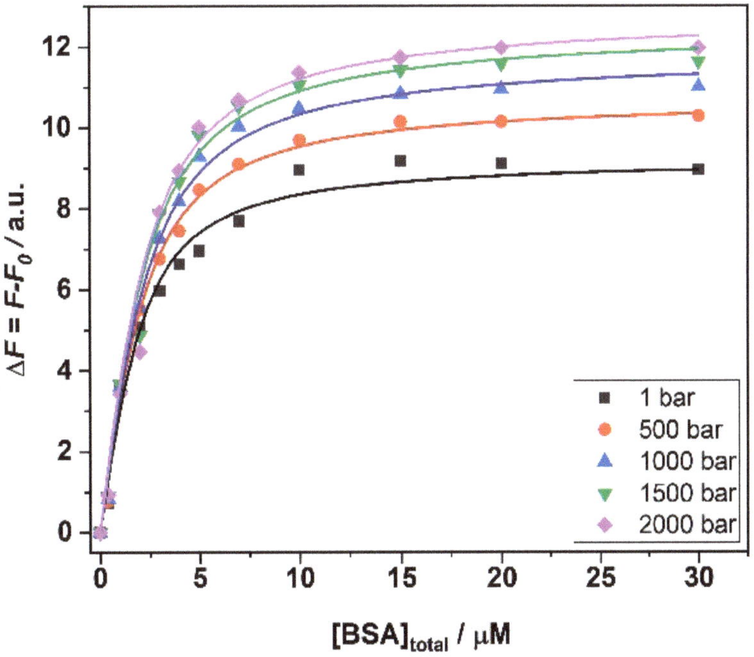

Figure 4. Binding isotherms for ANS/BSA complex formation obtained at T = 25 °C in the presence of 250 mM $MgCl_2$, at the indicated pressure values. The solid lines represent the best fit of experimental data according to an equivalent and independent binding sites model. All the experiments were performed in 10 mM Tris-HCl buffer. The binding isotherms were obtained by plotting $\Delta F = F - F_0$ (where F is the fluorescence intensity of ANS at the maximum in the presence of BSA, and F_0 is the intensity of ANS in the absence of BSA) as a function of the total BSA concentration.

Table 2. Binding constants (K_b) and stoichiometries (n) for the BSA:ANS complex formation in 10 mM Tris-HCl buffer, pH 7.4, in the presence of the indicated salts, temperatures, and pressures.

Solution Conditions	T/°C	p/bar	K_{b1}/M^{-1} ·10^6	K_{b2}/M^{-1} ·10^6	^1n
	5	1	1.0 ± 0.1	-	1:3
	5	500	1.0 ± 0.2	-	1:3
250 mM $MgCl_2$	5	1000	1.2 ± 0.3	-	1:3
	5	1500	1.8 ± 0.3	-	1:3
	5	2000	1.9 ± 0.3	-	1:3
	15	1	0.36 ± 0.13	-	1:3
	15	500	0.40 ± 0.16	-	1:3
250 mM $MgCl_2$	15	1000	0.41 ± 0.16	-	1:3
	15	1500	0.43 ± 0.17	-	1:3
	15	2000	0.45 ± 0.18	-	1:3
	25	1	4.9 ± 0.2	-	1:3
	25	500	4.3 ± 0.1	-	1:3
250 mM $MgCl_2$	25	1000	4.5 ± 0.1	-	1:3
	25	1500	4.9 ± 0.2	-	1:3
	25	2000	5.2 ± 0.1	-	1:3

Table 2. *Cont.*

Solution Conditions	T/°C	p/bar	K_{b1}/M^{-1}·10^6	K_{b2}/M^{-1}·10^6	^1n
250 mM $MgSO_4$	5	1	0.62 ± 0.15	-	1:3
	5	500	0.48 ± 0.07	-	1:3
	5	1000	0.47 ± 0.07	-	1:3
	5	1500	0.55 ± 0.20	-	1:3
	5	2000	0.44 ± 0.20	-	1:3
250 mM $MgSO_4$	15	1	0.39 ± 0.14	-	1:3
	15	500	0.40 ± 0.16	-	1:3
	15	1000	0.42 ± 0.15	-	1:3
	15	1500	0.43 ± 0.17	-	1:3
	15	2000	0.45 ± 0.18	-	1:3
250 mM $MgSO_4$	25	1	2.9 ± 0.3	-	1:3
	25	500	2.9 ± 0.3	-	1:3
	25	1000	2.7 ± 0.4	-	1:3
	25	1500	2.4 ± 0.7	-	1:3
	25	2000	2.2 ± 0.9	-	1:3
250 mM $Mg(ClO_4)_2$	5	1	0.19± 0.13	0.19 ± 0.13	1:2
	5	500	0.32 ± 0.25	0.40 ± 0.33	1:2
	5	1000	0.34 ± 0.26	0.34 ± 0.26	1:2
	5	1500	0.35 ± 0.19	0.52 ± 0.43	1:2
	5	2000	0.39 ± 0.07	0.66 ± 0.53	1:2
250 mM $Mg(ClO_4)_2$	15	1	0.15± 0.04	0.13 ± 0.13	1:2
	15	500	0.14 ± 0.01	0.15 ± 0.10	1:2
	15	1000	0.19 ± 0.02	0.19 ± 0.18	1:2
	15	1500	0.21 ± 0.02	0.21 ± 0.21	1:2
	15	2000	0.26 ± 0.01	0.24 ± 0.20	1:2
250 mM $Mg(ClO_4)_2$	25	1	0.59 ± 0.22	1.2 ± 0.1	1:2
	25	500	0.59 ± 0.17	1.1 ± 0.1	1:2
	25	1000	0.38 ± 0.10	1.2 ± 0.2	1:2
	25	1500	0.34 ± 0.03	1.2 ± 0.3	1:2
	25	2000	0.40 ± 0.05	0.89 ± 0.05	1:2

Note: ^1n represents the stoichiometry of binding as BSA:ANS.

An inspection of Table 2 reveals that pressure has an effect on the values of K_b that depends on the temperature and on the type of salt present in solution. It is important to note that BSA is stable in the whole pressure range covered and no unfolding and denaturation of the protein takes place [25–27]. Thus, variations observed in the values of K_b can most likely not be ascribed to protein conformational changes imposed by pressure. In the presence of $MgCl_2$, at 25 °C, only minor effects on the binding affinity were observed. The same holds true for T = 15 °C. Instead, the pressure effect seems more pronounced at T = 5 °C, were a clear increase of K_b was observed upon a pressure increase from 1 to 2000 bar. Thus, the application of pressure favors the formation of the complex at lower temperatures.

Instead, in the $MgSO_4$ containing buffer, at 25 °C, a slight decrease of the affinity is detected upon pressurization. The volume changes observed are very small (for comparison, the molar volume of one water molecule is about 18 mL mol^{-1}). The pressure effect seems to be slightly favorable for binding at 15 °C. At T = 5 °C, K_b decreases slightly with increasing pressure. Thus, depending on the temperature, the complex formation in the presence of $MgSO_4$ is slightly favored or disfavored. The changes are quite small or even negligible, however.

In the presence of $Mg(ClO_4)_2$, at T = 25 °C, the first binding constant of the two remaining binding sites, K_{b1}, decreases slightly with increasing pressure. Instead, the second binding mode, K_{b2}, does not seem to be significantly affected by pressure changes up to the 2000 bar regime. At 15 °C, K_{b1} and K_{b2} increase slightly upon pressurization.

Moreover, at the lowest temperature, at $T = 5$ °C, K_{b1} and K_{b2} increase with increasing pressure. Thus, the two binding modes respond to pressure in different ways, highlighting that the packing properties and hydration effects upon binding, which largely contribute to volume changes, are different for each binding site of the protein.

From the pressure dependence of the K_b values, the volume change upon binding, the protein–ligand binding volume ΔV_b, can be determined (for an in-depth discussion of pressure effects on ligand binding, please refer to Reference [28] and references therein):

$$\left[\frac{\partial \ln K_b}{\partial p}\right]_T = -\frac{\Delta V_b}{RT} \quad (1)$$

Here, $[\partial \ln K_b/\partial p]_T$ is the derivative of the logarithm of the binding constant (K_b) with respect to pressure (p) at constant temperature (T). R is the universal gas constant. ΔV_b is the binding volume defined as the difference between the partial molar volume of the complex (PL, where P is the protein and L the ligand) and the sum of the partial molar volumes of the uncomplexed state (P+L). Thus, the binding volume can be directly estimated by taking the slope of a plot of $\ln K_b$ vs. p, assuming that the volume change is independent of pressure in the (here rather small) pressure range covered. Figure 5A–D depict the plots of $\ln K_b$ vs. p obtained in the salt-containing media and at the three temperatures measured. All ΔV_b values obtained are collected in Table 3.

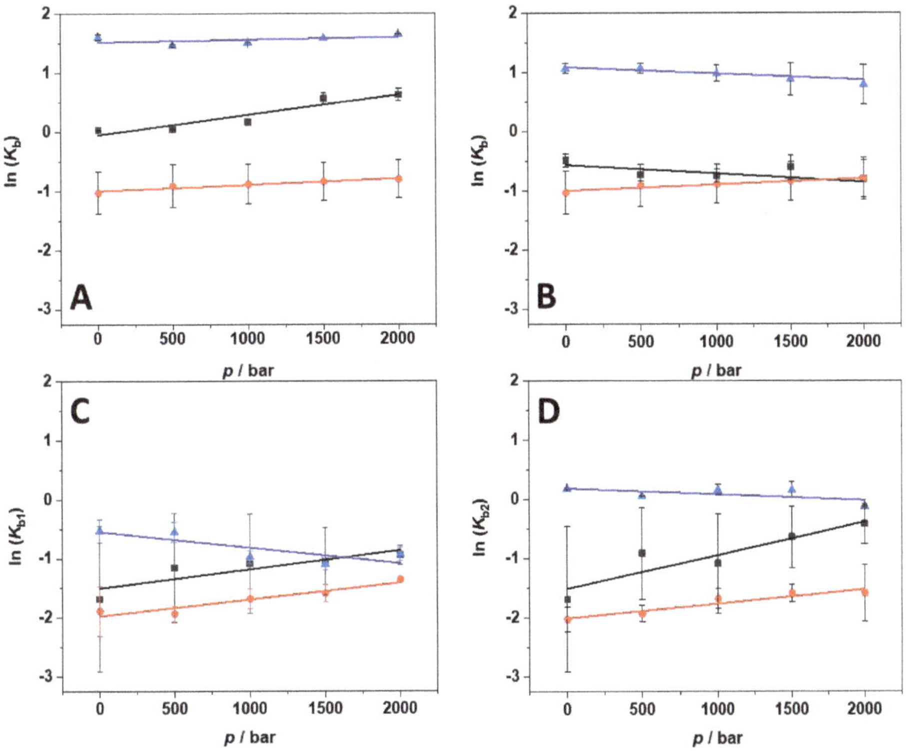

Figure 5. Pressure dependence of the binding constant (K_b) for the complex formation between BSA and ANS in the presence of 250 mM $MgCl_2$ (**A**), $MgSO_4$ (**B**), and $Mg(ClO_4)_2$ (**C**) and (**D**) at the temperatures of 5 °C (black squares), 15 °C (red circles), and 25 °C (blue triangles). The plot in (**C**) refers to the pressure dependence of the binding constant of the first binding site (K_{b1}), the plot in (**D**) to that of the second binding site (K_{b2}). From the slopes of $\ln(K_b)$ vs. p, the binding volume (ΔV_b) can be calculated by means of Equation (1).

Table 3. Binding volumes (ΔV_b) for the BSA:ANS complex formation at the indicated temperatures and in the presence of 250 mM $MgCl_2$, $MgSO_4$, and $Mg(ClO_4)_2$. The ΔV_b values are reported in mL mol^{-1} of protein.

T/°C	$MgCl_2$ ΔV_b/mL mol^{-1}	$MgSO_4$ ΔV_b/mL mol^{-1}	$Mg(ClO_4)_2$ ΔV_{b1}/mL mol^{-1}	$Mg(ClO_4)_2$ ΔV_{b2}/mL mol^{-1}
5	-7.9 ± 0.1	2.0 ± 1.0	-7.4 ± 2.4	-12.9 ± 3.2
15	-2.5 ± 0.4	-2.0 ± 1.0	-6.0 ± 1.0	-5.0 ± 1.0
25	-1.0 ± 1.0	3.6 ± 0.5	6.0 ± 2.0	2.0 ± 1.0

At $T = 25$ °C, the binding volume in the presence of $MgCl_2$ is close to zero, highlighting the negligible effect of pressure on the complex formation. Instead, in the sulfate-containing solution, the volume change is slightly positive, i.e., the application of pressure does not favor the interaction between the protein and the ligand. In the presence of perchlorate, the binding volumes of both binding sites are positive. However, $\Delta V_{b1} > \Delta V_{b2}$, indicating that the two binding sites are characterized by different packing and hydration properties. In the presence of $MgCl_2$, the decrease of temperature is accompanied by more negative ΔV_b values; this is to say, decreasing temperature and increasing pressure both favor the complex formation. Instead, in the $MgSO_4$-containing buffer, ΔV_b-changes with temperature are less pronounced. A small decrease of ΔV_b was observed, only. Interestingly, in the presence of $Mg(ClO_4)_2$, the temperature had a comparably strong impact on the volume changes. Both binding volumes become negative, reaching values of -7.4 and -12.9 mL mol^{-1} for the first and the second binding site, respectively. Thus, when magnesium perchlorate is present in solution, the combined increase of pressure and decrease of temperature strongly favor the complex formation. To highlight the changes of binding volume with temperature, ΔV_b (T) is shown for the different salts in Figure 6.

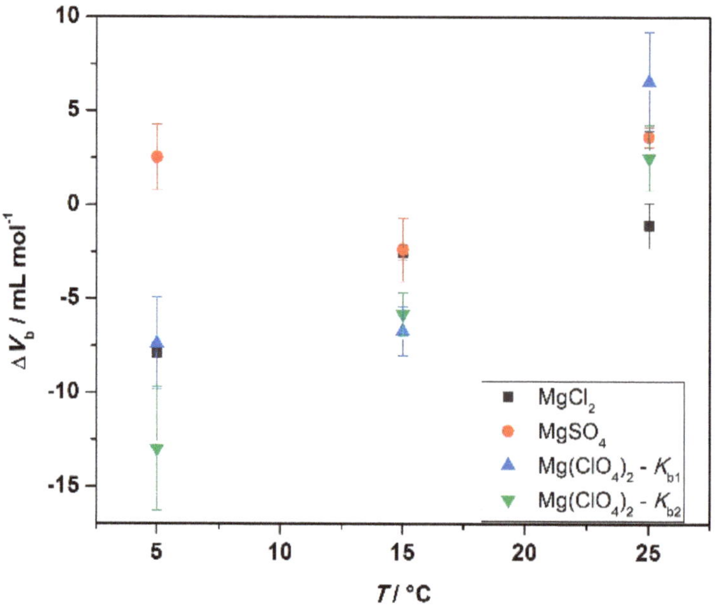

Figure 6. Plot of binding volumes, ΔV_b, as a function of temperature for the indicated 250 mM salt solutions.

4. Discussion

In this work, the combined effects of temperature and pressure on the binding characteristics of ANS to BSA were determined in the presence of Mars-relevant salts, including $MgCl_2$, $Mg(ClO_4)_2$, and $MgSO_4$. We found that the binding of the small aromatic ligand ANS to BSA depends significantly on the type of salt, i.e., the anion, on temperature, and on pressure. At ambient conditions (T = 25 °C and p = 1 bar), the presence of 250 mM $MgCl_2$ and $MgSO_4$ has no impact on the stoichiometry and no major effect on the binding strength of the complex formed. Both the binding stoichiometry and K_b are similar to those previously determined in neat buffer solution (three ANS molecules are bound to one BSA with a $K_b = 4.2 \cdot 10^6$ M^{-1} at 25 °C) [17].

Conversely, the presence of perchlorate perturbs the binding characteristics of ANS to BSA. Only two ANS molecules are now bound to BSA, and the two binding sites are characterized by different binding constants, i.e., the equivalence of binding sites is lost. This phenomenon could be due to the direct interaction of the perchlorate anion with BSA. Indeed, an interaction of perchlorate ions with charged residues of lysozyme was previously reported [29]. The interaction with BSA of other anions of such low charge density (e.g., iodide) was also reported [30]. Furthermore, owing to its low charge density, perchlorate has almost hydrophobic characteristics and can establish interactions with hydrophobic patches of proteins as well.

BSA is a heart-shaped protein of about 66 kDa with high homology with the human counterpart, HSA [24,31]. Its structure is composed by three domains, each of which is composed of two subdomains. A docking study performed on this system identified two potential binding sites for ANS in the subdomain IIIA and another one in the subdomain IB [17]. The two sites in the subdomain IIIA are buried in the inner core of the protein. Conversely, the other site is localized in the more solvent-exposed subdomain IB. Thus, it is possible that perchlorate can easily get access to the site in the subdomain IB, thereby completely hampering the binding of ANS to this site. The binding of perchlorate can occur through both hydrophobic and electrostatic interactions. Indeed, an inspection of the crystal structure revealed the presence of several positively charged residues (Lys, Arg, and His) that could establish interactions with anions such as perchlorate. Instead, the two sites in the subdomain IIIA are buried in the inner core of the protein. In this subdomain, some positively charged residues are also present. The loss of equivalence between the two different sites can most likely be ascribed to the interaction of perchlorate with one of the sites that, in this case, can partially occlude it, which leads to the observed decrease in the binding affinity ($K_{b1} = 5.9 \cdot 10^5$ M^{-1}, $K_{b2} = 1.2 \cdot 10^6$ M^{-1} at T = 25 °C).

A decrease of temperature, at ambient pressure, leads to an overall decrease of the binding constant of the ligand. Such a decrease could be due to an enhancement of the transient interactions of the salt anions and the protein in the binding area, and possibly also of the Mg^{2+} cation with the ligand, which decreases the activity (coefficient) of ANS. Indeed, the binding of anions such as chloride and perchlorate to carbonic anhydrase II, for example, is characterized by negative enthalpy changes [32], pointing out that a decrease of temperature should favor their binding process. It is important to recall that the binding of ANS to proteins is mainly but not exclusively due to hydrophobic interactions. The negatively charged sulfate moiety of ANS is able to establish electrostatic interactions with positively charged residues of the protein [33–35]. Consequentially, the presence of bound anions can partially affect the binding of ANS, leading to a reduction of the K_b-values with decreasing temperature. From the temperature dependence of K_b, it is possible to determine the enthalpy change for the binding process by means of the van't Hoff relation, assuming that the enthalpy change is independent of temperature [36]. Here, we found that the $\ln K_b$ vs. $1/T$ plots are non-linear for all solution conditions studied (data not shown). The non-linearity could be ascribed to the complexity of the systems where more than one ANS molecule is bound to BSA, with the binding sites having different binding enthalpies owing to their different chemical makeup. Further, competitive binding by salt anions such as SO_4^{2-} and ClO_4^{-} will be temperature-dependent as well.

Small but significant effects of pressure were observed for the binding process of ANS to BSA, with the effect being dependent both on the temperature and on the nature of the salt anion. Inspection of Table 3 and Figure 6 discloses several interesting points. In the presence of $MgCl_2$, the binding volume, ΔV_b, is close to zero at 25 °C; that is, there is no pressure effect on the complex formation at ambient temperature (up to 2 kbar). However, at lower temperatures, pressure favors the interaction, reaching a ΔV_b value of about -8 mL mol^{-1} at T = 5 °C, which translates to an increase of K_b by about a factor of two. A similar behavior was observed in the presence of $Mg(ClO_4)_2$, for which a negative ΔV_b was found for both binding sites at 5 °C. Negative ΔV_b-values imply that the partial molar volume of the complexed state (V_{PL}) is smaller than that the partial molar volumes of the uncomplexed state ($V_P + V_L$). A possible reason for such a negative binding volume could be dense packing and a decrease of void volume in the binding site upon ligand binding, which might be expected to be more pronounced at low temperatures, where the dynamics of the protein's surface groups is expected to be reduced. Upon ligand binding, in an induced-fit kind of scenario, tightening of the internal atomic packing of the protein molecule might take place, which leads to a decrease of the volume fluctuations of the protein and hence a decrease of the partial molar volume of the protein. A possible origin for a positive ΔV_b-value is most likely a change in the hydration of the protein binding site and/or the ligand(s). As hydration water of proteins generally has a slightly higher density compared to bulk water [37], dehydration results in a small volume increase of the system, with the effect being more pronounced at low temperature. In the presence of solutions of high ionic strength, where large electrostrictive effects prevail in bulk solution, in particular in the presence of small cations and anions of high charge density, such an effect might become less pronounced or even reversed, however. Positive ΔV_b-values could also be due to creation of void volume upon ligand binding if, for example, the binding site is partially obstructed by salt ions, which might be the case for the sulfate anion at low temperatures. Further, the strength of the binding of the anions to the protein might also be pressure sensitive. Application of high pressure could disfavor the binding of the salt anions to the proteins by weakening electrostatic interactions, which would allow an enhancement of the interaction between the ligand ANS and BSA, leading to an increase of K_b [38,39]. The sulfate and perchlorate data do not seem to support this idea, however.

5. Conclusions

In summary, we have found that the binding of a small aromatic ligand such as ANS to an archetypical multifunctional protein, BSA, depends not only significantly on temperature, but also on the type of salt and, to a lesser extent, on pressure. A significant decrease in the binding constant is observed at ambient conditions only in the presence of high concentrations the perchlorate. Interestingly, an increase in pressure and a decrease in temperature favor the binding process of the ligand, rendering the binding volume more negative.

Aside from advancing our general understanding of how ions influence protein–ligand interactions under non-standard temperatures and pressures, our work was specifically focused on ions found on Mars. Our motivation was to understand whether the more water-rich past of that planet, and the potentially more liquid, water-rich subsurface of the planet even today, hosts conditions theoretically conducive to life. In other words, do conditions such as high pressure and the presence of perchlorate ions render a planet uninhabitable with respect to known biochemistry? As our data show, chloride and sulfate ions do not significantly alter protein–ligand interactions under a range of temperature and pressure conditions. However, the chaotropic perchlorate ion does influence protein–ligand binding more profoundly, but it does not abolish it, implying that with respect to temperature, pressure and the presence of perchlorate ions, Martian conditions do not necessarily exclude protein–ligand interactions of the type examined here, but that modifications in binding sites could be required for life to theoretically persist under such geochemical conditions. We note that our data also imply that protein–ligand interactions would not necessarily be substantially altered in the high concentrations of sulfate ions associated with crustal fluids in the terrestrial deep subsurface, providing new insights into the environment for deep subsurface biochemistry on our own planet.

Supplementary Materials: The following are available online at https://www.mdpi.com/article/10.3390/biology10070687/s1. Figure S1: Job's plot for ANS:BSA complex formation obtained in the presence of 250 mM $MgCl_2$ at the temperature of (A) 5 °C and (B) 15 °C and at the pressure of 1 bar. The total concentration ([ANS] + [BSA]) was 35 μM. Figure S2: Job's plot for ANS:BSA complex formation obtained in the presence of 250 mM $MgSO_4$ at the temperature of (A) 5 °C and (B) 15 °C and at the pressure of 1 bar. The total concentration ([ANS] + [BSA]) was 35 μM. Figure S3: Job's plot for ANS:BSA complex formation obtained in the presence of 250 mM $Mg(ClO_4)_2$ at the temperature of (A) 5 °C and (B) 15 °C and at the pressure of 1 bar. The total concentration ([ANS] + [BSA]) was 35 μM. Figure S4: Far-UV CD spectra of BSA at the temperature of (A) 5 °C and (B) 15 °C, in the presence of 250 mM $MgCl_2$ (red spectrum), $MgSO_4$ (blue spectrum), and $Mg(ClO_4)_2$ (green spectrum). For reference, the CD spectrum of BSA in neat buffer condition (black spectrum) is also reported. All the spectra were acquired in 10 mM Tris-HCl buffer, pH 7.4, using a 0.01 cm path-length quartz cuvette.

Author Contributions: Conceptualization, R.W., R.O., and C.S.C.; methodology, R.W., R.O., and N.J.-A.; software, R.O. and N.J.-A.; validation, R.W., C.S.C., R.O., and N.J.-A.; formal analysis, N.J.-A.; investigation, R.O. and N.J.-A.; resources, R.W.; data curation, R.W., R.O., and N.J.-A.; writing—original draft preparation, R.O., N.J.-A., R.W., C.S.C., and S.G.; writing—review and editing, R.O., R.W., C.S.C., and S.G.; visualization, R.O., N.J.-A., and S.G.; supervision, R.W.; project administration, R.W.; funding acquisition, R.W. All authors have read and agreed to the published version of the manuscript.

Funding: R.W. acknowledges funding by the Deutsche Forschungsgemeinschaft (DFG, German Research Foundation) under Germany's Excellence Strategy—EXC 2033—390677874—RESOLV.

Institutional Review Board Statement: Not applicable.

Informed Consent Statement: Not applicable.

Data Availability Statement: The data presented in this study are available on request from the corresponding authors.

Conflicts of Interest: The authors declare no conflict of interest. The funders had no role in the design of the study; in the collection, analyses, or interpretation of data; in the writing of the manuscript, or in the decision to publish the results.

References

1. Cera, E.D. *Thermodynamic Theory of Site-Specific Binding Processes in Biological Macromolecules*, 1st ed.; Cambridge University Press: Cambridge, UK, 1995; ISBN 978-0-521-41659-7.
2. Protein-Ligand Interactions; Gohlke, H. (Eds.) *Methods and Principles in Medicinal Chemistry*; Wiley-VCH: Weinheim, Germany, 2012; ISBN 978-3-527-32966-3.
3. Pang, X.; Zhou, H.-X. Rate Constants and Mechanisms of Protein–Ligand Binding. *Annu. Rev. Biophys.* **2017**, *46*, 105–130. [CrossRef] [PubMed]
4. Woodbury, C.P., Jr. *Introduction to Macromolecular Binding Equilibria*; CRC Press: Boca Raton, FL, USA, 2019; ISBN 978-0-367-38832-4.
5. Du, X.; Li, Y.; Xia, Y.-L.; Ai, S.-M.; Liang, J.; Sang, P.; Ji, X.-L.; Liu, S.-Q. Insights into Protein–Ligand Interactions: Mechanisms, Models, and Methods. *Int. J. Mol. Sci.* **2016**, *17*, 144. [CrossRef]
6. Akasaka, K. (Ed.) *High Pressure Bioscience: Basic Concepts, Applications and Frontiers*; Subcellular Biochemistry; Springer: Dordrecht, The Netherlands, 2015; ISBN 978-94-017-9917-1.
7. Daniel, I.; Oger, P.; Winter, R. Origins of Life and Biochemistry under High-Pressure Conditions. *Chem. Soc. Rev.* **2006**, *35*, 858. [CrossRef] [PubMed]
8. Meersman, F.; Daniel, I.; Bartlett, D.H.; Winter, R.; Hazael, R.; McMillan, P.F. High-Pressure Biochemistry and Biophysics. *Rev. Miner. Geochem.* **2013**, *75*, 607–648. [CrossRef]
9. Roche, J.; Caro, J.A.; Norberto, D.R.; Barthe, P.; Roumestand, C.; Schlessman, J.L.; Garcia, A.E.; Garcia-Moreno, E.B.; Royer, C.A. Cavities Determine the Pressure Unfolding of Proteins. *Proc. Natl. Acad. Sci. USA* **2012**, *109*, 6945–6950. [CrossRef]

10. Winter, R. Interrogating the Structural Dynamics and Energetics of Biomolecular Systems with Pressure Modulation. *Annu. Rev. Biophys.* **2019**, *48*, 441–463. [CrossRef]
11. Osterloo, M.M.; Hamilton, V.E.; Bandfield, J.L.; Glotch, T.D.; Baldridge, A.M.; Christensen, P.R.; Tornabene, L.L.; Anderson, F.S. Chloride-Bearing Materials in the Southern Highlands of Mars. *Science* **2008**, *319*, 1651–1654. [CrossRef]
12. Gendrin, A. Sulfates in Martian Layered Terrains: The OMEGA/Mars Express View. *Science* **2005**, *307*, 1587–1591. [CrossRef]
13. Hecht, M.H.; Kounaves, S.P.; Quinn, R.C.; West, S.J.; Young, S.M.M.; Ming, D.W.; Catling, D.C.; Clark, B.C.; Boynton, W.V.; Hoffman, J.; et al. Detection of Perchlorate and the Soluble Chemistry of Martian Soil at the Phoenix Lander Site. *Science* **2009**, *325*, 64–67. [CrossRef]
14. Clifford, S.M.; Lasue, J.; Heggy, E.; Boisson, J.; McGovern, P.; Max, M.D. Depth of the Martian Cryosphere: Revised Estimates and Implications for the Existence and Detection of Subpermafrost Groundwater. *J. Geophys. Res.* **2010**, *115*, E07001. [CrossRef]
15. Orosei, R.; Lauro, S.E.; Pettinelli, E.; Cicchetti, A.; Coradini, M.; Cosciotti, B.; Di Paolo, F.; Flamini, E.; Mattei, E.; Pajola, M.; et al. Radar Evidence of Subglacial Liquid Water on Mars. *Science* **2018**, *361*, 490–493. [CrossRef]
16. Lauro, S.E.; Pettinelli, E.; Caprarelli, G.; Guallini, L.; Rossi, A.P.; Mattei, E.; Cosciotti, B.; Cicchetti, A.; Soldovieri, F.; Cartacci, M.; et al. Multiple Subglacial Water Bodies below the South Pole of Mars Unveiled by New MARSIS Data. *Nat. Astron.* **2021**, *5*, 63–70. [CrossRef]
17. Oliva, R.; Banerjee, S.; Cinar, H.; Ehrt, C.; Winter, R. Alteration of Protein Binding Affinities by Aqueous Two-Phase Systems Revealed by Pressure Perturbation. *Sci. Rep.* **2020**, *10*, 8074. [CrossRef]
18. Connors, K.A. *Binding Constants: The Measurement of Molecular Complex Stability*; Wiley: New York, NY, USA, 1987; ISBN 978-0-471-83083-2.
19. Ulatowski, F.; Dąbrowa, K.; Bałakier, T.; Jurczak, J. Recognizing the Limited Applicability of Job Plots in Studying Host–Guest Interactions in Supramolecular Chemistry. *J. Org. Chem.* **2016**, *81*, 1746–1756. [CrossRef]
20. Oliva, R.; Mukherjee, S.; Winter, R. Unraveling the Binding Characteristics of Small Ligands to Telomeric DNA by Pressure Modulation. *Sci. Rep.* **2021**, *11*, 9714. [CrossRef]
21. Cattoni, D.I.; Kaufman, S.B.; Flecha, F.L.G. Kinetics and Thermodynamics of the Interaction of 1-Anilino-Naphthalene-8-Sulfonate with Proteins. *Biochim. Biophys. Acta (BBA) Proteins Proteom.* **2009**, *1794*, 1700–1708. [CrossRef]
22. Kelly, S.M.; Jess, T.J.; Price, N.C. How to Study Proteins by Circular Dichroism. *Biochim. Biophys. Acta (BBA) Proteins Proteom.* **2005**, *1751*, 119–139. [CrossRef] [PubMed]
23. Pizzo, E.; Oliva, R.; Morra, R.; Bosso, A.; Ragucci, S.; Petraccone, L.; Del Vecchio, P.; Di Maro, A. Binding of a Type 1 RIP and of Its Chimeric Variant to Phospholipid Bilayers: Evidence for a Link between Cytotoxicity and Protein/Membrane Interactions. *Biochim. Biophys. Acta (BBA) Biomembr.* **2017**, *1859*, 2106–2112. [CrossRef] [PubMed]
24. Majorek, K.A.; Porebski, P.J.; Dayal, A.; Zimmerman, M.D.; Jablonska, K.; Stewart, A.J.; Chruszcz, M.; Minor, W. Structural and Immunologic Characterization of Bovine, Horse, and Rabbit Serum Albumins. *Mol. Immunol.* **2012**, *52*, 174–182. [CrossRef] [PubMed]
25. Hayakawa, I.; Kajihara, J.; Morikawa, K.; Oda, M.; Fujio, Y. Denaturation of Bovine Serum Albumin (BSA) and Ovalbumin by High Pressure, Heat and Chemicals. *J. Food Sci.* **1992**, *57*, 288–292. [CrossRef]
26. Masson, P.; Reybaud, J. Hydrophobic Interaction Electrophoresis under High Hydrostatic Pressure: Study of the Effects of Pressure upon the Interaction of Serum Albumin with a Long-Chain Aliphatic Ligand. *Electrophoresis* **1988**, *9*, 157–161. [CrossRef]
27. Aswal, V.K.; Chodankar, S.; Kohlbrecher, J.; Vavrin, R.; Wagh, A.G. Small-Angle Neutron Scattering Study of Protein Unfolding and Refolding. *Phys. Rev. E* **2009**, *80*, 011924. [CrossRef]
28. Oliva, R.; Jahmidi-Azizi, N.; Mukherjee, S.; Winter, R. Harnessing Pressure Modulation for Exploring Ligand Binding Reactions in Cosolvent Solutions. *J. Phys. Chem. B* **2021**, *125*, 539–546. [CrossRef]
29. Bye, J.W.; Falconer, R.J. Thermal Stability of Lysozyme as a Function of Ion Concentration: A Reappraisal of the Relationship between the Hofmeister Series and Protein Stability: Thermal Stability of Lysozyme. *Protein Sci.* **2013**, *22*, 1563–1570. [CrossRef] [PubMed]
30. Medda, L.; Monduzzi, M.; Salis, A. The Molecular Motion of Bovine Serum Albumin under Physiological Conditions is Ion Specific. *Chem. Commun.* **2015**, *51*, 6663–6666. [CrossRef] [PubMed]
31. Levi, V.; González Flecha, F.L. Labeling of Proteins with Fluorescent Probes: Photophysical Characterization of Dansylated Bovine Serum Albumin. *Biochem. Mol. Biol. Educ.* **2003**, *31*, 333–336. [CrossRef]
32. Fox, J.M.; Kang, K.; Sherman, W.; Héroux, A.; Sastry, G.M.; Baghbanzadeh, M.; Lockett, M.R.; Whitesides, G.M. Interactions between Hofmeister Anions and the Binding Pocket of a Protein. *J. Am. Chem. Soc.* **2015**, *137*, 3859–3866. [CrossRef] [PubMed]
33. Ory, J.J.; Banaszak, L.J. Studies of the Ligand Binding Reaction of Adipocyte Lipid Binding Protein Using the Fluorescent Probe 1,8-Anilinonaphthalene-8-Sulfonate. *Biophys. J.* **1999**, *77*, 1107–1116. [CrossRef]
34. Schonbrunn, E.; Eschenburg, S.; Luger, K.; Kabsch, W.; Amrhein, N. Structural Basis for the Interaction of the Fluorescence Probe 8-Anilino-1-Naphthalene Sulfonate (ANS) with the Antibiotic Target MurA. *Proc. Natl. Acad. Sci. USA* **2000**, *97*, 6345–6349. [CrossRef]
35. Matulis, D.; Lovrien, R. 1-Anilino-8-Naphthalene Sulfonate Anion-Protein Binding Depends Primarily on Ion Pair Formation. *Biophys. J.* **1998**, *74*, 422–429. [CrossRef]

36. Zhukov, A.; Karlsson, R. Statistical Aspects of van't Hoff Analysis: A Simulation Study. *J. Mol. Recognit.* **2007**, *20*, 379–385. [CrossRef] [PubMed]
37. Chalikian, T.V.; Macgregor, R.B. On Empirical Decomposition of Volumetric Data. *Biophys. Chem.* **2019**, *246*, 8–15. [CrossRef]
38. Mozhaev, V.V.; Heremans, K.; Frank, J.; Masson, P.; Balny, C. High Pressure Effects on Protein Structure and Function. *Proteins* **1996**, *24*, 81–91. [CrossRef]
39. Boonyaratanakornkit, B.B.; Park, C.B.; Clark, D.S. Pressure Effects on Intra- and Intermolecular Interactions within Proteins. *Biochim. Biophys. Acta (BBA) Protein Struct. Mol. Enzymol.* **2002**, *1595*, 235–249. [CrossRef]

biology

MDPI

Article

Kinetic Study of the Avocado Sunblotch Viroid Self-Cleavage Reaction Reveals Compensatory Effects between High-Pressure and High-Temperature: Implications for Origins of Life on Earth †

Hussein Kaddour [1,‡], Honorine Lucchi [2,‡], Guy Hervé [3], Jacques Vergne [4] and Marie-Christine Maurel [4,*]

1 Department of pharmacology, Renaissance School of Medicine, Stony Brook University, Stony Brook, NY 11794, USA; hussein.kaddour@stonybrook.edu
2 Société PYMABS, 5 rue Henri Auguste Desbyeres, 91000 Évry-Courcouronnes, France; honorine.lucchi@gmail.com
3 Laboratoire BIOSIPE, Institut de biologie Paris-Seine, Sorbonne Université, 7 quai Saint-Bernard, 75005 Paris, France; guy.herve@sorbonne-universite.fr
4 Institut de Systématique, Evolution, Biodiversité, (ISYEB), Sorbonne Université, Museum National d'Histoire Naturelle, CNRS, EPHE, F 75005 Paris, France; jvergne@mnhn.fr
* Correspondence: marie-christine.maurel@sorbonne-universite.fr; Tel.: +33-1-40-33-79-81
† This article is dedicated to the memory of Gaston Hui Bon Hoa. Together with Pierre Douzou, Gaston pioneered the use of high pressures and low temperatures in studying structure-function relationships in biomacromolecules.
‡ These authors contributed equally to this work.

Citation: Kaddour, H.; Lucchi, H.; Hervé, G.; Vergne, J.; Maurel, M.-C. Kinetic Study of the Avocado Sunblotch Viroid Self-Cleavage Reaction Reveals Compensatory Effects between High-Pressure and High-Temperature: Implications for Origins of Life on Earth. *Biology* **2021**, *10*, 720. https://doi.org/10.3390/biology10080720

Academic Editors: Dmitri Davydov and Christiane Jung

Received: 21 June 2021
Accepted: 25 July 2021
Published: 28 July 2021

Simple Summary: Viroids remain the smallest infectious agents ever discovered. They are found in plants and consist of single-stranded non-coding circular RNA. Due to their simplicity, viroids are considered relics of an ancient RNA World that may have originated in the deep seas near hydrothermal vents where temperature and pressure are both elevated. To test this hypothesis, a synthetic avocado sunblotch viroid, whose structure contain an autocatalytic hammerhead ribozyme, was subjected to increased pressure (from atmospheric pressure to 300 MPa) at different temperatures (0–65 °C) and the reaction rate constant of the catalytic activity was calculated for each condition. The results obtained allowed calculation of the positive activation volume of this viroid and revealed a compensatory effect between pressure and temperature. In conclusion, these results not only exemplify the plasticity of RNA and support the RNA World hypothesis, but also highlight the usefulness of the hydrostatic pressure in understanding the structure–function relationships of biomacromolecules.

Abstract: A high pressure apparatus allowing one to study enzyme kinetics under pressure was used to study the self-cleavage activity of the avocado sunblotch viroid. The kinetics of this reaction were determined under pressure over a range up to 300 MPa (1–3000 bar). It appears that the initial rate of this reaction decreases when pressure increases, revealing a positive $\Delta V\neq$ of activation, which correlates with the domain closure accompanying the reaction and the decrease of the surface of the viroid exposed to the solvent. Although, as expected, temperature increases the rate of the reaction whose energy of activation was determined, it appeared that it does not significantly influence the $\Delta V\neq$ of activation and that pressure does not influence the energy of activation. These results provide information about the structural aspects or this self-cleavage reaction, which is involved in the process of maturation of this viroid. The behavior of ASBVd results from the involvement of the hammerhead ribozyme present at its catalytic domain, indeed a structural motif is very widespread in the ancient and current RNA world.

Keywords: viroid; hydrostatic pressure; temperature; structure–activity relationship; RNA World

1. Introduction

Viroids are the smallest pathogens of plants characterized by a compact rod-like circular RNA 246–401 nucleotides long [1,2]. They have no envelope, no capsid, and they do not code for any protein. Viroids are divided into two families, the Pospiviroidae, and the Avsunviroidae family whose members possess a catalytic RNA with a hammerhead ribozyme (HHR) motif responsible for a crucial cleavage step during viroid replication, such as the avocado sunblotch viroid (ASBVd) [3]. Figure 1 shows the structure of ASBVd with the location of the HHR motif of about 35 nucleotides with a 3D structure composed of three helical junctions (I, II and III) and a core of invariant nucleotides required for its activity.

Chemically, metal ions are involved in HHR activity within the cleavage sites (C–U and C–G) [4]. Cleavage of HHR is a transesterification reaction that converts a $5', 3'$ diester to a $2', 3'$ cyclic phosphate diester via an SN2 mechanism [5]. During replication, (+) and (−) complementary strand sequences of Avsunviroidae are generated through the symmetric rolling circle mechanism. The analysis of the ASBVd contents in avocado extracts [6] revealed the presence of RNA of both polarities in multimeric forms, from monomers to octamers for ASBVd(+) and monomers to dimers for ASBVd(−). This difference in oligomeric sizes reveals a less efficient in vivo cleavage activity of ASBVd(+) than of ASBVd(−) that was observed by in vitro cleavage. The viroid moves within the cell due to intrinsic RNA signals but it is also likely that it recruits supporting protein or RNA factors. Due to the diversity of structures and dynamics that participate in viroid trafficking within the cell and between cells and during infectivity, it is of crucial interest to characterize the structural elements involved in viroid processing. Despite the large amount of information regarding the molecular biology of Avsunviroidae, much less is known regarding the structure and conformational aspects of the cleavage of minus and plus ASBVd strands and the catalytic role of Mg^{2+} in efficient self-cleavage of such viroids.

Over the last few decades, high hydrostatic pressure has been gaining attention as a key thermodynamic and kinetic parameter that brings insights into the structure–activity relationships in biomolecules, such as proteins and nucleic acids, but also as a tool that has been increasingly used in biotechnology [7,8]. Pressure increases the surface of these molecules, which is exposed to the solvent but the volume of their solution decreases. This is due to the electrostriction phenomenon in which water molecules come to pack around the ionized and polar groups presents at the surface of the macromolecule [9]. Pressure favors this process since the negative ΔV of electrostriction is -3 mL/mole of water [10]. Consequently, pressure tends to expose the charged groups to the solvent thus altering the tertiary structure of protein and to dissociate oligomeric proteins leading to the abolition of their biological role and to the inactivation of enzymes. In the case of nucleic acids, this methodology was applied to hairpin [11–13] and hammerhead [14] ribozymes, but not yet to complete genomes such as viroids. The previous studies focused only on the minimal self-cleaving sequence of RNA because of the technical difficulties, yet it is likely that sequences outside the catalytic core may affect the global conformational change and thus the fitness of the viroid in vivo. In this regard, Hui Bon Hoa et al. [15,16] studied the structures of both, ASBVd(−) and ASBVd(+) strands (Figure 1), by Raman spectroscopy and showed that both molecules exhibited a typical A-type RNA structure with an ordered double-helical content as expected. Nonetheless, small but specific differences between the two strands were found in the sugar puckering and base-stacking regions. Furthermore, both stands responded differently to deuteration and to the temperature increase, since both conditions differentially perturbed the double-helical content and the phosphodiester conformation of viroids, as revealed by the corresponding Raman spectral changes. These structural differences suggested that the rigidity and stability were higher and the D_2O accessibility to the H-bonding network was lower for ASBVd(+) compared to ASBVd(−), which correlated to the catalytic activity, ASBVd(−) being 3.5 times more active than ASBVd(+).

Another interesting aspect for the study of viroids' behavior under high pressures and high temperatures is that viroids are often deemed relics of the "RNA World" [17]. Indeed, viroids are functional nucleic acids that operate under unusual conditions [18] and might have once strived under conditions that are considered today to be extreme. Such conditions are also prevalent in terrestrial subsurface environments, which nurture a massive microbial reservoir, estimated at about 70% of the Earth's microbial life [19,20]. Some of these bacteria, for instance the subseafloor *Petrocella atlantisensis*, are able to strive in the laboratory, if cultured under high hydrostatic pressure [21]. It is also imaginable that such extreme conditions of high-pressure high-temperature are ordinary on other rocky planets, or even exoplanets. Furthermore the "intraterrestrial" life asked the question: would these intraterrestrials have appeared first? What if life was not born "on" Earth, but "in" Earth? Yet, how exactly viral and subviral particles behave under these conditions is unknown. In this investigation, pressure and temperature and their combination were used to obtain information concerning the activation volume and the activation energy associated to the formation of the transition state of the self-cleavage reaction of the full ASBVd(−) viroid.

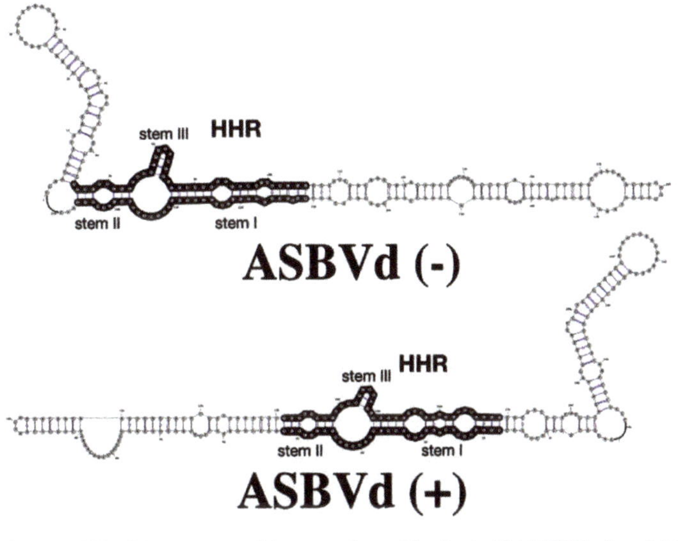

Figure 1. RNA 2D structures of the avocado sunblotch viroid (ABSVd(−)) and ASBVd(+) (top and bottom, respectively). The full-length genome of ASBVd can fold into 2D structures that preserve the hammerhead ribozyme (HHR) motif (regions in black) in both the (−) and (+) strands; the HHR motif of ASBVd(−) is more stable, with 3 base-pairs in stem III but only two base-pairs in ASBVd(+). (Reprinted with permission from ref. [22]. Copyright 2019 Marie-Christine Maurel).

2. Materials and Methods

2.1. In Vitro Synthesis of ASBVd(−)

Experiments were performed on synthetic linearized ASBVd(−) as follows: a previously cloned *pk*S plasmid with the ASBVd monomer between BamH1 and EcoR1 restriction sites [23,24] was subjected to a PCR amplification using 5′-TAATACGACTCACTATAGGA-AGAGATTGAAGACGAGTG-3′ and 5′-GATCACTTCGTCTCTTCAGG-3′, as forward and reverse primers, respectively, with the underlined sequence corresponding to the T7 promoter. After a clean-up step by an ethanol precipitation, verification of its size on a 2% agarose gel, and its quantification by ImageJ (NIH, Bethesda, Maryland, USA, https://imagej.nih.gov/ij/, accessed on 13 May 2021), the PCR product was used in an overnight in vitro RNA synthesis at 37 °C as previously detailed [16].

2.2. Kinetics Studies

All kinetics reactions, with the exception of one (at 0 °C and atmospheric pressure), were performed using a high-pressure high-temperature apparatus (Top-Industrie, France) as described previously [14]. Briefly, ASBVd(−) was denatured at 94 °C for 1 min and slowly (3 °C/min) renatured until reaching 23 °C, before dilution in the reaction buffer (50 mM HEPES, pH 7.5). The solution was loaded into the apparatus and equilibrated at the given pressure/temperature before starting the reaction by addition of 50 mM $MgCl_2$. Aliquots were withdrawn at appropriate times, quenched with stop solution (7 M urea, 0.01% xylene cyanol, and 50 mM EDTA). The reaction products were analyzed by a 10% denaturing PAGE and quantified using ImageJ as previously described [14]. The percentage of cleavage was plotted as a function of time and the plots were fitted to a single-exponential equation: $F = F_{max}(1 - e^{-k_{obs}t})$ where F is the percentage of the cleaved viroid at time t, F_{max}, the maximum percentage of cleaved viroid, and k_{obs}, the observed rate constants for cleavage. As the exact significance of the plateau observed is not known, k_{obs} was not deconvoluted into the rate constants for cleavage (k_{cleav}) and ligation (k_{lig}).

2.3. ASBVd(−) Structural Modeling

RNAfold WebServer [25,26] (http://rna.tbi.univie.ac.at/cgi-bin/RNAWebSuite/RNAfold.cgi, accessed on 23 May 2021) was used with the default parameters [27] and only the temperature was varied from 0 to 65 °C. To model the ASBVd(−) tertiary structure, the dot-bracket notations of the centroid secondary structures were input in the RNAComposer [28] and the CentroidFold secondary structure prediction method was selected. The pdb structures were visualized using iCn3D, a Web-based 3D Viewer for Sharing 1D/2D/3D Representations of Biomolecular Structures [29]. As for the ASBVd(−) solvent accessibility, it was predicted using RNASol an RNA solvent accessibility prediction WebServer [30].

3. Results

3.1. Influence of Pressure on the Reaction Rate

The self-cleavage activity was measured as indicated in "Materials and Methods" under a range of pressure going from 1 to 300 MPa and at 30 °C. The progress curves obtained are shown in Figure 2a where it can be seen that pressure had a significant negative effect on this reaction, 50% inhibition being observed at 300 MPa. The rate constants of this reaction were used to draw the variation of the Log of the rate constant as a function of pressure. This is shown in Figure 2b. The linear plot of such a representation allows the determination of the activation volume of the reaction, $\Delta V\neq$, since the slope of the line is equal to $-\Delta V\neq/RT$ [31]. In the present case, Figure 2b indicates that at low pressure this activation volume was 18.5 mL/mole and became 5 mL/mole at high pressure. Thus, it appears that pressures inferior to 100 MPa provoke a conformational change in the viroid that is less pronounced at higher pressures (150–300 MPa), although the additional effect was still measurable.

The fact that the slopes were negative indicates that during the formation of the transition state the surface of the viroid exposed to the solvent decreased together with the extent of the electrostriction, due to the exposure of charged and hydrophobic residues to the solvent. This is in accordance with the previous conclusion that the formation of the transition state of this viroid involves a domains' closure [32]. Thus, pressure had an effect on the initial conformation of the viroid in such a way that its conformation becomes closer to what it was in the transition state of the reaction. The above-described influence of pressure on the activity of the viroid is fully reversible.

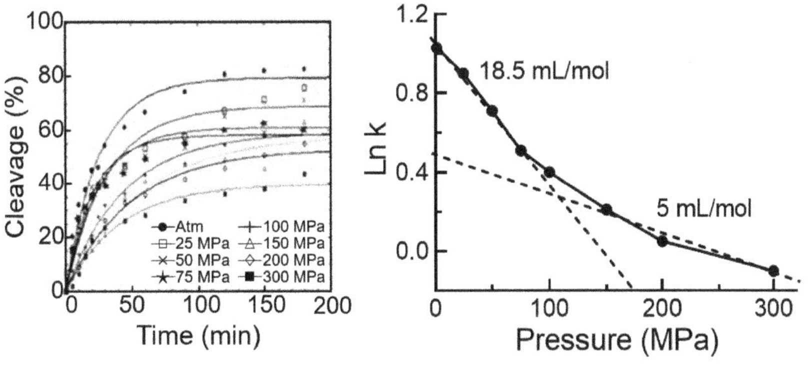

(a) (b)

Figure 2. Kinetics of the ASBVd(−) self-cleavage reaction. (**a**) Time course of the reaction at 30 °C and different pressures. (**b**) Plot of Ln k against pressure providing the activation volumes of the reaction.

3.2. *Influence of Temperature on the Reaction Rate*

The temperature dependence of the self-cleavage reaction is shown on Figure 3a. As expected, the temperature increased the rate of the reaction up to 55 °C then it decreased it, irrespective of the pressure. Since the rate of the self-cleavage reaction is independent of the viroid concentration, the initial rates of this reaction directly reflected the rate constants and were thus used here to draw the variation of Ln k as a function of pressure. That did not change the slope of the line obtained and allowed us to graph the Arrhenius plot, which provided a value of 64.9 KJ/mol for Ea, the activation energy of the reaction (Figure 3b).

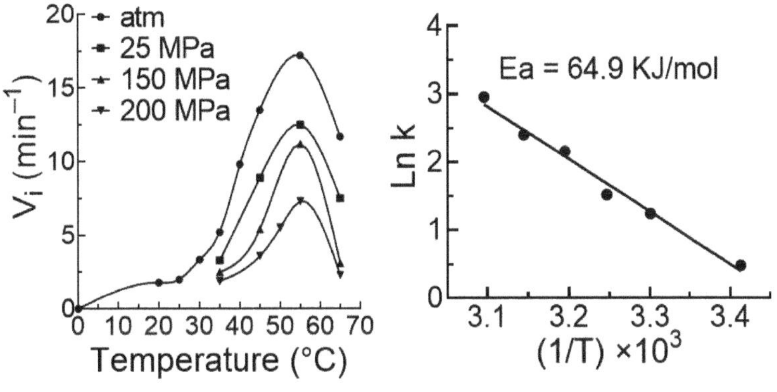

(a) (b)

Figure 3. Effects of temperature on the ASBVd(−) self-cleavage reaction. (**a**) Rates of reaction as a function of temperature at different pressures. (**b**) Corresponding Arrhenius plot at atmospheric pressure providing the energy of activation of the reaction.

3.3. *The 2D and 3D Structural Modeling of ASBVd(−) at Different Temperatures*

To gain additional insight into ASBVd(−) conformational changes during autocatalysis, 2D and 3D models depicting the secondary and tertiary structures of ASBVd(−) were simulated at the different experimental temperatures, ranging from 0 to 65 °C. In the 2D models, two prediction methods were used: the minimum free energy prediction and the thermodynamic prediction. The first method yields the "optimal secondary structure", which has the minimum free energy (MFE), and the second yields the "centroid secondary structure", which has the minimum total base-pair distance to all structures in the thermodynamic ensemble [27,33]. The MFE for both prediction methods are given in Table 1, showing an expected increase with the temperature.

Table 1. Minimum free energy (MFE) [1] of the different secondary structures of ASBVd(−) at different temperatures.

Temperature (°C)	Minimum Free Energy Prediction (kcal/mol)	Thermodynamic Ensemble Prediction (kcal/mol)
0	−118.4	−119.71
20	−83.78	−86.79
25	−75.16	−78.84
30	−66.63	−71.05
35	−58.54	−63.44
40	−50.75	−56.11
45	−43.13	−49.09
55	−28.64	−36.01
65	−17.16	−24.64

[1] Values determined using the RNAfold WebServer with the default parameters.

The MFE secondary structures, generally rod-like, did not significantly change between 0 and 45 °C, especially around the cleavage site (Figure 4). In fact, structures at 0–20–25 °C were identical, similarly for structures at 35–40–45 °C. Structures at 55 °C and 65 °C, although branched and different from those at lower temperatures, were also identical to each other.

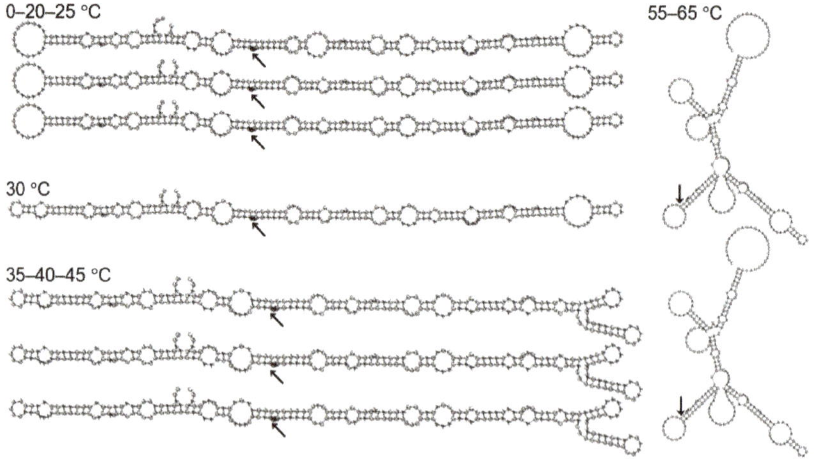

Figure 4. Optimal secondary structures of ASBVd(−) at different temperatures as determined using the RNAfold WebServer. Arrows denote C86, the cleavage site.

On the other hand, the centroid secondary structures were unique at each temperature and showed an expected gradual opening of the molecule, although the overall rod-like structure was persistent (Figure 5). Furthermore, the 3D tertiary structure, calculated using these centroid secondary structures as input, were also different at different temperatures (Figure 6). Specifically, at 0–30 °C the structures were largely twisted, at 35 °C both ends were antiparallel, at 40 °C a molecular closure in which the two ends came close to each occurred, and this was more pronounced at 55 °C. Interestingly at 45 °C, the viroid assumed a unique ohm-shape conformation in which the cleavage site pointed to the inside of the structure, an indication of a possible change in the solvent accessibility, and a novel active conformation for catalytic RNAs. Finally at 65 °C, the viroid assumed a partially open and less twisted structure, although the rod-like structure around the cleavage site was still maintained. In addition, ASBVd(−) accessibility to the solvent was also predicted and the result showed that, unsurprisingly, the cleavage site had the highest solvent accessible surface area among its surrounding nucleotides (Figure 7). Altogether, these results illustrated the importance of the conformational changes that accompany the RNA autocatalysis.

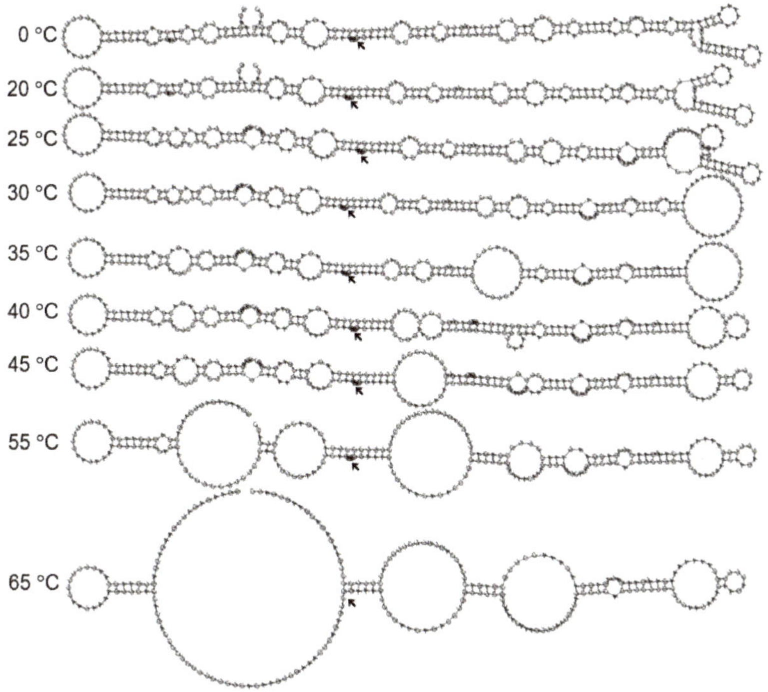

Figure 5. Centroid secondary structures of ASBVd(−) at different temperatures as determined using the RNAfold WebServer. Arrows denote C86, the cleavage site.

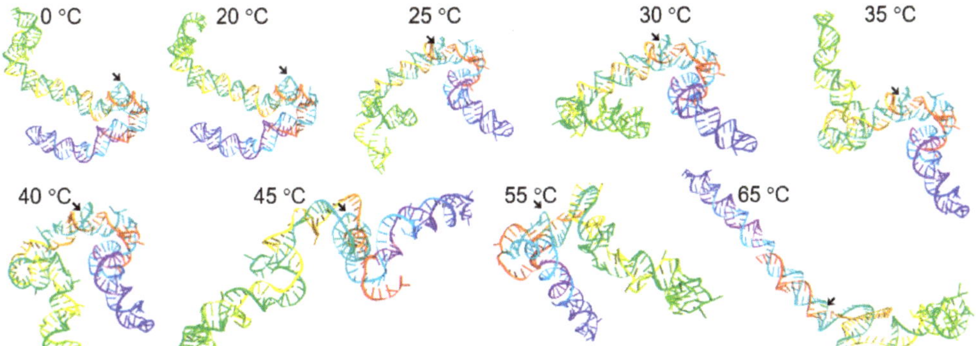

Figure 6. The 3D structures of ASBVd(−) at different temperatures as determined using the RNAComposer. The dot-bracket notations of the centroid secondary structures shown in Figure 5 were used as input and the CentroidFold secondary structure prediction method was selected. Arrows denote C86, the cleavage site. The nucleotides are rainbow-colored (3′-red, orange, yellow, green, turquoise, blue, indigo, and violet-5′). 3′ and 5′ indicate the 3′-OH and 5′-phosphate extremities of the viroid.

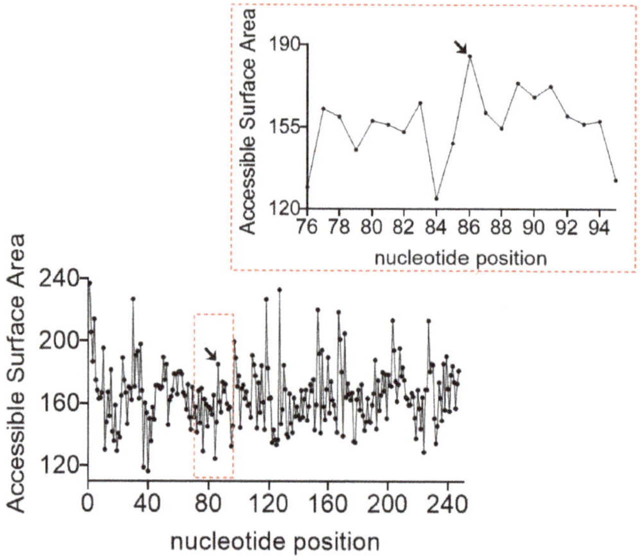

Figure 7. Accessible surface area of ASBVd(−) nucleotides as determined using the RNASol Web-Server. The inset is the enlarged graph around the cleavage site, denoted with an arrow.

3.4. Reciprocal Effects of Pressure and Temperature on the Activation Energy

Pressure had no influence on the temperature dependence of the self-cleavage reaction as explained below. This temperature dependence was determined under pressures going from 1 to 200 MPa. As shown in Figure 3a the temperature dependence profiles were exactly the same at all pressures. The rate of reaction was measured at four pressures and three temperatures. The results are shown in Figure 8. Although accurate energy of activation cannot be calculated on three points, the interesting observation is that the plots of Ln k f(1/T) obtained at various pressures were nearly parallels, indicating that the energy of activation of the reaction was not significantly affected by pressure.

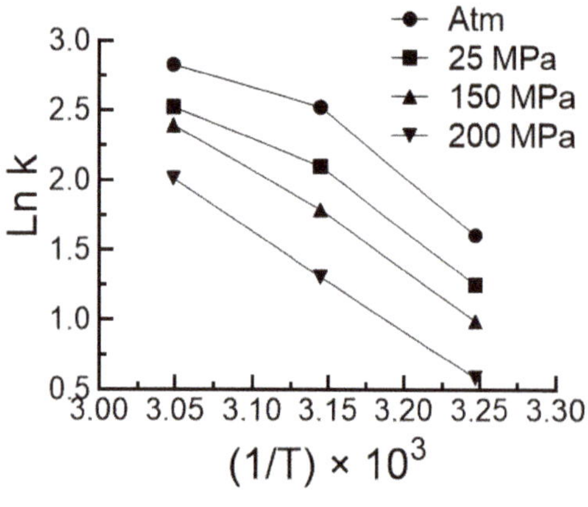

Figure 8. Arrhenius plots of the autocleavage reaction of ASBVd(−) at different pressures.

Pressure and temperature exert reciprocal compensatory effects. This is visualized in Figure 9. This property illustrates the adaptability of RNA molecules and viroids in particular. It might have played an important role in the early development of life, particularly in the environment of the deep-sea vents, which have been proposed to be the cradle of life [34].

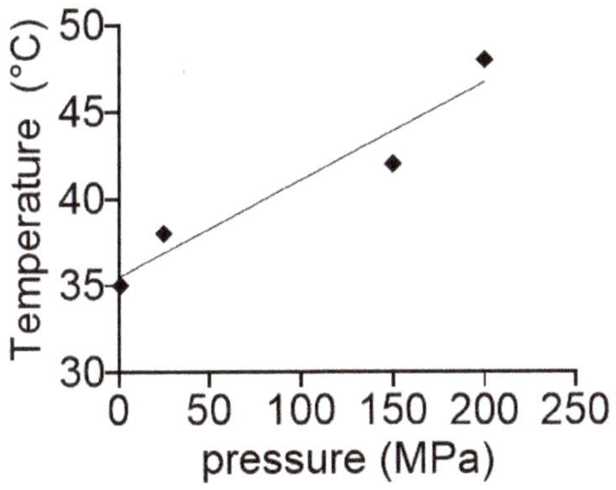

Figure 9. Reciprocal compensatory effects of pressure and temperature in the ASBVd(−) autocatalytic reaction. The plot was determined by estimating the temperature required at each pressure to achieve a 5% cleavage of the viroid in 1 min.

4. Discussion

The importance of hydrostatic pressure and temperature as critical physical parameters in the understanding of the structure–function relationships of enzymes has long been established [35–39]. Regarding small autocatalytic RNAs, or ribozymes, the conformational changes accompanying the catalytic activity have also been characterized. For instance, a hairpin ribozyme requires a $\Delta V\neq$ ranging between 23 and 34 mL/mole depending on the particular RNA [11–13]. The hairpin ribozyme $\Delta V\neq$ was about 2–3 fold larger than that of a viroid-derived hammerhead ribozyme, ranging between 3 and 12 mL/mole and reflecting the presence in the solution of two isomer populations with different conformations [14]. In this study, ASBVd(−) also exhibited at least two conformers with measurable $\Delta V\neq$ of 5 and 18.5 mL/mole (Figure 2b). The fact that $\Delta V\neq$ of the entire ASBVd(−) was similar to that of the minimal ribozymic motif suggests that the measured activation volume corresponds exclusively to a local conformational change near the catalytic site and the viroid region outside the catalytic core does not play a significant role in the catalytic reaction. This explanation is in-line with the hypothesis that the viroid sequences outside the catalytic core have essentially evolved to stabilize its overall structure and optimize its activity.

Another interesting observation is that a relatively slow ASBVd(−) autocatalytic reaction had a $\Delta V\neq$ comparable to that of a fast-cleaving minimal hammerhead ribozyme, indicating that $\Delta V\neq$ alone does not necessarily correlate with enzymatic activity, and rather depends on the structural moieties of the molecule. For instance, the lower activity of ASBVd(−) compared to the minimal hammerhead and hairpin ribozymes may be due to the relatively larger size of the viroid requiring more Mg^{2+} ions to shield the phosphate groups, before triggering the specific chemical reaction of cleavage. Furthermore, it is possible that large regions outside the catalytic site might be at play, in such a way that despite the large conformational changes, the overall $\Delta V\neq$ is compensated and, hence, small. In this regard, ASBVd(−) tertiary structure modeling at different temperatures, revealed that, indeed, both ends of the rod-like structure of the viroid were involved in large conformational changes in a way that the structure bent around the cleavage site at 55 °C, where the viroid was most active. This molecular closure was similar to that of the small ribozymes.

The temperature-dependent activity is extensively studied in the case of small ribozymes [40–44]. However, little is known about the temperature dependence of viroids self-cleavage activity. It is shown here that, as expected, ASBVd(−) autocatalytic activity increased with temperature up to 55 °C and then rapidly dropped above 55 °C, and that also occurred at different pressures (Figure 3a). With this strong dependency on temperature, one could expect that the energy of activation would change under pressure. For instance, the higher the pressure, the slower the catalytic reaction will be, and, as a consequence, the higher the activation energy. However, this was not the case (Figure 8). A possible explanation could be that the domain closure contributes poorly to the energy of activation, which could be essentially linked to the chemistry of the reaction. By contrast, pressure and temperature have had compensatory effects on the autocatalytic reaction (Figure 9). This finding has direct relevance to the possible sites of the origins of life on Earth, where viroids may have evolved [45], and suggests that near hydrothermal vents environments, where pressure and temperature are high [46], may elicit a comparable activity to that occurring at warm ponds on the early Earth's surface [47]. The significance of these results also extend to the extant biology where ribozymes are omnipresent and ultraconserved, particularly in the human genome [48].

5. Conclusions

In summary, the present study reported measurable compensatory effects between pressure and temperature on the self-cleavage activity of ASBVd(−). We conclude that viroids, despite their simplicity, exhibit exceptional plasticity and adaptability to a wide array of physical conditions that may have once existed on early Earth.

Author Contributions: Conceptualization, G.H. and M.-C.M.; methodology, J.V. and G.H.; software, H.K.; validation, G.H., M.-C.M., J.V. and H.K.; experimental investigation, H.K. and H.L.; writing—review and editing, G.H., M.-C.M., J.V. and H.K. All authors have read and agreed to the published version of the manuscript.

Funding: This research received no external funding.

Institutional Review Board Statement: Not applicable.

Informed Consent Statement: Not applicable.

Data Availability Statement: The data presented herein are available from the corresponding author upon a reasonable request.

Acknowledgments: This article is dedicated to the memory of Gaston Hui Bon Hoa. Together with Pierre Douzou, Gaston pioneered the use of high pressures and low temperatures in studying structure-function relationships in biomacromolecules. Julie Renard is acknowledged for her participation through her short training in the laboratory.

Conflicts of Interest: The authors declare no conflict of interest.

References

1. Adkar-Purushothama, C.R.; Perreault, J.-P. Current overview on viroid–host interactions. *WIREs RNA* **2020**, *11*, e1570. [CrossRef] [PubMed]
2. Flores, R.; Gas, M.-E.; Molina, D.; Hernández, C.; Daròs, J.-A. Analysis of viroid replication. In *Plant Virology Protocols*; Springer: Totowa, NJ, USA, 2008; pp. 167–183.
3. Ding, B. The Biology of Viroid-Host Interactions. *Annu. Rev. Phytopathol.* **2009**, *47*, 105–131. [CrossRef]
4. Maurel, M.-C.; Leclerc, F.; Hervé, G. Ribozyme Chemistry: To be or not to be under high pressure. *Chem. Rev.* **2019**, *120*, 4898–4918. [CrossRef] [PubMed]
5. Leclerc, F.; Karplus, M. Two-metal-ion mechanism for hammerhead-ribozyme catalysis. *J. Phys. Chem. B* **2006**, *110*, 3395–3409. [CrossRef] [PubMed]
6. Navarro, J.-A.; Daròs, J.-A.; Flores, R. Complexes containing both polarity strands of avocado sunblotch viroid: Identification in chloroplasts and characterization. *Virology* **1999**, *253*, 77–85. [CrossRef] [PubMed]
7. Silva, J.L.; Oliveira, A.C.; Vieira, T.C.R.G.; de Oliveira, G.A.P.; Suarez, M.C.; Foguel, D. High-Pressure Chemical Biology and Biotechnology. *Chem. Rev.* **2014**, *114*, 7239–7267. [CrossRef] [PubMed]
8. Winter, R. Interrogating the Structural Dynamics and Energetics of Biomolecular Systems with Pressure Modulation. *Annu. Rev. Biophys.* **2019**, *48*, 441–463. [CrossRef]
9. Han, T.; Liu, H.; Wang, J.; Gao, C.; Han, Y. Electrostrictive Effect of Materials under High Pressure Revealed by Electrochemical Impedance Spectroscopy. *J. Phys. Chem. C* **2021**, *125*, 8788–8793. [CrossRef]
10. Hills, G.; Kinnibrugh, D. The pressure coefficient of the hydrogen electrode reaction. *J. Electrochem. Soc.* **1966**, *113*, 1111. [CrossRef]

11. Tobe, S.; Heams, T.; Vergne, J.; Herve, G.; Maurel, M.-C. The catalytic mechanism of hairpin ribozyme studied by hydrostatic pressure. *Nucleic Acids Res.* **2005**, *33*, 2557–2564. [CrossRef]
12. Hervé, G.; Tobé, S.; Heams, T.; Vergne, J.; Maurel, M.-C. Hydrostatic and osmotic pressure study of the hairpin ribozyme. *Biochim. Biophys. Acta (BBA)-Proteins Proteom.* **2006**, *1764*, 573–577. [CrossRef]
13. Ztouti, M.; Kaddour, H.; Miralles, F.; Simian, C.; Vergne, J.; Hervé, G.; Maurel, M.C. Adenine, a hairpin ribozyme cofactor–high-pressure and competition studies. *FEBS J.* **2009**, *276*, 2574–2588. [CrossRef] [PubMed]
14. Kaddour, H.; Vergne, J.; Hervé, G.; Maurel, M.C. High-pressure analysis of a hammerhead ribozyme from Chrysanthemum chlorotic mottle viroid reveals two different populations of self-cleaving molecule. *FEBS J.* **2011**, *278*, 3739–3747. [CrossRef] [PubMed]
15. Gaston, H.B.H. Application of NIR Raman Spectroscopy to Probe the Flexibility of RNA Structure. In *RNA Spectroscopy: Methods and Protocols*; Arluison, V., Wien, F., Eds.; Springer: New York, NY, USA, 2020; pp. 149–164.
16. Hui-Bon-Hoa, G.; Kaddour, H.; Vergne, J.; Kruglik, S.G.; Maurel, M.-C. Raman characterization of Avocado Sunblotchviroid and its response to external perturbations and self-cleavage. *BMC Biophys.* **2014**, *7*, 2. [CrossRef]
17. Diener, T.O. *The Viroids*; Springer Science & Business Media: Boston, MA, USA, 2012.
18. Chang, T.; He, S.; Amini, R.; Li, Y. Functional Nucleic Acids under Unusual Conditions. *ChemBioChem* **2021**, *22*, 2368–2383. [CrossRef]
19. Magnabosco, C.; Lin, L.H.; Dong, H.; Bomberg, M.; Ghiorse, W.; Stan-Lotter, H.; Pedersen, K.; Kieft, T.L.; van Heerden, E.; Onstott, T.C. The biomass and biodiversity of the continental subsurface. *Nat. Geosci.* **2018**, *11*, 707–717. [CrossRef]
20. Paul, B.G.; Bagby, S.C.; Czornyj, E.; Arambula, D.; Handa, S.; Sczyrba, A.; Ghosh, P.; Miller, J.F.; Valentine, D.L. Targeted diversity generation by intraterrestrial archaea and archaeal viruses. *Nat. Commun.* **2015**, *6*, 6585. [CrossRef]
21. Quéméneur, M.; Erauso, G.; Frouin, E.; Zeghal, E.; Vandecasteele, C.; Ollivier, B.; Tamburini, C.; Garel, M.; Ménez, B.; Postec, A. Hydrostatic Pressure Helps to Cultivate an Original Anaerobic Bacterium From the Atlantis Massif Subseafloor (IODP Expedition 357): Petrocella atlantisensis gen. nov. sp. nov. *Front. Microbiol.* **2019**, *10*, 1479. [CrossRef] [PubMed]
22. Maurel, M.-C.; Leclerc, F.; Vergne, J.; Zaccai, G. RNA Back and Forth: Looking through Ribozyme and Viroid Motifs. *Viruses* **2019**, *11*, 283. [CrossRef] [PubMed]
23. Delan-Forino, C.; Deforges, J.; Benard, L.; Sargueil, B.; Maurel, M.-C.; Torchet, C. Structural Analyses of Avocado sunblotch viroid Reveal Differences in the Folding of Plus and Minus RNA Strands. *Viruses* **2014**, *6*, 489–506. [CrossRef]
24. Delan-Forino, C.; Maurel, M.-C.; Torchet, C. Replication of avocado sunblotch viroid in the yeast Saccharomyces cerevisiae. *J. Virol.* **2011**, *85*, 3229–3238. [CrossRef]
25. Gruber, A.R.; Lorenz, R.; Bernhart, S.H.; Neuböck, R.; Hofacker, I.L. The vienna RNA websuite. *Nucleic Acids Res.* **2008**, *36*, W70–W74. [CrossRef]
26. Lorenz, R.; Bernhart, S.H.; Zu Siederdissen, C.H.; Tafer, H.; Flamm, C.; Stadler, P.F.; Hofacker, I.L. ViennaRNA Package 2.0. *Algorithms Mol. Biol.* **2011**, *6*, 26. [CrossRef] [PubMed]
27. Mathews, D.H.; Disney, M.D.; Childs, J.L.; Schroeder, S.J.; Zuker, M.; Turner, D.H. Incorporating chemical modification constraints into a dynamic programming algorithm for prediction of RNA secondary structure. *Proc. Natl. Acad. Sci. USA* **2004**, *101*, 7287–7292. [CrossRef]
28. Popenda, M.; Szachniuk, M.; Antczak, M.; Purzycka, K.J.; Lukasiak, P.; Bartol, N.; Blazewicz, J.; Adamiak, R.W. Automated 3D structure composition for large RNAs. *Nucleic Acids Res.* **2012**, *40*, e112. [CrossRef] [PubMed]
29. Wang, J.; Youkharibache, P.; Zhang, D.; Lanczycki, C.J.; Geer, R.C.; Madej, T.; Phan, L.; Ward, M.; Lu, S.; Marchler, G.H.; et al. iCn3D, a web-based 3D viewer for sharing 1D/2D/3D representations of biomolecular structures. *Bioinformatics* **2020**, *36*, 131–135. [CrossRef] [PubMed]
30. Sun, S.; Wu, Q.; Peng, Z.; Yang, J. Enhanced prediction of RNA solvent accessibility with long short-term memory neural networks and improved sequence profiles. *Bioinformatics* **2019**, *35*, 1686–1691. [CrossRef]
31. Heremans, K. High pressure effects on proteins and other biomolecules. *Annu. Rev. Biophys. Bioeng.* **1982**, *11*, 1–21. [CrossRef]
32. Leclerc, F.; Zaccai, G.; Vergne, J.; Řihovà, M.; Martel, A.; Maurel, M.-C. Self-assembly Controls Self-cleavage of HHR from ASBVd (−): A Combined SANS and Modeling Study. *Sci. Rep.* **2016**, *6*, 30287. [CrossRef] [PubMed]
33. Ding, Y.; Chan, C.Y.; Lawrence, C.E. RNA secondary structure prediction by centroids in a Boltzmann weighted ensemble. *RNA* **2005**, *11*, 1157–1166. [CrossRef]
34. Daniel, I.; Oger, P.; Winter, R. Origins of life and biochemistry under high-pressure conditions. *Chem. Soc. Rev.* **2006**, *35*, 858–875. [CrossRef]
35. Dufour, E.; Hervé, G.; Haertle, T. Hydrolysis of β-lactoglobulin by thermolysin and pepsin under high hydrostatic pressure. *Biopolym. Orig. Res. Biomol.* **1995**, *35*, 475–483. [CrossRef]
36. Northrop, D.B. Effects of high pressure on enzymatic activity. *Biochim. Biophys. Acta (BBA)-Protein Struct. Mol. Enzymol.* **2002**, *1595*, 71–79. [CrossRef]
37. Guy, H.I.; Schmidt, B.; Hervé, G.; Evans, D.R. Pressure-induced dissociation of carbamoyl-phosphate synthetase domains: The catalytically active form is dimeric. *J. Biol. Chem.* **1998**, *273*, 14172–14178. [CrossRef] [PubMed]
38. Eisenmenger, M.J.; Reyes-De-Corcuera, J.I. High pressure enhancement of enzymes: A review. *Enzym. Microb. Technol.* **2009**, *45*, 331–347. [CrossRef]

39. Hervé, G.; Evans, H.G.; Fernado, R.; Patel, C.; Hachem, F.; Evans, D.R. Activation of latent dihydroorotase from Aquifex aeolicus by pressure. *J. Biol. Chem.* **2017**, *292*, 629–637. [CrossRef] [PubMed]
40. Peracchi, A. Origins of the temperature dependence of hammerhead ribozyme catalysis. *Nucleic Acids Res.* **1999**, *27*, 2875–2882. [CrossRef] [PubMed]
41. Hertel, K.J.; Uhlenbeck, O.C. The internal equilibrium of the hammerhead ribozyme reaction. *Biochemistry* **1995**, *34*, 1744–1749. [CrossRef]
42. Feig, A.L.; Ammons, G.E.; Uhlenbeck, O.C. Cryoenzymology of the hammerhead ribozyme. *RNA* **1998**, *4*, 1251–1258. [CrossRef] [PubMed]
43. Takagi, Y.; Taira, K. Temperature-dependent change in the rate-determining step in a reaction catalyzed by a hammerhead ribozyme. *FEBS Lett.* **1995**, *361*, 273–276. [CrossRef]
44. El-Murr, N.; Maurel, M.-C.; Rihova, M.; Vergne, J.; Hervé, G.; Kato, M.; Kawamura, K. Behavior of a hammerhead ribozyme in aqueous solution at medium to high temperatures. *Naturwissenschaften* **2012**, *99*, 731–738. [CrossRef] [PubMed]
45. Moelling, K.; Broecker, F. Viroids and the Origin of Life. *Int. J. Mol. Sci.* **2021**, *22*, 3476. [CrossRef] [PubMed]
46. Martin, W.; Baross, J.; Kelley, D.; Russell, M.J. Hydrothermal vents and the origin of life. *Nat. Rev. Microbiol.* **2008**, *6*, 805–814. [CrossRef]
47. Damer, B.; Deamer, D. The Hot Spring Hypothesis for an Origin of Life. *Astrobiology* **2019**, *20*, 429–452. [CrossRef] [PubMed]
48. De La Peña, M.; García-Robles, I. Intronic hammerhead ribozymes are ultraconserved in the human genome. *EMBO Rep.* **2010**, *11*, 711–716. [CrossRef]

biology

MDPI

Article

Pressure Perturbation Studies of Noncanonical Viral Nucleic Acid Structures

Judit Somkuti, Orsolya Réka Molnár, Anna Grád and László Smeller *

Department of Biophysics and Radiation Biology, Semmelweis University, 1094 Budapest, Hungary; somkuti.judit@med.semmelweis-univ.hu (J.S.); molnar.orsolya@med.semmelweis-univ.hu (O.R.M.); grad.anna@med.semmelweis-univ.hu (A.G.)
* Correspondence: smeller.laszlo@med.semmelweis-univ.hu

Simple Summary: It is well known that nucleic acids adopt a double-helical structure that is essential in the storage and replication of genetic code. However, noncanonical structures of DNA are less explored. The most important of these structures are the G-quadruplexes, which are formed by guanine-rich sequences of the genome. These G-quadruplexes were found in several crucial positions of the genome; they regulate important processes such as cell proliferation and death. Here we are investigating the quadruplex structures appearing in the genome of the hepatitis B, whose infection is among the ten leading causes of death. Our unique approach—the high-pressure technique—allowed us to characterize the stability of these quadruplexes in wide temperature and pressure ranges. Pressure experiments gave us the volume changes occurring at the unfolding, e.g., the embedded volume of the folded structure. Volumetric parameters are especially important because the space available for molecules is quite limited in the crowded environment of the cell. We also investigated how the stability of the viral quadruplexes can be increased by the binding of TMPyP4, a special ligand developed for cancer therapy.

Abstract: G-quadruplexes are noncanonical structures formed by guanine-rich sequences of the genome. They are found in crucial loci of the human genome, they take part in the regulation of important processes like cell proliferation and cell death. Much less is known about the subjects of this work, the viral G-quadruplexes. We have chosen three potentially G-quadruplex-forming sequences of hepatitis B. We measured the stability and the thermodynamic parameters of these quadruplexes. We also investigated the potential stabilization of these G-quadruplexes by binding a special ligand that was originally developed for cancer therapy. Fluorescence and infrared spectroscopic measurements were performed over wide temperature and pressure ranges. Our experiments indicate the small unfolding volume change of all three oligos. We found a difference between the unfolding of the 2-quartet and the 3-quartet G-quadruplexes. All three G-quadruplexes were stabilized by TMPyP4, which is a cationic porphyrin developed for stabilizing the human telomere.

Keywords: G-quadruplex; hepatitis B; DNA; oligo; FRET; FTIR; spectroscopy; pressure; volume change; TMPyP4

Citation: Somkuti, J.; Molnár, O.R.; Grád, A.; Smeller, L. Pressure Perturbation Studies of Noncanonical Viral Nucleic Acid Structures. *Biology* **2021**, *10*, 1173. https://doi.org/10.3390/biology10111173

Academic Editors: Dmitri Davydov and Christiane Jung

Received: 29 September 2021
Accepted: 8 November 2021
Published: 12 November 2021

1. Introduction

Guanine-rich nucleic acid sequences can form non-canonical structures. One of the most important among these structures are the four-stranded G-quadruplex (GQs), in which four guanines are arranged in one plane. They are connected by Hoogsteen-type hydrogen bonds instead of the Watson–Crick-type ones (Figure 1), and they are stabilized by eight hydrogen bonds. A GQ is typically composed of two or three G-quartets. A central metal ion is essential, as it is necessary to stabilize the structure. GQs can have a number of different conformations they can be formed by one, two or four different strands. The monomers are the most important forms, in these structures one nucleic acid chain is folded to form the GQ. As for the orientation of the strands, they can appear in parallel, antiparallel or hybrid forms [1,2]. GQs, in vitro and in vivo, can interact with various ions and molecules that give them special biological significance. In vivo, GQs take part in the regulation of gene expression; in vitro, they are used in analytical biochemistry [3]. Their in-vivo relevance is mostly related to the stabilization of the DNA or RNA. GQs came into the focus of the research, when their abundance in the telomere region of the human genome was reported [4,5]. Formation of GQs in this region inhibits the telomerase activity. Additionally, they were found in the promoter region of several oncogenes [6,7], which made them a potential target for cancer treatment [4,8]. Recently, potentially GQ-forming sequences were found in several viral genomes, and it opens the possibility to target viral GQs using molecules developed for cancer research. Additionally, an interaction between viral proteins and GQs was also reported recently, which underlines the importance of GQs in viral research [9].

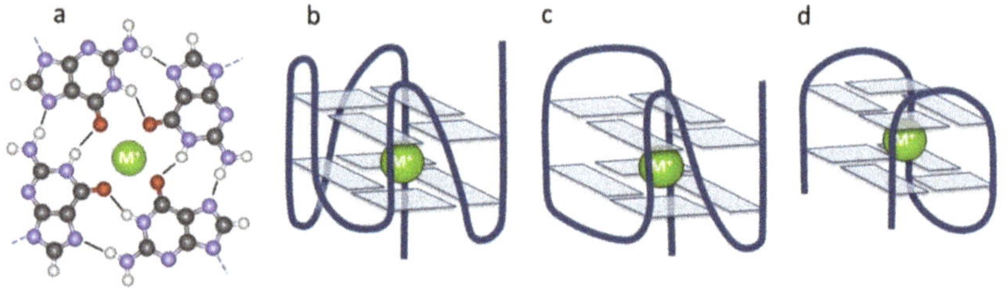

Figure 1. (**a**) Structure of a G-quartet formed by four guanine bases. The figure was made by the Viewerlite 4.2 program, selecting one quartet from the 2HY9 pdb structure. (**b–d**) Typical structures of a two-quartet GQ. The panels show the parallel, hybrid and basket forms respectively.

In this paper we report the evaluation of three GQ-forming sequence of the hepatitis B virus (HBV). HBV is one of the most frequent chronic viral infections, around 350–400 million people are currently infected worldwide [10]. HBV infection was among the ten leading causes of death in 2010 [11]. HBV has a small circular DNA genome with a length of approximately 3.2 kilobase pairs [10–13]. HBV has four overlapping reading frames that encode seven proteins (including S for surface or envelope gene, C for the core gene and P for the polymerase gene) [12,14].

Lavezzo et al. [15] were searching for potential GQ-forming sequences in genomes of several viruses. For the HBV, the highest G-score was associated to the GGC TGG GGC TTG GTC ATG GGC CAT CAG (NC_003977.2:1204..1230 (+strand)) sequence, which can be found in the coding region of the polymerase protein.

Several other potential GQ-forming sequences with slightly lower score were also identified. Biswas et al. [12] found a conserved sequence containing GGG tetrads in the promoter region of the envelope-coding gene, the S protein of the virus. This GGG AGT GGG AGC ATT CGG GCC AGG G sequence is also worthy of investigation. Another promising GQ-prone sequence might be the GGG TGG CTT TGG GGC ATG G (NC_003977.2 NC_003977.2:1886..1904 (+strand)) which can be found in the C protein's signaling region in the virus.

In experimental practice, pressure is a highly overlooked variable of thermodynamics, although it is equally important as temperature [16–22]. The low number of high-pressure studies can be partially explained by technical difficulties. Experiments performed at few kilobars are considered by some as non-physiological. Of course, high temperatures or a few moles of GuHCl—which are frequently used in stability studies of macromolecules—are not physiological either. However, high-pressure experiments give the unique possibility of revealing the volumetric properties of the system under study.

The usefulness of high-pressure experiments has been proven in a wide range of publications [22–30]. According to the Le Chatelier's principle, the pressurized system prefers the state that has the smallest volume. This is how protein unfolding is induced by pressure [31–33]. Typically 5 kbar pressure is enough to unfold an average protein, like myoglobin [34], although there are much more stable ones as well [35]. Intermolecular interactions are even more sensitive to pressure; typically 2 kbar leads to disaggregation of oligomeric structures [29,34,36]. Lipid-phase transition lines are also shifting with pressure, which is again a nice example for the Le Chatelier's principle: pressure stabilizes the more tightly packed gel phase [37,38].

Nucleic acids were treated as pressure insensitive for a long time. The unwinding of the double helix structures is hardly influenced by pressure, but noncanonical structures, like GQs and i-motifs show volume changes during their unfolding [22,26,39–41]. Therefore, they are appropriate for such high-pressure studies that can provide volumetric data. The volume change of the folded GQ structure allows characterization of the tightness and stability of this noncanonical form.

This paper focuses on the stability and volumetric parameters of the above mentioned three GQ-prone sequences of the hepatitis B virus. The investigation of these structures is of vital importance for designing methods wherein the life cycle of the virus is influenced by targeting these noncanonical structure-forming parts of the genome.

2. Materials and Methods

Three oligonucleotides—named HepB1, HepB2 and HepB3—were investigated. Their sequences are: HepB1: GGC TGG GGC TTG GTC ATG GGC CAT CAG, HepB2: GGG AGT GGG AGC ATT CGG GCC AGG G HepB3: TTG GGT GGC TTT GGG GCA TGG AC. The oligonucleotides were purchased from IDT (Coralville, IA, USA) and Sigma-Aldrich Kft (Budapest, Hungary).

For the fluorescence studies, the oligos were labeled with the FRET pair FAM and TAMRA. (FRET: Förster resonance energy transfer, FAM: Carboxyfluorescein CAS Number: 3301-79-9, TAMRA^{TM}: Tetramethylrhodamine) The labeling was performed by IDT or Sigma-Aldrich, where the oligos were synthetized. The oligos were obtained from the manufacturers in lyophilized form.

For the fluorescence experiments, the HepB_FRET samples were first dissolved in MilliQ water in a concentration of 100 µM, according to the suggestion of IDT. This stock solution was kept frozen and diluted with an appropriate buffer during sample preparation. The final concentration of the oligos in the samples was 1 µM, unless stated otherwise. For the heating experiments, 100 mM K-phosphate buffer (pH 7.4) was used, because of its insensitivity to temperature changes. For experiments with Li^+ and Rb^+, Tris buffer was used. TMPyP4 (meso-5,10,15,20-Tetrakis-(N-methyl-4-pyridyl)porphine) was purchased from Merck KGaA, (Darmstadt, Germany) and ChemCruz (Dallas, TX, USA).

In the infrared experiments much higher concentration of HepB was required. The oligos were dissolved in D_2O-based Bis-Tris buffer (100 mM, pD 7.4) in a concentration of 20 mg/mL. The metal ion concentrations were 100 mM. All chemicals not specified above differently were purchased from Sigma-Aldrich.

Fluorescence experiments were performed as described earlier in details [25,42]. Fluorolog-FL3 fluorimeter (Horiba Jobin Yvon, Longjumeau, France) was used mainly for the temperature scans. It was equipped with a programmable temperature-controlled cell (DI instruments, Budapest, Hungary). An HH802U thermometer and the corresponding software from Omega were used to record the temperature by a thermocouple directly in the cuvette (Omega Engineering Inc., Norwalk, CT, USA). The temperature was increased by 0.2 °C/min. Spectra were recorded every 5 min, resulting in spectra of ca. 1 °C intervals. Fluorescence intensity was divided with the signal of the reference diode of the spectrometer in order to standardize the experiments. For the high-pressure experiments, a homemade reflection-mode diamond cell was adopted for the sample holder. The pressure was measured by recording the ruby fluorescence. A small ruby chip was placed into the pressure cell, and it was excited by a green HeNe laser (Coherent, Santa Clara, CA,

USA). The emitted light was detected by a CCD camera (Andor, Belfast, UK) attached to a THR1000 monochromator (Jobin Yvon, Longjumeau, France).

FTIR spectra were measured with a Bruker Vertex 80v spectrometer. A total of 256 spectra were averaged at a 2 cm^{-1} resolution. D_2O buffer was used as solvent, in order to avoid the large absorption band of water around 1640 cm^{-1}. The samples were measured in a temperature-controlled diamond anvil cell (Diacell, Leicester, UK). The pressure was measured using the 983 cm^{-1} line of $BaSO_4$ [43]. The experiments were performed by increasing the temperature with a rate of 12 °C/hour at constant pressure. Spectra were recorded in 5 min intervals, i.e., in ca. 1 °C steps.

CD (circular dichroism) spectra were recorded with Jasco J-720 spectrometer in a 1 mm cuvette with 0.1 nm steps. The spectra were smoothed with Fourier filter.

The transition temperature was determined by fitting the temperature dependence of spectral parameters by the following sigmoidal function:

$$y(T) = a + bT + \frac{\Delta a + \Delta bT}{1 + \exp\left(\frac{\Delta H}{R}\left(\frac{1}{T} - \frac{1}{T_m}\right)\right)} \tag{1}$$

Here, y is the physical parameter to be fitted (e.g., fluorescence intensity, ratio of fluorescence intensities at two different wavelengths or absorbance at certain wavenumber of the infrared spectrum), a and b are the parameters describing the linear dependence of $y(T)$ below the transition, T is the thermodynamic temperature, Δa and Δb are the changes of a and b during the transition, ΔH is the enthalpy change, R is the universal gas constant, and T_m is the transition midpoint.

The Clausius–Clapeyron equation was used to calculate the volume changes taking place during the pressure experiments:

$$\Delta V = \frac{\Delta H}{T_m}\frac{dT_m}{dp} \tag{2}$$

It has to be mentioned, that in this paper the volume change is defined as the unfolding volume, that means $\Delta V = V_{unfolded} - V_{folded}$.

3. Results and Discussion

3.1. Temperature Stability of HepB1-3 Detected by FRET

Figure 2a–c shows the change of the fluorescence spectra of the three oligos during the temperature scan. All the oligos were labeled by FRET pair, and K^+ ions were present to stabilize the GQs. An increase of the donor fluorescence intensity at 520 nm can be observed while the fluorescence of the acceptor is decreasing. The intensity at the acceptor position seems to be constant in case of HepB1, but this is due to the emission of the donor at 580 nm. Indeed, the high temperature spectra contain purely the donor emission, and the acceptor emission is completely lost. For comparison, a spectrum of GQ with FAM labeling only is shown in Figure 2d. In this case energy transfer is not possible, so it shows the spectrum of the donor without energy transfer. This spectrum is quite similar to the high temperature spectra on Figure 2a–c. Consequently, we can state the absence of—or at least a considerable reduced—energy transfer in the high-temperature spectra of HepB1-3. The increase of the donor fluorescence and the simultaneous decrease of the acceptor fluorescence clearly indicates the unfolding of the GQ structure at high temperatures. The Förster distance of the FAM-TAMRA FRET pair is 5.5 nm. In case of the folded GQ, the distance between the quartets is around 0.3 nm, while the width of the structure is around 2.5 nm. The distance between the first and last phosphorus atoms is around 2.5 nm in a three-quartet hybrid GQ. Since a 3D structure is not available for any HepB variants, these values were calculated using the 2HY9.pdb structure, which is a hybrid-form GQ found in human telomere sequences [44]. In this form the two terminal bases are at the different sides of the three-dimensional structure, having the biggest possible distance from each other. This means, that the highest possible distance in the two terminal bases in the folded

GQ is much smaller than the Förster distance of the FRET pair we used. Therefore, the energy transfer in the low temperature spectra shows unequivocally a folded GQ form. Our HepB1, HepB2 and HepB3 oligos had 27, 25 and 23 bases respectively. The contour lengths of oligos containing 27, 25 and 23 bases were 8.1, 7.5 and 6.9 nm, which, together with the lengths of the linker of the chromophores (ca. 2 and 1 nm), were definitely larger than the Förster distance of the FAM-TAMRA pair. This means the loss of the energy transfer, i.e., the high intensity of the donor fluorophore is a clear sign of the unfolding of the GQ structure.

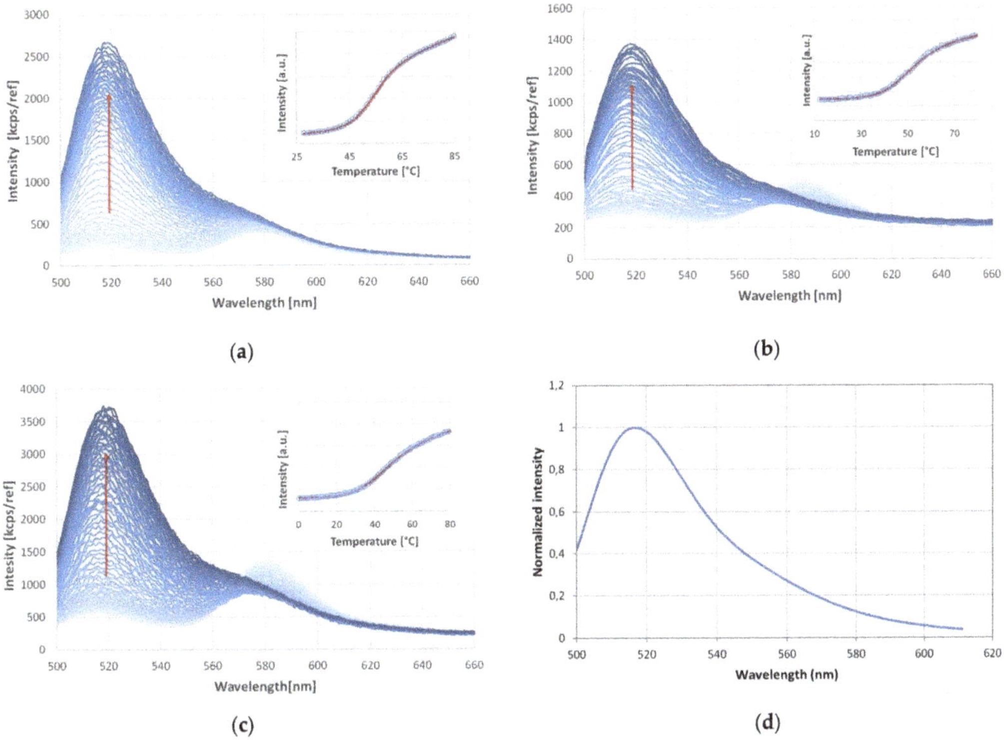

Figure 2. Fluorescence spectra of (**a**) HepB1, (**b**) HepB2, (**c**) HepB3 and (**d**) human telomere (Htel) at atmospheric pressure. The HepB oligos are labeled by the FRET pair FAM (as donor) and TAMRA (as acceptor), Htel was labeled only with FAM. The fluorescence intensity is divided with the signal of the reference diode of the spectrometer in order to standardize the experiments. The lowest temperature spectrum has the lightest color while the high temperature one is dark. Additionally a red arrow shows the direction of the spectral changes during temperature increase. The inserts in (**a**–**c**) show the fit of the donor intensity with the function of Equation (1). The oligos were measured in presence of 140 mM K-phosphate buffer (pH 7.4). The oligo labeled with FAM only can be seen in panel (**d**) to show the case, when there is no energy transfer.

The folded state can be characterized by the relative FRET efficiency (E_{rel}) [45]. It is defined as:

$$E_{rel} = I_a/(I_a + I_d) \quad (3)$$

where I_a and I_d are the fluorescence intensities at the acceptor and donor positions. Since the donor also emits slightly at the acceptor position, the value 0.11 means complete absence of the FRET.

The E_{rel} values are summarized in Table 1. All the folded values are around 0.65. The small variation of E_{rel} suggests that the folded forms have the same or at least similar folded conformation. In our earlier circular dichroism spectroscopic studies, we found a hybrid structure for the potassium-stabilized HepB1 [46]. We measured the CD spectra of HepB2 and HepB3 in presence of K^+ ion. These spectra are shown in the Supplementary Materials (Figure S1a,b). Based on these spectra we can rationalize the hybrid structure for all the HepB variants in the presence of K^+ ion [47,48]. The small E_{rel} values at high temperatures indicate the single-stranded (unfolded) conformation. Oliva et al. [45] measured $E_{rel} = 0.33$ for the unfolded Htel, which was shorter than our oligos. Their E_{rel} value for the folded hybrid form was a bit higher than our values, but HepB1 was proven to form a hybrid structure in presence of potassium ion. The discrepancy can be explained, again, by the different oligo lengths.

Table 1. Relative fluorescence efficiency values of HepB oligos in folded and unfolded conformations. All experiments were performed in presence of potassium ion.

Oligo Name	Relative FRET Efficiency E_{rel}	
	Folded	**Unfolded**
HepB1	0.65	0.21
HepB2	0.64	0.27
HepB3	0.69	0.24

We evaluated the donor emission intensity to characterize the unfolding quantitatively. The donor intensity versus temperature is plotted in the inserts. A sigmoid curve (Equation (1)) was fitted, which was obtained from the two state thermodynamics. These are shown in the inserts. The transition temperatures were 53.8, 51.9 and 41.4 °C for HepB1, HepB2 and HepB3 respectively. It is noteworthy that HepB1 is the most stable, although HepB2 would be able to form a three-quartet GQ, which is considered more stable than the two-quartet one. Transition temperatures around 50 °C are typical for two-quartet GQs. As for the unfolding temperature of the two-quartet thrombin-binding aptamer (TBA), 53 °C was measured [41], while the three-quartet Htel unfolds at around 65 °C [42,49]. This means that either HepB2 does not form a three-quartet GQ, or it was somehow destabilized. Guedin et al. [50] investigated the effect of the loop length, and they found a clear destabilization caused by long loops. Since HepB2 has a long loop in the middle, this can be the reason for its low stability. The low stability of HepB3 may be surprising at the first sight, but it can only form two G-quartets; if we compare it with HepB1—which also has a two-quartet structure—HepB1 is more stable. We can hypothesize, that the last guanine of the HepB1 sequence can turn back and it can form a stability-increasing structure with two other guanines. This is not possible in case of HepB3, which results its lower stability.

3.2. Stabilizing Effect of Monovalent Cations

All the GQs have to be stabilized by metal ions that are located in the middle of the G-quartet, or in between of the quartets, depending on the geometrical constraints. We investigated four ions of the first column of the periodic table, namely: Li^+, Na^+, K^+, Rb^+. They have different ionic radii, which would predict differences in their stabilizing ability. We measured the temperature stability (i. e. the transition temperature, T_m) for all the HepB oligos in the presence of all four ions. The results can be seen in Table 2.

Table 2. Transition temperature (T_m) of the three studied HepB oligos in presence of different cations. The order of stabilizing ability is indicated as well.

Oligo	Li^+	Na^+	K^+	Rb^+	Stabilizing Order
HepB1	58.5	56.6	53.8	54.4	$Li^+ > Na^+ > Rb^+ \gtrsim K^+$
HepB2	46.9	51.0	51.9	45.6	$K^+ > Na^+ > Li^+ \gtrsim Rb^+$
HepB3	49.4	48.1	41.4	44.4	$Li^+ > Na^+ > Rb^+ > K^+$

$\gtrsim$ means a little bit larger.

As it can be seen, there is a difference between the values of HepB2 and the other GQs. This can be explained by the different sequences, which result in different structures. HepB2 contains four GGG repeats, while in the other two sequences there are GG sequences as well. This means, that HepB1 and HepB3 can only form a two-quartet GQ, while in HepB2 a three-quartet structure can be formed. Moreover, different cations can stabilize different conformations. In our earlier study we have shown, that HepB1 forms parallel structure in the presence of Li^+, Na^+ and Rb^+, while K^+ induces a hybrid structure. There is no common rule for the order of stabilization among the monovalent cations. Earlier studies suggested that K^+ is the most potent stabilizer, followed by Na^+ and Rb^+ ions [51–53]. Li^+ was reported to be too small to considerably stabilize the GQ form. Our results show somehow different order in stabilization. This can be explained by the fact, that earlier studies mainly focused on three-quartet GQ-forming, while HepB1 and HepB3—where the order of the stabilizing ions is different from the conventional one—can only form two-stage GQs. In case of two-stage GQs lithium is the most potent stabilizer. This implies a more closely packed structure, which can be stabilized by a relatively small ion, too. However, the differences in the stabilizing abilities of the ions are quite small. This fact suggests that the main factor in the stability of the quadruplexes is not the size of the central ion, but the hydrogen bonds stabilizing the GQ structure.

3.3. Pressure Experiments

3.3.1. FRET Experiments under Pressure

Volumetric characterization of the GQs can be obtained from the pressure dependence of the system. The experiments described hereafter were performed in the presence of potassium ions, since this is the one that is present in highest concentration in vivo. The temperature unfolding experiments described above were also repeated at different elevated pressures. Unfortunately, this work is not as straightforward as it could be, using the pure thermodynamic description. This is due to the pH-dependence of the GQs. Although they are quite pH-insensitive, the slight pH-induced shift in the unfolding temperature can also lead to the distortion of the analysis.

This result inspired us to control and take into account the pH-alterations more carefully than is usually done. All of the experiments were pH-corrected, which means, that the pH was calculated for the actual pressure and temperature of the transition point. We used the dpH/dT values from Good et al. [54] This allowed us to perform a three dimensional fit afterwards, using the following function:

$$T_m = a + b \cdot \mathrm{pH} + c \cdot p. \tag{4}$$

This way we obtained the pH- and pressure dependence of the unfolding temperature. Since the pH-dependence is not important, from the point of view of our volumetric study, and the three-dimensional plots are difficult to interpret, we made a pH-correction. (See the three-dimensional fits in Figures S2–S4) We corrected all the measurement points to the physiological pH value, pH = 7.4. Plots of the corrected T_m values as function of the pressure are shown in Figure 3. A linear fit was applied to the points to obtain the dT_m/dp value, which was used to determine the volume change values. The slope of the line is actually the same as the *c* value deriving from the 3D fit (Equation (4)).

The volume change of the unfolding can be obtained from the slope of these lines using Equation (2). This also requires the ΔH values, which were obtained from the fit of the donor emission intensity data to Equation (1). The entropy changes decreased slightly with the pressure, therefore the value extrapolated to zero pressure was used. The ΔH values are: 192 ± 4 kJ/mol for HepB1, 124 ± 10 kJ/mol for HepB2 and 82 ± 9 kJ/mol for HepB3. The smaller enthalpy changes are reflected in the transition curves too; they are much less sharp, in the cases of HepB2 and HepB3, compared with HepB1.

Using these values, we can calculate the volume changes for each oligo.

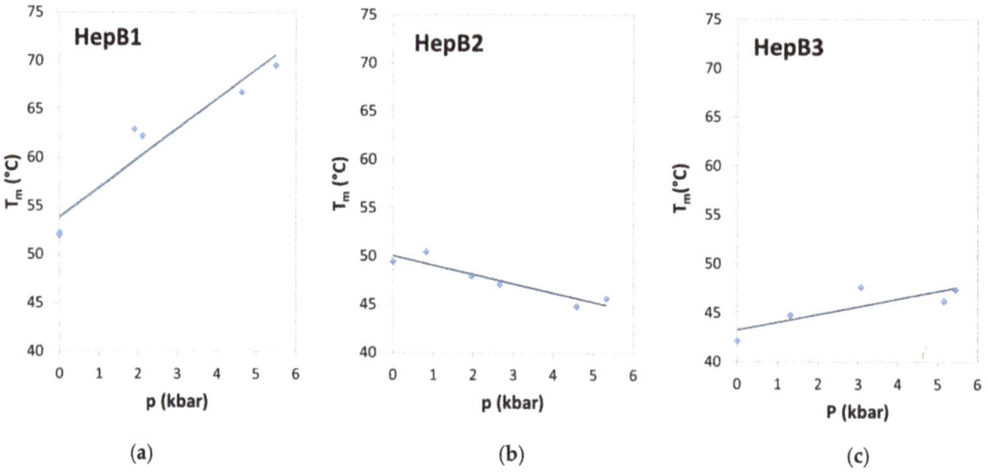

Figure 3. Pressure dependence of the unfolding temperature values for the three HepB variants. (**a**) HepB1, (**b**) HepB2, (**c**) HEpB3. The temperature values are pH-corrected as described in the text.

3.3.2. Unfolding of GQ as Seen from the Infrared Spectroscopy

FTIR spectra were recorded in the diamond anvil cell (DAC). The transmission cell has two diamond windows and requires a very small sample volume (few × 10 nl). However, the concentration of the sample should be much higher compared with the fluorescence experiments, in order to obtain good quality spectra. This is because the absorption of water in the infrared range limits the path length.

The infrared spectrum contains absorption bands belonging to the molecular vibrations. The most conformation-sensitive vibration in the HepB GQs is the one in the range of 1660–1680. This band comes mainly from the $C_6 = O_6$ carbonyl vibration of the guanine base [42,55]. Since this takes part in the Hoogsteen-type hydrogen bond network, unfolding of the GQ alters the vibrational frequency [56]. Figure 4 shows this spectral region in case of HepB1 at a few selected temperatures. The position of the band is at 1660–1665 cm^{-1} for free guanine, it is near 1672 cm^{-1} in case of Hoogsteen-type hydrogen bonding, and it is at 1689 cm^{-1} in the Watson–Crick type double helix [42,57]. The presence of the 1672 cm^{-1} band in the low-temperature spectra is clear, and its disappearance in high-temperature spectra is also unequivocal. Simultaneously, the absorption in the middle of the 1660 cm^{-1} band is increasing. To determine the transition temperature, we fitted the absorbance values at 1660 cm^{-1} with Equation (1). We performed the same experiments at different pressure values. The transition temperatures are plotted against pressure in Figure 5. The ΔV value was obtained using calculations similar to the ones used for the fluorescence experiments earlier (see Table 3).

The other two HepB variants seemed to have different structure at high concentration needed for the infrared measurements. Their stability was considerably higher even at atmospheric pressure. This could be the sign of the stacking aggregation [58] or formation of the intermolecular GQs, which can be formed by two or four oligos. Therefore, we do not report their pressure behavior, here. The volume-change values obtained from the fluorescence and infrared experiments are in agreement in case of HepB1. One can, however, observe a slight curvature in both the fluorescence and infrared phase boundaries. This curvature points toward the possibility of the elliptic boundary, which is typical in case of proteins [16,19,59]. A similar phase diagram has been suggested by Chalikian and Macgregor [22] on the basis of theoretical calculations, but this is the first example, where such curved phase boundary is measured experimentally. Unfortunately, the experimental points cover only a small fraction of the ellipse; therefore, the fitting of the elliptic phase boundary is not possible. This is why we used the simple linear fit. Most probably, the rest of the ellipse lies out of the relevant and experimentally reachable region of the p-T diagram, if we take into account the freezing curve of the water [16,60].

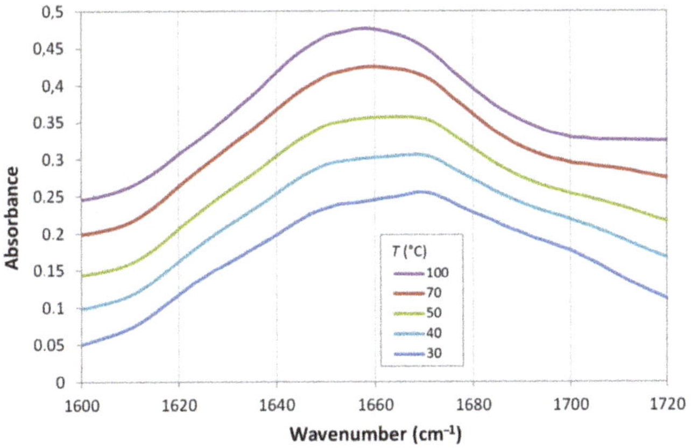

Figure 4. Infrared spectrum of HepB1 in the range of the C=O vibration at selected temperatures.

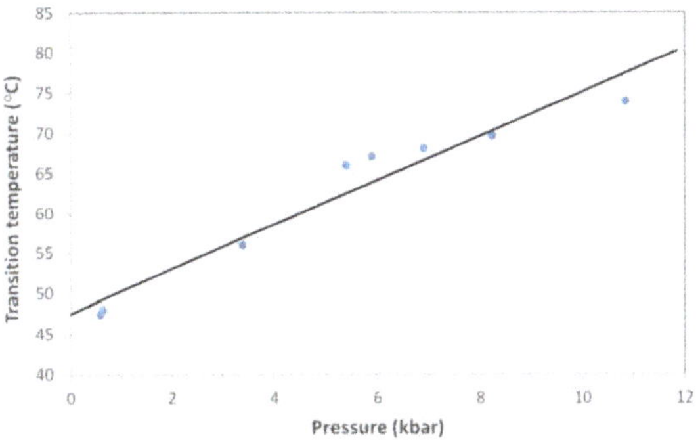

Figure 5. Transition temperatures of HepB1 versus pressure determined by FTIR spectroscopy.

Table 3. Pressure dependence of unfolding temperature and the calculated volume-change values for the HepB oligos in the presence of potassium ions.

Oligo Name	Technique	dT_m/dp (°C/kbar)	dV (cm^3/mol)
HepB1	FRET	3.04 ± 0.58	17.8 ± 3.8
	IR	2.75 ± 0.28	16.1 ± 2.0
HepB2	FRET	−0.96 ± 0.22	−3.7 ± 0.6
HepB3	FRET	0.79 ± 0.38	2.0 ± 1.1

3.3.3. Volume Changes at the Unfolding of HepB GQs

As was mentioned at the end of Materials and Methods, ΔV is defined as the unfolding volume change. This is important to clarify, because not all the publications follow this convention. Positive ΔV means that the unfolded state has a larger volume compared with the folded one. This means that pressure favors the folded state. If the sample is pressurized, the unfolding temperature raises, i.e., $dT_m/dp > 0$. The phase diagram looks like the one in Scheme 1a. If the phase boundary is crossed in the direction of the unfolding, a positive experimental ΔV can be obtained. If ΔV is negative, i.e., the folded state is more compact than the unfolded one; the phase-boundary line has a negative slope, $dT_m/dp < 0$ (Scheme 1b). All these considerations are valid only if the unfolding is an endothermic reaction, as it is in the case of GQs [61].

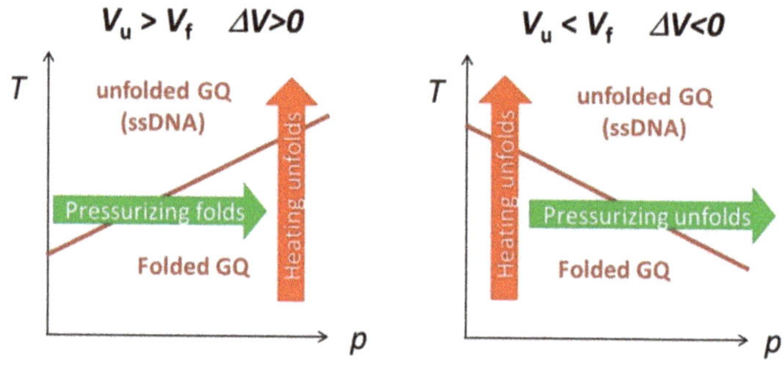

(**a**) (**b**)

Scheme 1. Shape of the temperature–pressure phase diagram, in the cases of different signs of the unfolding volume ΔV. (**a**) $\Delta V > 0$ and (**b**) $\Delta V < 0$. V_f and V_u are the volumes of the folded and unfolded molecules respectively.

A further important remark is that we always measure the volume change of our sample during the unfolding. ΔV is not only the volume change of the GQ itself, volume changes in the hydration shell contribute to it, as well.

As was mentioned earlier, the double-helix DNA does not really respond to pressure, due to its almost-zero unwinding volume. However, in GQs clear pressure effect has been measured for several different forms [25,42,49,62]. The rehydration of the coordinated cations and the volume changes of the DNA molecule itself are believed to be responsible for the volume change during the unfolding [49]. Measurements performed earlier using the thrombin binding aptamer (TBA) showed negative unfolding volume change [41]: $\Delta V = -55 \pm 4$ cm^3/mol. For Htel, -92 ± 5 cm^3/mol was measured by Takahashi et al. [62]. These authors observed reduction of the ΔV in the presence of crowding agents such as polyethylene glycol. Considerably smaller value (-43 ± 7 cm^3/mol) was measured by Li et al. [49]. In our earlier experiments, we investigated four human GQs—c-MYC, KIT, VEGF and Htel—wherein we obtained $\Delta V = -17 \pm 1, -6 \pm 1, -18 \pm 5, -19 \pm 3$ cm^3/mol values respectively [25,42]. The variation in the experimental values points to the importance of slight environmental parameters like crowding, concentration, etc. We have also noticed (looking into the details of the presumably multistep process) that different experimental techniques can provide slightly different transition temperatures.

As mentioned earlier, the rehydration of the central ions was suggested to be responsible for the pressure sensitivity of GQs. Rehydration decreases the volume of the system, since the hydration shell is denser than the bulk water. It could not be, however, the only contribution, because similar values were measured for the GQs containing the same number of quartets, consequently the same number of stabilizing ion. Chalikian's group studied the volumetric aspects of the GQ folding in the case of Htel [63]. They distinguished four terms in the volume change:

$$\Delta V = \Delta V_M + \Delta V_T + \Delta V_H + nV_{K+} \quad (5)$$

where ΔV is the measured unfolding volume change, ΔV_M is the molecular volume, i.e., the volume impenetrable to other molecules, ΔV_T is the thermal volume, which is a result of molecular vibrations and imperfect packing, ΔV_H is the volume change due to the uptake of water molecules into the hydration shell, and V_{K+} is the partial molar volume of the K^+ ion. (Our equation differs from the Equation (4) of ref [63] since they study the folding, while we describe the unfolding volume changes.)

Their calculations based on Htel experiments show more than ten-times higher hydration volume change (779 cm^3/mol), compared with the experimental value (69 cm^3/mol). This was compensated however by high thermal volume of the opposite sign. ΔV_M and V_{K+} are small (6 and 6.3 cm^3/mol, respectively) compared with the other two terms. This means that the volume change of GQs is a delicate balance between hydration and thermal volumes.

According to the results of our pressure experiments we obtained both negative and positive volume changes. As it was mentioned earlier, HepB1 and HepB3 can form two-quartet GQs, while HepB2 is able to form three G-quartets. This correlates with the signs of the volume change values, which is negative only in case of the three-quartet GQ. The positive unfolding volumes in case of HepB1 and HepB3 are unusual for the GQs. There is however a unique feature in these sequences: they contain longer G repeats with three and four guanines. Since there are only two quartets, not all of the guanines of such long G repeats can participate in the stabilization of the GQ form; they might even destabilize the GQ structure and can be responsible for the positive volume changes.

3.4. Stabilization of the HepB GQs with TMPyP4

The cationic porphyrin compound TMPyP4 was developed to stabilize the human telomere GQ, in order to inhibit the telomerase enzyme, which elongates the telomere region of the DNA, contributing to the immortality of cancer cells. We investigated whether this porphyrin molecule is able to stabilize the GQs in the genome of the hepatitis B virus. The porphyrin was added to the FRET-labeled GQs at a four-fold excess. The unfolding temperature increased considerably for all the HepB variants. In some cases, the transition shifted out of our experimental range, which only allowed us to obtain a lower estimate for the stabilization. Table 4 shows the extent of stabilization.

Table 4. Temperature stabilization of HepB variants by the cationic porphyrin TMPyP4. All experiments were performed in the presence of potassium ion.

	Oligo Name		
	HepB1	**HepB2**	**HepB3**
ΔT_m (°C) = $T_{m,HepB+TMPyP4} - T_{m,HepB}$	23	>36	>47

As can be seen, all the HepB GQs are considerably stabilized by the binding of TMPyP4. One can, however, ask as to whether the ligand binds to the unlabeled oligos, too, or only to the FRET-labeled ones. The binding of TMPyP4 to the unlabeled HepB GQs can be proven by a competitive binding assay, similar to the one described by Luo [64]. The principle is, briefly: 1. The unfolding temperature of a FRET-labeled oligo is measured (T_{m1}). 2. The increased unfolding temperature (T_{m2}), in presence of the ligand, is determined. 3. Finally, the sample containing both the labeled and unlabeled oligo, together with the ligand, is measured. If the ligand binds to the unlabeled oligo, the fluorescence curve in the third and first experiments are similar, the T_{m3} is near to T_{m1} rather than to T_{m2}. The results are shown in Figures S5–S7. Our results show clearly that TMPyP4 binds to all tree unlabeled oligos, however, with different strength. HepB2 binds TMPyP4 with smaller affinity than the others, as can be seen from the results of the competitive study.

The stabilization of HepB oligos by TMPyP4 points toward practical applications: TMPyP4 can shift the equilibrium between the double helix and the GQ form and might hinder the transcription and the proliferation of the virus.

4. Conclusions

We found that all of the three potential GQ-forming sequences of the hepatitis B virus fold into a GQ structure. They can be stabilized by Li^+, Na^+, K^+, and Rb^+. Lithium is the most potent stabilizer for the two-quartet GQs, formed by the HepB1 and HepB3 oligos. This suggests that these GQs have a more closely packed structure that allows the stabilization by the small Li^+ ion. Pressure studies resulted in a positive unfolding volume for HepB1, while, for HepB2 and HepB3, we obtained small negative and positive values. Volumetric parameters are important factors in crowded environment, which is typical for biological systems. Under this molecular crowding condition, the available volume is limited, which can shift the folding equilibrium of GQs. All the HepB oligos were stabilized by TMPyP4, which was developed to increase the stability of the human telomere GQ. The stabilization effect was very pronounced—more than 20 °C—which points toward practical applications: TMPyP4 might shift the equilibrium between the double helix and the GQ form and might hinder the transcription of the virus. This might have a medical importance, since the stabilization of GQs in the viral DNA shifts the equilibrium between the double helix and the GQ form, which is believed to influence the transcription of the genome.

Supplementary Materials: The following are available online at https://www.mdpi.com/article/10.3390/biology10111173/s1, Figure S1: CD spectra of HepB2 (a) and HepB3 (b) in presence of K^+ ion. Figures S2–S4: Three dimensional fits of unfolding parameters of HepB1, HepB2 and HepB3 in the pressure-temperature-pH parameter space. Figures S5–S7: Competitive binding assays of HepB1, HepB2 and HepB3.

Author Contributions: Conceptualization, L.S.; investigation: O.R.M., J.S., A.G.; formal analysis: O.R.M., J.S., L.S., A.G.; resources, L.S.; writing—original draft preparation, L.S.; writing—review and editing, L.S.; visualization, O.R.M., J.S., L.S.; supervision, L.S.; funding acquisition, L.S. All authors have read and agreed to the published version of the manuscript.

Funding: This research was funded by the National Research, Development and Innovation Office of Hungary, NKFI K-124697.

Institutional Review Board Statement: Not applicable.

Informed Consent Statement: Not applicable.

Data Availability Statement: The data presented in this study are available on request from the corresponding authors.

Acknowledgments: The authors thank Peter Horváth for his help in the CD experiments.

Conflicts of Interest: The authors declare no conflict of interest. The funders had no role in the design of the study; in the collection, analyses, or interpretation of data; in the writing of the manuscript, or in the decision to publish the results.

References

1. Fry, M. Tetraplex DNA and its interacting proteins. *Front. Biosci. Landmark* **2007**, *12*, 4336–4351. [CrossRef] [PubMed]
2. Burge, S.; Parkinson, G.N.; Hazel, P.; Todd, A.K.; Neidle, S. Quadruplex DNA: Sequence, topology and structure. *Nucleic Acids Res.* **2006**, *34*, 5402–5415. [CrossRef] [PubMed]
3. Kosman, J.; Juskowiak, B. Peroxidase-mimicking DNAzymes for biosensing applications: A review. *Anal. Chim. Acta* **2011**, *707*, 7–17. [CrossRef] [PubMed]
4. Neidle, S. Human telomeric G-quadruplex: The current status of telomeric G-quadruplexes as therapeutic targets in human cancer. *FEBS J.* **2009**, *277*, 1118–1125. [CrossRef] [PubMed]
5. Neidle, S.; Parkinson, G.N. The structure of telomeric DNA. *Curr. Opin. Struct. Biol.* **2003**, *13*, 275–283. [CrossRef]
6. Siddiqui-Jain, A.; Grand, C.L.; Bearss, D.; Hurley, L.H. Direct evidence for a G-quadruplex in a promoter region and its targeting with a small molecule to repress c-MYC transcription. *Proc. Natl. Acad. Sci. USA* **2002**, *99*, 11593–11598. [CrossRef]
7. Seenisamy, J.; Rezler, E.M.; Powell, T.J.; Tye, D.; Gokhale, V.; Joshi, C.S.; Siddiqui-Jain, A.; Hurley, L.H. The Dynamic Character of the G-Quadruplex Element in the c-MYC Promoter and Modification by TMPyP4. *J. Am. Chem. Soc.* **2004**, *126*, 8702–8709. [CrossRef]
8. Balasubramanian, S.; Hurley, L.H.; Neidle, S. Targeting G-quadruplexes in gene promoters: A novel anticancer strategy? *Nat. Rev. Drug Discov.* **2011**, *10*, 261–275. [CrossRef]
9. Lavigne, M.; Helynck, O.; Rigolet, P.; Boudria-Souilah, R.; Nowakowski, M.; Baron, B.; Brülé, S.; Hoos, S.; Raynal, B.; Guittat, L.; et al. SARS-CoV-2 Nsp3 unique domain SUD interacts with guanine quadruplexes and G4-ligands inhibit this interaction. *Nucleic Acids Res.* **2021**, *49*, 7695–7712. [CrossRef]

10. Liaw, Y.F.; Chu, C.M. Hepatitis B virus infection. *Lancet* **2009**, *373*, 582–592. [CrossRef]
11. Trepo, C.; Chan, H.L.Y.; Lok, A. Hepatitis B virus infection. *Lancet* **2014**, *384*, 2053–2063. [CrossRef]
12. Biswas, B.; Kandpal, M.; Vivekanandan, P. A G-quadruplex motif in an envelope gene promoter regulates transcription and virion secretion in HBV genotype B. *Nucleic Acids Res.* **2017**, *45*, 11268–11280. [CrossRef]
13. Lin, C.-L.; Kao, J.-H. The clinical implications of hepatitis B virus genotype: Recent advances. *J. Gastroenterol. Hepatol.* **2011**, *26*, 123–130. [CrossRef] [PubMed]
14. Seeger, C.; Mason, W.S. Hepatitis B virus biology. *Microbiol. Mol. Biol. Rev.* **2000**, *64*, 51. [CrossRef] [PubMed]
15. Lavezzo, E.; Berselli, M.; Frasson, I.; Perrone, R.; Palù, G.; Brazzale, A.R.; Richter, S.N.; Toppo, S. G-quadruplex forming sequences in the genome of all known human viruses: A comprehensive guide. *PLoS Comput. Biol.* **2018**, *14*, e1006675. [CrossRef] [PubMed]
16. Smeller, L. Pressure-temperature phase diagrams of biomolecules. *Biochim. Biophys. Acta* **2002**, *1595*, 11–29.
17. Meersman, F.; Dobson, C.M.; Heremans, K. Protein unfolding, amyloid fibril formation and configurational energy landscapes under high pressure conditions. *Chem. Soc. Rev.* **2006**, *35*, 908–917. [CrossRef]
18. Sebert, P. (Ed.) *Comparative High Pressure Biology*; CRC Press-Taylor & Francis Group: Boca Raton, FL, USA, 2010; pp. 1–555.
19. Smeller, L. Protein Denaturation on p-T Axes—Thermodynamics and Analysis. *High Press. Biosci.* **2015**, *72*, 19–39.
20. Winter, R. Interrogating the Structural Dynamics and Energetics of Biomolecular Systems with Pressure Modulation. *Annu. Rev. Biophys.* **2019**, *48*, 441–463. [CrossRef] [PubMed]
21. Roche, J.; Royer, C.A. Lessons from pressure denaturation of proteins. *J. R. Soc. Interface* **2018**, *15*, 21. [CrossRef]
22. Chalikian, T.V.; Macgregor, R.B. Volumetric Properties of Four-Stranded DNA Structures. *Biology* **2021**, *10*, 813. [CrossRef]
23. Meersman, F.; McMillan, P.F. High hydrostatic pressure: A probing tool and a necessary parameter in biophysical chemistry. *Chem. Commun.* **2013**, *50*, 766–775. [CrossRef] [PubMed]
24. Somkuti, J.; Bublin, M.; Breiteneder, H.; Smeller, L. Pressure-Temperature Stability, Ca2+ Binding, and Pressure-Temperature Phase Diagram of Cod Parvalbumin: Gad m 1. *Biochemistry* **2012**, *51*, 5903–5911. [CrossRef] [PubMed]
25. Molnár, O.R.; Somkuti, J.; Smeller, L. Negative volume changes of human G-quadruplexes at unfolding. *Heliyon* **2020**, *6*, e05702. [CrossRef]
26. Somkuti, J.; Molnár, O.R.; Smeller, L. Revealing unfolding steps and volume changes of human telomeric i-motif DNA. *Phys. Chem. Chem. Phys.* **2020**, *22*, 23816–23823. [CrossRef]
27. Meersman, F.; Dobson, C.M. Probing the pressure-temperature stability of amyloid fibrils provides new insights into their molecular properties. *Biochim. Biophys. Acta* **2006**, *1764*, 452–460. [CrossRef] [PubMed]
28. Jahmidi-Azizi, N.; Oliva, R.; Gault, S.; Cockell, C.; Winter, R. The Effects of Temperature and Pressure on Protein-Ligand Binding in the Presence of Mars-Relevant Salts. *Biology* **2021**, *10*, 687. [CrossRef] [PubMed]
29. Dirix, C.; Meersman, F.; MacPhee, C.E.; Dobson, C.M.; Heremans, K. High hydrostatic pressure dissociates early aggregates of TTR105-115, but not the mature amyloid fibrils. *J. Mol. Biol.* **2005**, *347*, 903–909. [CrossRef] [PubMed]
30. Roche, J.; Royer, C.A.; Roumestand, C. Exploring Protein Conformational Landscapes Using High-Pressure NMR. *Methods Enzym.* **2018**, *614*, 293–320.
31. Williamson, M.P.; Kitahara, R. Characterization of low-lying excited states of proteins by high-pressure NMR. *Biochim. Biophys. Acta* **2018**, *1867*, 350–358. [CrossRef] [PubMed]
32. Somkuti, J.; Mártonfalvi, Z.; Kellermayer, M.; Smeller, L. Different pressure-temperature behavior of the structured and unstructured regions of titin. *Biochim. Biophys. Acta* **2013**, *1834*, 112–118. [CrossRef]
33. Dubois, C.; Planelles-Herrero, V.; Tillatte-Tripodi, C.; Delbecq, S.; Mammri, L.; Sirkia, E.; Ropars, V.; Roumestand, C.; Barthe, P. Pressure and Chemical Unfolding of an α-Helical Bundle Protein: The GH2 Domain of the Protein Adaptor GIPC1. *Int. J. Mol. Sci.* **2021**, *22*, 3597. [CrossRef] [PubMed]
34. Smeller, L.; Rubens, P.; Heremans, K. Pressure Effect on the Temperature-Induced Unfolding and Tendency to Aggregate of Myoglobin. *Biochemistry* **1999**, *38*, 3816–3820. [CrossRef]
35. Scheyhing, C.H.; Meersman, F.; Ehrmann, M.A.; Heremans, K.; Vogel, R.F. Temperature-pressure stability of green fluorescent protein: A Fourier transform infrared spectroscopy study. *Biopolymers* **2002**, *65*, 244–253. [CrossRef] [PubMed]
36. Ostermeier, L.; de Oliveira, G.A.; Dzwolak, W.; Silva, J.L.; Winter, R. Exploring the polymorphism, conformational dynamics and function of amyloidogenic peptides and proteins by temperature and pressure modulation. *Biophys. Chem.* **2020**, *268*, 106506. [CrossRef] [PubMed]
37. Kriegler, S.; Herzog, M.; Oliva, R.; Gault, S.; Cockell, C.S.; Winter, R. Structural responses of model biomembranes to Mars-relevant salts. *Phys. Chem. Chem. Phys.* **2021**, *23*, 14212–14223. [CrossRef] [PubMed]
38. Winter, R. *Pressure Effects on Artificial and Cellular Membranes, in High Pressure Bioscience: Basic Concepts, Applications and Frontiers*; Akasaka, K., Matsuki, H., Eds.; Springer: Berlin/Heidelberg, Germany, 2015; pp. 345–370.
39. Takahashi, S.; Sugimoto, N. Pressure-dependent formation of i-motif and G-quadruplex DNA structures. *Phys. Chem. Chem. Phys.* **2015**, *17*, 31004–31010. [CrossRef]
40. Fan, H.Y.; Shek, Y.L.; Amiri, A.; Dubins, D.N.; Heerklotz, H.; MacGregor, R.B.; Chalikian, T.V. Volumetric Characterization of Sodium-Induced G-Quadruplex Formation. *J. Am. Chem. Soc.* **2011**, *133*, 4518–4526. [CrossRef]
41. Takahashi, S.; Sugimoto, N. Effect of pressure on the stability of G-quadruplex DNA: Thermodynamics under crowding conditions. *Angew. Chem. Int. Ed. Engl.* **2013**, *52*, 13774–13778. [CrossRef] [PubMed]

42. Somkuti, J.; Adányi, M.; Smeller, L. Self-crowding influences the temperature—Pressure stability of the human telomere G-quadruplex. *Biophys. Chem.* **2019**, *254*, 106248. [CrossRef] [PubMed]
43. Wong, P.T.T.; Moffat, D.J. A New Internal Pressure Calibrant for High-Pressure Infrared Spectroscopy of Aqueous Systems. *Appl. Spectrosc.* **1989**, *43*, 1279–1281. [CrossRef]
44. Dai, J.; Punchihewa, C.; Ambrus, A.; Chen, D.; Jones, R.A.; Yang, D. Structure of the intramolecular human telomeric G-quadruplex in potassium solution: A novel adenine triple formation. *Nucleic Acids Res.* **2007**, *35*, 2440–2450. [CrossRef] [PubMed]
45. Oliva, R.; Mukherjee, S.; Winter, R. Unraveling the binding characteristics of small ligands to telomeric DNA by pressure modulation. *Sci. Rep.* **2021**, *11*, 9714. [CrossRef]
46. Orsolya Réka Molnár, A.V.; Somkuti, J.; Smeller, L. Characterization of a G-quadruplex from hepatitis B virus and its stabilization by binding TMPyP4, BRACO19 and PhenDC3. *Sci. Rep.* **2021**, in press.
47. Largy, E.; Mergny, J.-L.; Gabelica, V. Role of Alkali Metal Ions in G-Quadruplex Nucleic Acid Structure and Stability. *Alkali Metal Ions* **2016**, *16*, 203–258.
48. Ambrus, A.; Chen, D.; Dai, J.; Bialis, T.; Jones, R.A.; Yang, D. Human telomeric sequence forms a hybrid-type intramolecular G-quadruplex structure with mixed parallel/antiparallel strands in potassium solution. *Nucleic Acids Res.* **2006**, *34*, 2723–2735. [CrossRef]
49. Li, Y.Y.; Dubins, D.N.; Le, D.M.N.T.; Leung, K.; Macgregor, R.B. The role of loops and cation on the volume of unfolding of G-quadruplexes related to HTel. *Biophys. Chem.* **2017**, *231*, 55–63. [CrossRef] [PubMed]
50. Guédin, A.; Gros, J.; Alberti, P.; Mergny, J.-L. How long is too long? Effects of loop size on G-quadruplex stability. *Nucleic Acids Res.* **2010**, *38*, 7858–7868. [CrossRef] [PubMed]
51. Bhattacharyya, D.; Arachchilage, G.M.; Basu, S. Metal Cations in G-Quadruplex Folding and Stability. *Front. Chem.* **2016**, *4*, 38. [CrossRef] [PubMed]
52. Venczel, E.A.; Sen, D. Parallel and antiparallel G-DNA structures from a complex telomeric sequence. *Biochemistry* **1993**, *32*, 6220–6228. [CrossRef] [PubMed]
53. Sen, D.; Gilbert, W. A sodium-potassium switch in the formation of four-stranded G4-DNA. *Nature* **1990**, *344*, 410–414. [CrossRef] [PubMed]
54. Good, N.E.; Winget, G.D.; Winter, W.; Connolly, T.N.; Izawa, S.; Singh, R.M.M. Hydrogen Ion Buffers for Biological Research. *Biochemistry* **1966**, *5*, 467–477. [CrossRef]
55. Banyay, M.; Sarkar, M.; Gräslund, A. A library of IR bands of nucleic acids in solution. *Biophys. Chem.* **2003**, *104*, 477–488. [CrossRef]
56. Mondragón-Sánchez, J.A.; Liquier, J.; Shafer, R.H.; Taillandier, E. Tetraplex Structure Formation in the Thrombin-Binding DNA Aptamer by Metal Cations Measured by Vibrational Spectroscopy. *J. Biomol. Struct. Dyn.* **2004**, *22*, 365–373. [CrossRef] [PubMed]
57. Taillandier, E.; Liquier, J. Infrared-Spectroscopy of DNA. *Methods Enzymol.* **1992**, *211*, 307–335. [PubMed]
58. Li, Y.Y.; Abu-Ghazalah, R.; Zamiri, B.; MacGregor, R.B., Jr. Concentration-dependent conformational changes in GQ-forming ODNs. *Biophys. Chem.* **2016**, *211*, 70–75. [CrossRef]
59. Panick, G.; Vidugiris, G.J.A.; Malessa, R.; Rapp, G.; Winter, R.; Royer, C.A. Exploring the Temperature-Pressure Phase Diagram of Staphylococcal Nuclease. *Biochemistry* **1999**, *38*, 4157–4164. [CrossRef] [PubMed]
60. Eisenberg, D.S.; Kauzmann, W. *The Structure and Properties of Water*; Oxford University Press: Oxford, UK, 2005; p. 296.
61. Basu, A.; Kumar, G.S. Calorimetric investigation on the interaction of proflavine with human telomeric G-quadruplex DNA. *J. Chem. Thermodyn.* **2016**, *98*, 208–213. [CrossRef]
62. Takahashi, S.; Bhowmik, S.; Sugimoto, N. Volumetric analysis of formation of the complex of G-quadruplex DNA with hemin using high pressure. *J. Inorg. Biochem.* **2017**, *166*, 199–207. [CrossRef]
63. Shek, Y.L.; Noudeh, G.D.; Nazari, M.; Heerklotz, H.; Abu-Ghazalah, R.M.; Dubins, D.N.; Chalikian, T.V. Folding thermodynamics of the hybrid-1 type intramolecular human telomeric G-quadruplex. *Biopolymers* **2013**, *101*, 216–227. [CrossRef]
64. Luo, Y.; Granzhan, A.; Verga, D.; Mergny, J. FRET—MC: A fluorescence melting competition assay for studying G4 structures in vitro. *Biopolymers* **2020**, *112*, ebip23415. [CrossRef] [PubMed]

biology

MDPI

Review

Volumetric Properties of Four-Stranded DNA Structures

Tigran V. Chalikian * and Robert B. Macgregor, Jr.

Department of Pharmaceutical Sciences, Leslie Dan Faculty of Pharmacy, University of Toronto, 144 College Street, Toronto, ON M5S 3M2, Canada; rob.macgregor@utoronto.ca
* Correspondence: t.chalikian@utoronto.ca; Tel.: +1-416-946-3715; Fax: +1-416-978-8511

Simple Summary: The volumetric properties of biomolecules define their pressure stability, while also characterizing their intrinsic and hydration properties. In this paper, we review the recent progress in volumetric investigations of G-quadruplexes and *i*-motifs, four-stranded secondary structures of DNA that have been found in the cell and implicated in regulatory genomic functions. Although the volumetric studies of G-quadruplexes and *i*-motifs are still in their nascent state, the data on volume, expansibility, and compressibility accumulated to date have begun to provide insights into the balance of forces governing the stability of these non-canonical structures. We present the available volumetric data and discuss how they can be rationalized in terms of intra-and intermolecular interactions involving G-quadruplexes and *i*-motifs including their solute-solvent interactions.

Abstract: Four-stranded non-canonical DNA structures including G-quadruplexes and *i*-motifs have been found in the genome and are thought to be involved in regulation of biological function. These structures have been implicated in telomere biology, genomic instability, and regulation of transcription and translation events. To gain an understanding of the molecular determinants underlying the biological role of four-stranded DNA structures, their biophysical properties have been extensively studied. The limited libraries on volume, expansibility, and compressibility accumulated to date have begun to provide insights into the molecular origins of helix-to-coil and helix-to-helix conformational transitions involving four-stranded DNA structures. In this article, we review the recent progress in volumetric investigations of G-quadruplexes and *i*-motifs, emphasizing how such data can be used to characterize intra-and intermolecular interactions, including solvation. We describe how volumetric data can be interpreted at the molecular level to yield a better understanding of the role that solute–solvent interactions play in modulating the stability and recognition events of nucleic acids. Taken together, volumetric studies facilitate unveiling the molecular determinants of biological events involving biopolymers, including G-quadruplexes and *i*-motifs, by providing one more piece to the thermodynamic puzzle describing the energetics of cellular processes in vitro and, by extension, in vivo.

Keywords: G-quadruplex; *i*-motif; volumetric properties; pressure-temperature phase diagram; thermodynamics

Citation: Chalikian, T.V.; Macgregor, R.B., Jr. Volumetric Properties of Four-Stranded DNA Structures. *Biology* **2021**, *10*, 813. https://doi.org/10.3390/biology10080813

Academic Editor: Dmitri Davydov

Received: 15 July 2021
Accepted: 19 August 2021
Published: 22 August 2021

1. Introduction

DNA molecules rich in guanine are prone to folding into four-stranded G-quadruplex structures, while cytosine-rich molecules tend to fold into four-stranded *i*-motif structures at slightly acidic pH [1–9]. G-quadruplexes are formed by stacking of two or more G-tetrads on top of each other. A G-tetrad represents a cyclic planar construct in which four guanine bases are linked together via Hoogsteen hydrogen bonds as shown in Figure 1a. The stacking results in the formation of a central cavity in which mono- or divalent cations are coordinated to the O6 atoms of guanines [1–3,7,10–12]. Sodium and potassium are the two biologically most relevant cations stabilizing G-quadruplex structures. The four consecutive G-runs involved in the formation of stacked tetrads in an intramolecular G-quadruplex are connected to each other via three single stranded linkers known as loops.

The polarity of the loops defines the specific topology assumed by the G-quadruplex. G-quadruplexes can assume a parallel, antiparallel, or hybrid topologies with the molecularity ranging from mono to tetra (Figure 1b) [7,8,13].

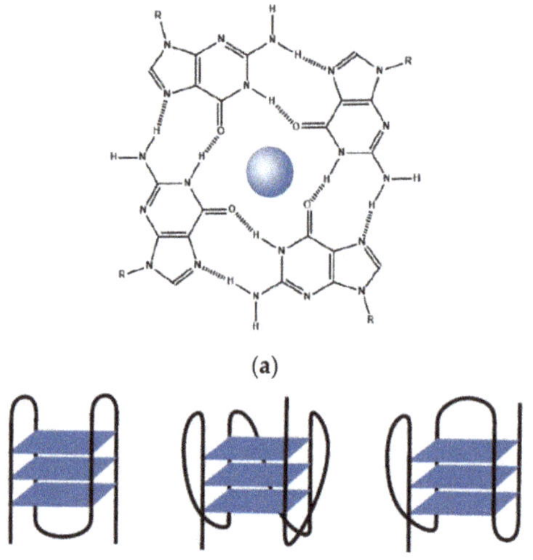

(a) (b)

Figure 1. (**a**) Structure of a G-quartet with a coordinated ion; (**b**) Schematic representation of antiparallel, parallel, and hybrid intramolecular G-quadruplexes.

Cytosine-rich DNA molecules can fold into the four-stranded *i*-motif conformation in which two parallel duplexes interact in an anti-parallel manner through mutual intercalation of hemiprotonated cytosine base pairs (Figure 2a,b) [4–6,14–16]. Although *i*-motif structures are favored at slightly acidic pH, they may exist at neutral pH, making the study of *i*-motifs biologically relevant [4,14,17–20]. In fact, there is increasing evidence suggesting that four-stranded nucleic acid structures, including G-quadruplex and *i*-motif structures, exist in the cell and are involved in regulation of genomic events including telomere control, gene expression, and DNA replication [10,21–30]. The existence of *i*-motifs in vivo may be related to an increase in the pK_a of cytosine protonation in the crowded environment of the cell [31]. In addition, given the excluded volume effect, crowders may stabilize the compact *i*-motif conformation relative the extended unfolded conformation [31].

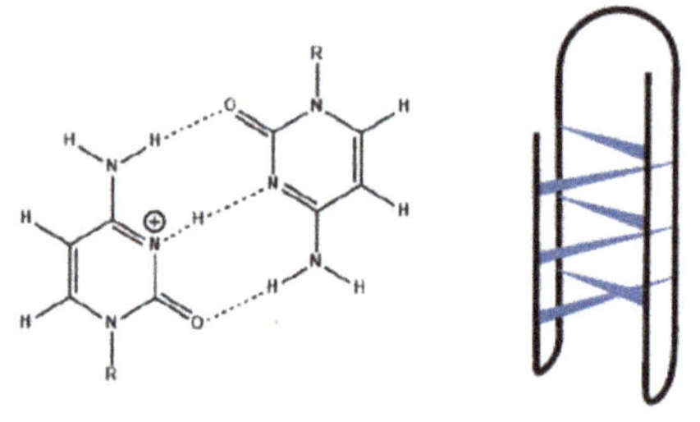

(a) (b)

Figure 2. (**a**) A hemiprotonated cytosine-cytosine$^+$ base pair; (**b**) Schematic representation of an *i*-motif structure.

The thermodynamic and kinetic properties of interconversions between the duplex, tetraplex, and single-stranded conformations will necessarily constrain and define the role these structures play in vivo [7,32,33]. The stability characteristics of G-quadruplex and *i*-motif structures have been extensively and systematically studied by varying parameters such as temperature, pH, salt, and the concentration of cosolvent [4,5,7,31,32,34–42]. These studies have provided a wealth of information about the modulation of the differential free energy of the folded and unfolded conformations of the two tetrahelical DNA structures as a function of temperature, pH, salt, and the identity and concentration of cosolvents [32]. Comparative analyses of thermodynamic data have provided valuable insights into the contributions of intra- and intermolecular interactions (e.g., counterion-DNA interactions) and individual structural features (e.g., the length and nucleotide content of loops) to the stability of G-quadruplexes and *i*-motifs [32].

The volumetric data obtained from pressure-dependent measurements complement the stability data afforded by more conventional temperature-, pH-, salt-, and cosolvent-dependent studies [43–49]. Analysis of the effect of hydrostatic pressure on the equilibrium between the folded and unfolded DNA structures yield molar changes in volume, expansibility, and compressibility that accompany formation of the folded structures. The volumetric properties of solutes are determined by the entire ensemble of intra- and intermolecular interactions involving the solute, including solute–solvent interactions, and volume and energy fluctuations of the solute molecule [45–47,50–55]. The volumetric characteristics of G-quadruplexes and *i*-motifs reflect their structural and hydration properties, which differ significantly from those of other nucleic acid secondary structures, such as the B-form DNA duplex. The four-stranded structures are globular in shape with a surface charge density lower than that of other DNA structures; in addition, the G-quadruplex exhibits a compressible and expandable internal cavity [34,35,56,57].

In this work, we describe the current state of the art and give an overview of the studies that have dealt with the volumetric characterization of G-quadruplex and *i*-motif structures. We begin by defining volumetric properties. Next, we outline the experimental methods that have been used in volumetric investigations and explain how macroscopic volumetric properties can be rationalized to gain microscopic insights. We subsequently proceed to reviewing published data on changes in volume, expansibility, and compressibility accompanying conformational transitions involving tetraplex DNA structures. Finally, we discuss the use of volumetric properties to construct the pressure–temperature diagram of G-quadruplex stability.

2. Definitions and Experimental Methods

2.1. Observables

The partial molar volume of a solute, V°, is the pressure slope of its chemical potential, μ:

$$V^\circ = \left(\frac{\partial \mu}{\partial P}\right)_T = \lim_{C\to 0}\left(\frac{\partial V}{\partial N}\right)_{T,P} \quad (1)$$

where P is the pressure; T is the temperature; V is the volume of solution; N is the number of moles of a solute in solution; and C is the concentration of a solute.

The partial molar expansibility of a solute is the temperature derivative of its partial molar volume:

$$E^\circ = \left(\frac{\partial V^\circ}{\partial T}\right)_P = \left(\frac{\partial^2 \mu}{\partial P \partial T}\right) = \lim_{C\to 0}\left(\frac{\partial \alpha V}{\partial N}\right)_{T,P} \quad (2)$$

where $\alpha = \frac{1}{V}\left(\frac{\partial V}{\partial T}\right)_P$ is the coefficient of thermal expansibility of solution; and $E = \alpha V$ is the expansibility of solution.

The partial molar isothermal compressibility of a solute is the negative pressure derivative of partial molar volume:

$$K^\circ{}_T = \left(\frac{\partial V^\circ}{\partial P}\right)_T = -\left(\frac{\partial^2 \mu}{\partial P^2}\right)_T = \lim_{C\to 0}\left(\frac{\partial \beta_T V}{\partial N}\right)_{T,P} \quad (3)$$

where $\beta_T = -\frac{1}{V}(\frac{\partial V}{\partial P})_T$ is the coefficient of isothermal compressibility of solution; and $K_T = \beta_T V$ is the isothermal compressibility of solution.

The partial molar adiabatic compressibility of a solute is given by:

$$K^\circ{}_S = \lim_{C\to 0}\left(\frac{\partial \beta_S V}{\partial N}\right)_{T,P} \quad (4)$$

where $\beta_S = -\frac{1}{V}(\frac{\partial V}{\partial P})_S$ is the coefficient of adiabatic compressibility of solution; S is the entropy; and $K_S = \beta_S V$ is the adiabatic compressibility of solution.

Partial molar isothermal and adiabatic compressibilities are related to each other via the relationship [58,59]:

$$K^\circ{}_T = K^\circ{}_S + \frac{T\alpha_0^2}{\rho_0 C_{P0}}\cdot\left(\frac{2E^\circ}{\alpha_0} - \frac{C^\circ{}_P}{\rho_0 c_{P0}}\right) \quad (5)$$

where α_0, ρ_0, and c_{P0} are the coefficient of thermal expansion, density, and specific heat capacity of the neat solvent, respectively; and $C^\circ{}_P$ is the partial molar heat capacity of a solute.

According to scaled particle theory, the partial molar volume, V°, can be broken down into the following terms [60,61]:

$$V^\circ = V_C + V_I + \beta_{T0}RT \quad (6)$$

where V_C is the volume of the cavity comprising a solute; it is given by $V_C = V_M + V_T$; V_M is the molecular volume of a solute; V_T is the void volume around a solute (the thermal volume); V_I is the interaction volume that is a change in solvent volume under the influence of solute-solvent interactions; and β_{T0} is the coefficient of isothermal compressibility of solvent.

Interaction volume, V_I is related to the properties of water of solute hydration via $V_I = n_h(V^\circ{}_h - V^\circ{}_0)$, where n_h is the hydration number (the number of water molecules influenced by the solute), and $V^\circ{}_h$ and $V^\circ{}_0$ are the partial molar volumes of water of hydration and bulk water, respectively.

The partial molar expansibility, E°, and adiabatic compressibility, $K^\circ{}_S$, of a solute are related to its intrinsic and hydration properties as follows:

$$E^\circ = E_M + n_h(E^\circ{}_h - E^\circ{}_0) \quad (7)$$

$$K^\circ{}_S = K_M + n_h(K^\circ{}_{Sh} - K^\circ{}_{S0}) \quad (8)$$

where E_M and K_M are, respectively, the intrinsic expansibility and compressibility of the solute molecule; $E^\circ{}_h$ and $E^\circ{}_0$ are the partial molar expansibilities of water of hydration and bulk water, respectively; and $K^\circ{}_{Sh}$ and $K^\circ{}_{S0}$ are the partial molar adiabatic compressibilities of water of hydration and bulk water, respectively.

The volumetric properties of a solute can be expressed more rigorously based on the concepts of statistical thermodynamics in which water of hydration is represented by a heterogeneous network of solvent molecules with varying affinities for the solute [62–64]. The statistical thermodynamic formalism has been extended to the analysis of the volumetric properties of solutes in binary solvents consisting of water and water-miscible cosolvents [51,65].

2.2. Experimental Techniques

Differential measurements of density of solution and solvent have been widely employed to measure the partial molar volume, V°, of solutes and changes in volume, ΔV, accompanying their binding events and conformational transitions [66–77]. The partial molar volume, V°, of a solute can be determined from density data as follows:

$$V^\circ = \frac{M}{\rho_0} - \frac{\rho - \rho_0}{\rho_0 C} = \frac{M}{\rho} - \frac{\rho - \rho_0}{\rho\rho_0 m} \quad (9)$$

where ρ and ρ_0 are the densities of solution and solvent, respectively; M is the molecular mass of a solute; and C and m are the molar and molal concentrations of a solute, respectively.

If measurements of volume are carried out as a function of temperature, the resulting data can be used to determine the partial molar expansibility, $E°$, of a solute or a change in expansibility, ΔE, accompanying a reaction involving a solute such as a conformational transition or ligand binding [78]. Pressure-perturbation calorimetry (PPC) offers an alternative way to determine the partial molar expansibility, $E°$, of a solute as a function of temperature [79–83]. If a change in temperature within the experimental range causes a conformational transition of the solute, the measured $E°(T)$ profile will display a characteristic peak. Given $E° = (\frac{\partial V°}{\partial T})_P$ [see Equation (2)], a change in volume, ΔV, accompanying the conformational transition equals the area under the peak:

$$\Delta V = \int_{T_1}^{T_2} E^o(T)dT \quad (10)$$

A combination of density and sound velocity measurements can be used to determine the partial molar adiabatic compressibility, $K°_S$, of solutes and changes in adiabatic compressibility, ΔK_S, accompanying binding events and conformational transitions [84,85]. Sound velocity, U, in a medium is related to its density, ρ, and coefficient of adiabatic compressibility, β_S, via the Newton-Laplace equation: $U^2 = (\rho\beta_S)^{-1}$. Differentiation of this equation with respect to the concentration of a solute yields the following relationship for its partial molar adiabatic compressibility for the limit of infinite dilution [84,86,87]:

$$K°_S = \beta_{S0}\left(2V° - 2[U] - \frac{M}{\rho_0}\right) \quad (11)$$

where β_{S0} is the coefficient of adiabatic compressibility of solvent; $[U] = \frac{U-U_0}{U_0 C}$ is the relative molar sound velocity increment of a solute; U and U_0 are the sound velocities in solution and solvent, respectively.

Pressure-dependent measurements of conformation-sensitive spectroscopic parameters (typically, light absorption, fluorescence, NMR, and, more recently, circular dichroism) have been used to monitor pressure-induced shifts in the conformational equilibria of proteins and nucleic acids [88–91]. Provided that the solute population is restricted to two conformations (folded and unfolded), such measurements enable one to determine the equilibrium constant, K, as a function of pressure. In turn, the pressure dependence of K can be used to calculate a change in volume, ΔV, accompanying the conformational transition:

$$\Delta V = -RT\left(\frac{\partial lnK}{\partial P}\right)_T \quad (12)$$

Alternatively, ΔV can be determined from the Clausius–Clapeyron relation:

$$\frac{dT_M}{dP} = T_M\frac{\Delta V}{\Delta H} \quad (13)$$

where T_M is the transition temperature; and ΔH is the transition enthalpy.

3. Differential Volume of Four-Stranded and Single-Stranded Conformations

3.1. G-quadruplexes

Table 1 presents a compilation of literature data on changes in volume accompanying unfolding transitions of G-quadruplexes differing in topology and sequence. Inspection of Table 1 reveals that G-quadruplex-to-single strand transitions are accompanied by negative changes in volume, ΔV [48,92–97]. To rationalize a change in volume accompanying G-quadruplex unfolding, one needs to carefully consider the entire set of molecular interactions that may contribute to the change. Equation (6) can be modified to analyze the molecular origins underlying the negative values of ΔV observed for G-quadruplex unfolding:

$$\Delta V = \Delta V_M + \Delta V_T + \Delta V_I + n_{M+} V_{M+} \quad (14)$$

where n_{M+} is the number of stabilizing cations released from the central cavity to the bulk; and V_{M+} is the partial molar volume of the stabilizing cation.

The differential molecular, ΔV_M, and thermal, ΔV_T, volumes of the G-quadruplex and coiled states of DNA can be computed from the X-ray or NMR structure of the G-quadruplex conformation and the molecular dynamics-simulated single-stranded conformations. A change in thermal volume, ΔV_T, is related to a change in solvent-accessible surface area, ΔS_A, via $\Delta V_T = \delta \Delta S_A$, where δ = 0.5 Å is the thickness of the thermal volume [98].

Table 1. Changes in volume, ΔV, accompanying the unfolding transitions of G-quadruplexes differing in sequence, topology, and stabilizing cation determined at temperature, T.

Sequence (DNA)	Topology	Cation	T, °C	ΔV, cm^3 mol^{-1}
d($G_2T_2G_2TGT$-$G_2T_2G_2$) (TBA) [a]	Antiparallel	K^+	58.1 ± 1.4	−54.6 ± 4.2
d[A(G_3T_2A)$_3G_3$](Tel22) [b]	Antiparallel	Na^+	54.6 ± 0.9	−38.4 ± 10.1
d[A(G_3T_2A)$_3G_3$](Tel22) [c]	Antiparallel	Na^+	40.0 ± 0.6	−66 ± 3
d[A(G_3T_2A)$_3G_3$](Tel22) [b]	Hybrid	K^+	64.6 ± 2.2	−42.7 ± 6.7
d[TGA(G_3TG_3TA)$_2$A](c-MYC) [d]	Parallel	K^+	83.4 ± 1.1	−16.9 ± 1.8
d($AG_3AG_3CGCTG_3$-AG_2AG_3) (KIT) [d]	Parallel	K^+	58.5 ± 0.4	−6.2 ± 0.9
d($T_2G_4CG_3C_2G_5C$-G_4T_2) (VEGF) [d]	Parallel	K^+	78.8 ± 1.1	−18.1 ± 4.6
d[A_3(G_3T_2A)$_3G_3A_2$](Tel26) [e]	Hybrid	K^+	25.0	−69 ± 7
d[TGA(G_3TG_3TA)$_2$A](c-MYC) [f]	Parallel	K^+	25.0	−34 ± 15

[a] from ref. [94]; [b] from ref. [97]; [c] from ref. [92]; [d] from ref. [96]; [e] from ref. [93]; [f] from ref. [99].

Table 2 shows the computed changes in intrinsic (molecular) volume, ΔV_M, and solvent accessible surface area, ΔS_A, associated with the unfolding transitions of three G-quadruplex structures, specifically, the Na^+-stabilized antiparallel human telomeric G-quadruplex Tel22 [d(A(G_3T_2A)$_3G_3$)], the K^+-stabilized hybrid human telomeric G-quadruplex Tel26 [d(A_3(G_3T_2A)$_3G_3A_2$)], and the K^+-stabilized parallel c-MYC G-quadruplex [d($TGAG_3TG_3TAG_3TG_3T_2$)]. It is tempting to ascribe the negative change in volume to the presence of the intramolecular cavity within the G-quadruplex, which makes it distinct from other secondary structures (e.g., double- and triple-stranded DNA). However, elimination of the central cavity due to unfolding provides just one of the negative contributions to the change in volume. This source of negative volume change must be considered in concert with other contributions such as the release of counterions and changes in hydration and thermal volume.

Table 2. Changes in volume, ΔV (cm^3 mol^{-1}), determined at 25 °C, intrinsic volume, ΔV_M (cm^3 mol^{-1}), solvent accessible surface area, ΔS_A (Å^2), thermal volume, ΔV_T (cm^3 mol^{-1}), and interaction volume, ΔV_I, accompanying G-quadruplex unfolding transitions.

G-Quadruplex	ΔV	ΔV_M	ΔS_A	$\Delta V_T = \delta \Delta S_A$	ΔV_I [a]
Tel22	−67	−233 [b]	1230 [b]	370	−186
Tel26	−69	−4 [c]	2348 [c]	707	−779
c-MYC	−34	2 [d]	879 [d]	265	−306

[a] $\Delta V_I = \Delta V - (\Delta V_M + \Delta V_T + n_{M+} V_{M+})$; [b] computed based on PDB entry 143D [92]; [c] computed based on PDB entry 2HY9 [93]; [d] computed based on PDB entry 1XAV [34].

The release of cations internally bound inside the central cavity contributes to the volumetric properties of G-quadruplex transitions. The $n_{M+} V_{M+}$ term in Equation (14) serves to take this contribution into account. On the other hand, G-quadruplex unfolding is not accompanied by a pronounced release of externally bound (condensed) counterions [34,35,56]. In this respect, G-quadruplexes are distinct from other DNA structures, such as the double-stranded B-DNA. Depending on the specific G-quadruplex topology and loop and flanking sequences, the unfolding transition may lead to a very slight release, no release, or significant uptake of external counterions [34,35,56]. Thus, the uptake or release of these counterions should contribute only modestly to the observed changes in volume.

Inspection of data in Table 2 reveals a change in molecular volume, ΔV_M, which involves the contribution due to the elimination of the central cavity, is not the main component of the experimentally measured change in volume accompanying the unfolding transitions of G-quadruplexes. The thermal, ΔV_T, and interaction, ΔV_I, contributions are large and play a decisive role in determining the magnitude and the sign of the overall change in volume, ΔV, associated with G-quadruplex unfolding.

Changes in volume, ΔV, accompanying G-quadruplex unfolding transitions have been combined with structural data on ΔV_M and ΔS_A to estimate the values of ΔV_I and changes in hydration, Δn_h [92,93]. The estimates of Δn_h were 103, 432, and 170 for the Tel22, Tel26, and c-MYC G-quadruplexes, respectively [92,93]. Thus, G-quadruplex-to-coil transitions are all accompanied by an increase in hydration with a considerable uptake of water from the bulk. The estimated changes in hydration represent the differential hydration of the folded and unfolded states. A recent crystallographic study revealed elaborate, topology-dependent, organized networks of water molecules in the grooves and loop regions of G-quadruplexes [100]. It was found that the primary sphere water molecules make direct contacts with groove and loop atomic groups, thereby contributing to the stability of the specific G-quadruplex topology and loop conformations [100]. Disruption of such water networks contributes to the changes in hydration that are observed in and evaluated from the results of volumetric measurements.

3.2. Influence of the Bases in the Loops

The Sugimoto and Macgregor groups simultaneously published systematic studies of the extent to which the loops of G-quadruplex structures influence the effect of hydrostatic pressure on the stability of these tetrahelical structures [97,101]. The experimental space in such measurements is very large; for each simple, monomolecular oligonucleotide that can fold into a G-quadruplex, there are three different loops, each of which can have a different sequence and number of bases (or other linking moieties). In this respect, loops are highly polymorphic; and we are still a long way from an understanding of how the loops influence molar changes in volume that accompany folding of intramolecular G-quadruplexes.

Two systems have been studied; these are the thrombin binding aptamer (TBA) and the human telomeric sequence (Tel22) [97,101]. In order to attempt to isolate the factors that arise solely from the loops, the sequence of the loops has been systematically altered while preserving the topology of the folded structure [97,101]. The original and altered G-quadruplex-forming oligonucleotides that have been investigated are shown in Tables 3 and 4. In addition to nucleic acid base substitutions, Takahashi and Sugimoto examined the behavior of TBA derivatives in which the loops were replaced by a 12-carbon methylene linker, $(\text{-CH}_2\text{-})_{12}$ [101]. These substitutions remove the ability of the bases in the loops to stack with the G-tetrads in TBA.

Table 3. Molar chanes in volume (ΔV) accompanying the unfolding transitions of thrombin binding aptamer (TBA) and thrombin binding aptamers with altered loops determined from the pressure dependences of the unfolding temperature, T_M. The values were calculated from analysis of the effect of hydrostatic pressure on the thermal unfolding of the G-quadruplex using the Clapeyron equation. For TBA 1LC12 and TBA 2LC12, a 12-carbon methylene chain replaces the nucleobases in the respective loops. The changes in the original TBA sequence are underlined.

DNA	Sequence	T_M, °C [e]	ΔV, cm^3 mol^{-1}
TBA [a,c]	d($G_2T_2G_2TGTG_2T_2G_2$)	52.6 ± 3.4	−54.6 ± 4.2
TBA T3A [b,c]	d($G_2\underline{A}TG_2TGTG_2T_2G_2$)	45.1 ± 0.1	−75.5 ± 2.2
TBA G8T [b,c]	d($G_2T_2G_2T\underline{T}TG_2T_2G_2$)	47.1 ± 6.6	−41.1 ± 2.4
TBA 1LC12 [b,c]	d[$G_2\underline{\text{-}(CH_2)_{12}\text{-}}G_2TGTG_2T_2G_2$]	49.0 ± 3.9	−57.8 ± 8.4
TBA 2LC12 [b,c]	d[$G_2T_2G_2\underline{\text{-}(CH_2)_{12}\text{-}}G_2T_2G_2$]	36.5 ± 0.6	−103.4 ± 8.0
TBA [a,d]	d($G_2T_2G_2TGTG_2T_2G_2$)	59.3 ± 2.3	−12.9 ± 0.9
TBA T3A [b,d]	d($G_2\underline{A}TG_2TGTG_2T_2G_2$)	56.7 ± 2.2	−14.7 ± 4.9
TBA G8T [b,d]	d($G_2T_2G_2T\underline{T}TG_2T_2G_2$)	54.5 ± 0.7	−13.2 ± 2.1
TBA 1LC12 [b,d]	d[$G_2\underline{\text{-}(CH_2)_{12}\text{-}}G_2TGTG_2T_2G_2$]	56.6 ± 6.0	−9.7 ± 5.2
TBA 2LC12 [b,d]	d[$G_2T_2G_2\underline{\text{-}(CH_2)_{12}\text{-}}G_2T_2G_2$]	62.4 ± 0.3	−5.6 ± 1.7

[a] from ref. [94]; [b] from ref. [101]; [c] the solutions contained 30 mM Tris-HCl at pH 7.0 and 100 mM KCl; [d] the solutions contained 30 mM Tris-HCl at pH 7.0, 100 mM KCl, and 40 wt% PEG200; [e] the unfolding transition at atmospheric pressure.

Table 4. Volume changes associated with the unfolding of the original and modified human telomeric G-quadruplexes in the presence of Na^+ or K^+ at 57 °C, ΔV_{57} (cm^3 mol^{-1}), presented by Li et al. [97]. The changes to the original Tel22 sequence are underlined. Values were obtained by analyzing the effect of hydrostatic pressure on the equilibrium between the folded and unfolded states of the respective G-quadruplexes assuming a two-state monomolecular reaction. The values were extrapolated to a common temperature of 57 °C which corresponds to the average T_M of the G-quadruplexes studied. All samples contained 10 mM Tris at pH 7.4, 0.1 mM EDTA, and either 100 mM NaCl or 100 mM KCl.

DNA	Sequence	(ΔV, cm^3 mol^{-1})	
		Na^+	K^+
Tel22	d($AG_3T_2AG_3T_2AG_3T_2AG_3$)	−38.4 ± 10.1	−42.7 ± 6.7
L1AAT	d($AG_3\underline{AAT}G_3T_2AG_3T_2AG_3$)	−29.4 ± 5.6	−38.0 ± 7.3
L2AAT	d($AG_3T_2AG_3\underline{AAT}G_2T_2AG_3$)	−29.8 ± 10.1	−35.6 ± 8.0
L3AAT	d($AG_3T_2AG_3T_2AG_3\underline{AAT}G_3$)	−34.5 ± 1.1	−27.2 ± 6.4
L1TTT	d($AG_3\underline{TTT}G_3T_2AG_3T_2AG_3$)	−35.2 ± 3.0	−35.2 ± 3.9
L2TTT	d($AG_3T_2AG_3\underline{TTT}G_3T_2AG_3$)	−26.2 ± 8.0	−30.5 ± 11.1
L3TTT	d($AG_3T_2AG_2T_2AG_3\underline{TTT}G_3$)	−38.6 ± 4.0	−21.9 ± 7.9
L1AAA	d($AG_3\underline{AAA}G_3T_2AG_3T_2AG_3$)	−37.7 ± 9.0	−37.7 ± 4.8
L2AAA	d($AG_3T_2AG_3\underline{AAA}G_3T_2AG_3$)	−30.2 ± 13.1	−37.8 ± 1.0
L3AAA	d($AG_3T_2AG_3T_2AG_3\underline{AAA}G_3$)	−41.4 ± 6.8	−31.7 ± 1.0

Inspection of the data in Tables 3 and 4 reveals that the response of the TBA- and Tel22-based systems to hydrostatic pressure is qualitatively similar. The unfolding transitions of the studied G-quadruplexes shift to lower temperatures with increasing pressure regardless of the sequence of the loops, even when a (-CH_2-)$_{12}$ linker substitutes the bases of the loops; changes in volume, ΔV, accompanying unfolding of the G-quadruplexes are all negative.

However, the magnitude of ΔV depends on the nature of the substitution. In some cases, the substitution leads to a greater pressure sensitivity, while, in other cases, it does not result in an appreciable change in ΔV. Note that Takahashi and Sugimoto [101] reported their ΔV values at the T_M of G-quadruplex unfolding, whereas the data reported by Li et al. [97] were extrapolated to a common temperature of 57 °C (near the transition temperatures). Although the T_M values of the G-quadruplexes in the two studies appear to be similar, a more accurate picture of the role of the loops in the volume change of G-quadruplex unfolding would emerge if the values of ΔV from the two studies are extrapolated to the same temperature.

Takahashi and Sugimoto have also studied the pressure dependence of the stability of the TBA-based G-quadruplexes in aqueous solutions containing ethylene glycol, PEG200, and PEG4000 [94,95,101]. The values of ΔV for the TBA G-quadruplex and its derivatives in the presence of PEG200 are shown in Table 3. The purpose of including cosolvents is to study the role of solvation of the loops in the observed pressure dependences. Independent of the type of the cosolvent, the effect of pressure on the stability was significantly reduced in solutions containing cosolvents relative to the values of ΔV obtained in an aqueous buffer. For example, a change in volume, ΔV, accompanying the unfolding of TBA G-quadruplex decreases from -54.6 cm^3 mol^{-1} in water to -12.9 cm^3 mol^{-1} in PEG200 [94]. This finding was rationalized in terms of changes in interaction volume, ΔV_I, in Equation (14); it appears that the effect of the loop sequence on the molar changes in volume arises predominantly from the differential hydration of the loops.

It is apparent that other factors such as topological differences (i.e., parallel, anti-parallel, etc.) may also contribute to the observed behavior. In addition, it seems reasonable to propose that the stacking of the G-tetrads or the stacking of the bases in the loops with the G-tetrads might also significantly contribute to the molar volume change of unfolding. The role of the stacking of the G-tetrads has not been directly assessed to date. The data originating from the -$(CH_2)_{12}$-substituted oligonucleotides provide insights into how the stacking of the bases in the loops with the two terminal G-tetrads influence the volume change. Currently, however, it is difficult to assign with any degree of confidence the differential volumetric properties of the oligonucleotide constructs with and without the -$(CH_2)_{12}$- links to any one specific molecular interaction. Additional measurements are required in order to parse the roles of stacking and folding topology in the pressure-dependent stability of G-quadruplexes.

3.3. *i-Motifs*

Table 5 lists changes in volume, ΔV, measured for heat-induced and pH-induced *i*-motif-to-coil transitions. In contrast to G-quadruplexes, which are characterized by large negative changes in volume upon unfolding, *i*-motif-to-single strand transitions exhibit near-zero changes in volume [57,102,103]. Because of the small value of the volume change, the stability of *i*-motifs is nearly insensitive to hydrostatic pressure. In agreement with this expectation, the transition temperatures of the heat-induced *i*-motif-to-coil transitions do not change or change very weakly with pressure [57,102,103]. When treating the volumetric properties of *i*-motif structures derived from measurements at high pressures, it is important to account for the pressure-induced changes in the pH of the solution, as the stability of an *i*-motif critically depends on pH. It is easy to confound the resulting pH-induced change in *i*-motif stability for its pressure dependence with the resulting change in volume.

Table 5. Changes in volume, ΔV, and adiabatic compressibility, ΔK_S, accompanying the unfolding transitions of *i*-motif structures determined at temperature, T.

Sequence (DNA)	pH	T, °C	ΔV, cm^3 mol^{-1}	ΔK_S, 10^{-4} cm^3 mol^{-1}bar^{-1}
d($C_3TA_2)_3C_3$ (Tel22-iM) [a]	4.6	36	~0	
d($C_3TA_2)_3C_3$ (Tel22-iM) [b]	5.15	45.5	-11 ± 2	
d($T_2AC_3AC_3TAC_3A$-C_3TCA) (c-MYC-iM) [c]	5.0	25.0	~0	~0

[a] from ref. [102]; [b] from ref. [103]; [c] from ref. [57].

In the absence of structural data on *i*-motifs, one cannot reliably estimate the magnitude or even the sign of ΔV_M in Equation (14). As mentioned above, the value of ΔV_T correlates with a change in solvent-accessible surface area, S_A, of the DNA associated with the *i*-motif-to-coil transition. Since the *i*-motif conformation is more compact than the unfolded conformation (ΔS_A is negative), the change, ΔV_T, should be negative. The magnitude and the sign of ΔV_I are more difficult to assess. On the one hand, polar groups of hemiprotonated cytosine residues that are hydrogen-bonded with water in the coil state become buried within the interior of the *i*-motif, thereby diminishing the extent of solute−solvent interactions. On the other hand, the proximity of negatively charged phosphate groups within *i*-motif conformation should increase the charge density and enhance the volume-reducing effect of solute−solvent interactions, ΔV_I. The experimentally measured value of $\Delta V \approx 0$ suggests a near perfect compensation between the ΔV_M, ΔV_T, and ΔV_I terms in Equation (14).

4. Differential Expansibility

Table 6 presents changes in expansibility, ΔE, associated with G-quadruplex-to-coil transitions of the Tel22 and Tel26 telomeric sequences. The partial molar expansibilities, $E°$, of the two G-quadruplexes increase upon unfolding. The relationship for ΔE can be obtained by modifying Equation (7):

$$\Delta E = \Delta E_M + \Delta n_h(E°_h - E°_0) + n_{M+}E_{M+} + \Delta E_{rel} \quad (15)$$

where E_{M+} is the is the partial molar expansibility of the stabilizing cation; ΔE_{rel} is the change in the relaxation contribution, $E_{rel} = (\langle\Delta H\Delta V\rangle - \langle\Delta H\rangle\langle\Delta V\rangle)/RT^2$; $\langle\Delta H\rangle$ and $\langle\Delta V\rangle$ are, respectively, the ensemble average changes in enthalpy and volume relative to a "ground state" conformation.

Table 6. Changes in adiabatic compressibility, ΔK_S, and expansibility, ΔE, accompanying the unfolding transitions of G-quadruplexes varying in sequence, topology, and stabilizing cation at 25 °C.

Sequence (DNA)	Topology	Cation	ΔK_S, 10^{-4} cm^3 mol^{-1}bar^{-1}	ΔE, cm^3 mol^{-1}K^{-1}
d[A($G_3T_2A)_3G_3$](Tel22) [a]	Antiparallel	Na^+	-236 ± 20	0.87 ± 0.16
d[$A_3(G_3T_2A)_3G_3A_2$](Tel26) [b]	Hybrid	K^+	-332 ± 18	0.92 ± 0.07
d[TGA($G_3TG_3TA)_2A$](c-MYC) [c]	Parallel	K^+	-304 ± 26	

[a] from ref. [92]; [b] from ref. [93]; [c] from ref. [99].

The intrinsic term in Equation (15) is given by $\Delta E_M = \alpha_{MU}V_{MU} - \alpha_{MF}V_{MF}$, where α_{MU} and α_{MF} are the intrinsic coefficients of thermal expansibility of the unfolded (coil) and folded (G-quadruplex) states, respectively; and V_{MU} and V_{MF} are the intrinsic volumes of the unfolded (coil) and folded (G-quadruplex) states, respectively. The intrinsic coefficient of thermal expansibility of the unfolded state, α_{MU}, is close to zero. There are currently no data on the value of α_{MF}; however, one would expect the intrinsic coefficient of thermal expansibility of the folded state, α_{MF}, to be a sizeable quantity owing to the expandable central cavity. Therefore, ΔE_M should be negative for G-quadruplex unfolding. In the absence of data, it seems reasonable to propose that the value of α_{MF} is on the order of the intrinsic coefficient of thermal expansibility of globular proteins. In common with G-quadruplexes, globular proteins are characterized by potentially expandable internal voids [104,105]. The average intrinsic coefficient of thermal expansibility of globular proteins is ~1×10^{-4} K^{-1} [50].

The relaxation component, ΔE_{rel}, originates from the existence of a broadly distributed isoenergetic population of unfolded conformations differing in enthalpy and volume. An increase in temperature shifts the population of coil-like conformations towards the species with a greater enthalpy, which would result in a positive or negative value of ΔE_{rel} depending on the sign of the volume difference between the high and low enthalpy subpopulations [93].

At room temperature, all low molecular weight model compounds studied to date exhibit positive partial molar expansibilities, $E°$ [106–113]. The intrinsic expansibility, E_M, of low molecular weight compounds is close to zero. Hence, according to Equation (7), the positive values of $E°$ of small molecules are suggestive of the positive values of the differential expansibility of water of hydration and bulk water, $(E°_h - E°_0)$, for all functional groups independent of their chemical nature. The hydration term in Equation (15), $\Delta n_h(E°_h - E°_0)$, is positive given the positive values of Δn_h (water is taken up by the hydration shell of the DNA upon its G-quadruplex-to-coil transition) and $(E°_h - E°_0)$.

5. Differential Compressibility

5.1. G-quadruplexes

Table 6 presents changes in adiabatic compressibility, ΔK_S, accompanying unfolding transitions of the Tel22, Tel26, and c-MYC G-quadruplexes. The partial molar adiabatic compressibilities, $K°_S$, of the three G-quadruplexes all decrease upon their unfolding. The relationship for ΔK_S can be obtained by modifying Equation (8):

$$\Delta K_S = \Delta K_M + \Delta n_h(K°_{Sh} - K°_{S0}) + n_{M+}K_{SM+} + \Delta K_{Srel} \tag{16}$$

where K_{SM+} is the partial molar adiabatic compressibility of the stabilizing ion. The relaxation contribution in Equation (16) is given by $K_{Srel} = (\langle\Delta V^2\rangle - \langle\Delta V\rangle^2)/RT$, where $\langle\Delta V\rangle$ is the ensemble average changes in volume relative to a "ground state" conformation. The intrinsic compressibility, K_M, of a solute is given by $K_M = \beta_M V_M$, where β_M is the intrinsic coefficient of adiabatic compressibility.

Owing to the presence of the central cavity, a G-quadruplex possesses a compressible interior that is absent in its unfolded state. In other words, the value of β_M of the native G-quadruplex is sizeable, but reduces to near zero in the unfolded state, which is devoid of a compressible interior. There are no estimates of the value of β_M for G-quadruplexes. However, given the structural similarity of G-quadruplexes and globular proteins, the β_M of a G-quadruplex can be expected to be on the order of 25×10^{-6} bar^{-1}, the average coefficient of adiabatic compressibility of a globular protein [46,50,114–116]. Further studies, particularly, the pressure-dependent NMR characterization of native G-quadruplexes, may help evaluate the value of $\beta_M = -\frac{1}{V_M}\left(\frac{\partial V_M}{\partial P}\right)_T$, which, in turn, would assist in a more reliable estimate of the molecular determinants of changes in compressibility accompanying conformational transitions involving G-quadruplexes.

For nucleic acids, the hydration term, $\Delta n_h(K°_{Sh} - K°_{S0})$, in Eq.(16) is negative given the positive sign of Δn_h and the negative sign of $(K°_{Sh} - K°_{S0})$ [44,47,117–119]. The volumetric properties of water of hydration of nucleic acids are dominated by the hydration of charged and clustered polar groups, which exhibit partial molar adiabatic compressibilities, $K°_{Sh}$, of water of hydration lower than that of bulk water, $K°_{S0}$ [45,120]. In contrast, isolated polar groups and nonpolar groups may exhibit partial molar compressibilities that are greater than that of bulk water [45,120]. Currently, it is difficult to come up with a reliable estimate of the value of $(K°_{Sh} - K°_{S0})$ for parsing the measured changes in compressibility, ΔK_S, in terms of specific components using Equation (16). For charged solutes, such as DNA, the partial molar adiabatic compressibility, $K°_{Sh}$, of water of hydration is ~25% smaller than that of bulk water [64]. However, the functional groups that become solvent exposed and subsequently solvated when a G-quadruplex unfolds are not all charged. In contrast, many of them are polar uncharged or even nonpolar; for example, the functional groups of nucleic acid bases that, due to their participation in base pairing and stacking interactions in the folded state, are shielded from the solvent, but become solvent-exposed and hydrated when the structure unfolds. Consequently, there is no clarity about the specific value of $(K°_{Sh} - K°_{S0})$ that should be used in the analysis.

The relaxation component, ΔK_{rel}, originates from the broadly distributed ensemble of nearly isoenergetic unfolded single-stranded conformations that vary in volume. An increase in pressure shifts the ensemble of unfolded conformations towards the species with smaller volumes that gives rise to an additional positive contribution to the observed change in compressibility associated with G-quadruplex unfolding [93].

5.2. *i*-Motifs

There is only a single work that reports a change in adiabatic compressibility, ΔK_S, accompanying the helix-to-coil transition of an *i*-motif [57]. For the c-MYC *i*-motif, the value of ΔK_S for the pH-induced helix-to-coil transition at 25 °C is nearly zero (see Table 5) [57].

As mentioned above, the intrinsic compressibility term, K_M, in Equation (16) represents the compressibility of the water-inaccessible interior core of the solute. While the intrinsic compressibility, K_M, of the ensemble of unfolded conformations is close to zero, that of the folded *i*-motif conformation is less certain and, in principle, may be significant. The sign and the magnitude of hydration contribution to compressibility in Equation (16), $\Delta n_h(K_h - K_0)$, is also unclear. The differential partial molar compressibility of hydration and bulk water, $(K_h - K_0)$, is negative for the unfolded, coil-like state. On the other hand, in the folded *i*-motif conformation, the value of $(K_h - K_0)$ may be more negative relative to the coil state (because the negatively charged phosphates are brought closer together), it may be the same, or it may be less negative (e.g., due to a more effective mutual neutralization of the positively charged cytosines and negatively charged phosphates). Should the change in intrinsic compressibility, ΔK_M, in Equation (16) be near zero, that is the interior of the *i*-motif conformation is rigid, the observation that $\Delta K_S \approx 0$ suggests the similarity of the hydration of the *i*-motif and coil states with $\Delta\Delta K_h \approx 0$. Although the current data do not enable us to discriminate between the various scenarios, the observed $\Delta K_S \approx 0$ is an indication of a near-perfect offsetting of the ΔK_M and $\Delta\Delta K_h$ terms in Equation (16). In addition, it should be noted that there may be a relaxation component in analogy with G-quadruplexes.

In the aggregate, the current volumetric data on *i*-motifs collected to date suggest that fortuitous compensations between the intrinsic and hydration contributions to volume and compressibility result in ΔV and ΔK_S of zero. A compressibility change of zero implies that the compensations leading to ΔV being zero are not restricted to ambient pressure, but also act at elevated pressures.

6. Pressure-Temperature Phase Diagram

The stability of a G-quadruplex (or any other biopolymer) as a function of temperature and pressure can be presented analytically as follows [121–126]:

$$\begin{aligned}\Delta G(P,T) = \Delta H_M\left(1 - \tfrac{T}{T_M}\right) + \Delta C_P\left(T - T_M - T ln\tfrac{T}{T_M}\right)\\ +[\Delta V(T_R) + \Delta E(T - T_R)](P - P_R) - 0.5\Delta K_T\left(P^2 - {P_R}^2\right)\end{aligned} \quad (17)$$

where ΔH_M is the differential enthalpy of the folded and unfolded states at the transition temperature, T_M, and reference pressure, P_R; ΔC_P is the differential heat capacity of the folded and unfolded states; $\Delta V(T_R)$ is the differential volume of the folded and unfolded states at the reference temperature, T_R, and pressure, P_R; and ΔE and ΔK_T are, respectively, the differential expansibility and isothermal compressibility of the folded and unfolded states.

The relationship for pressure-temperature phase diagram can be derived by equating Equation (17) to zero and solving it with respect to the denaturation pressure, P_M:

$$\Delta H_M\left(1-\frac{T}{T_M}\right)+\Delta C_P\left(T-T_M-Tln\frac{T}{T_M}\right)+[\Delta V(T_R)+\Delta E(T-T_R)](P-P_R)-0.5\Delta K_T\left(P^2-{P_R}^2\right)=0 \quad (18)$$

The reference pressure, P_R, is generally set equal to ambient pressure (1 bar). It can be ignored relative to pressures, P_M, at which proteins and nucleic acids denature. The latter are, typically, on the order of ~1 kbar and higher:

$$0.5\Delta K_T{P_M}^2-[\Delta V(T_R)+\Delta E(T-T_R)]P_M-\Delta H_M\left(1-\frac{T}{T_M}\right)-\Delta C_P\left(T-T_M-Tln\frac{T}{T_M}\right)=0 \quad (19)$$

Solving Equation (19) with respect to P_M, one obtains the following:

$$P_M=\frac{\Delta V(T_R)+\Delta E(T-T_R)\pm\sqrt{D}}{\Delta K_T} \quad (20)$$

where $D=[\Delta V(T_R)+\Delta E(T-T_R)]^2+2\Delta K_T\left[\Delta H_M\left(1-\frac{T}{T_M}\right)-\Delta C_P\left(T-T_M-Tln\frac{T}{T_M}\right)\right]$.

Equation (20) has been used to compute the pressure-temperature phase diagram of the c-MYC G-quadruplex [99]. In the computation, the change in heat capacity, ΔC_P, has been evaluated based on the results reported by Majhi et al. [127].

Figure 3 presents the pressure–temperature stability phase diagram for the c-MYC G-quadruplex [99]. As is seen from Figure 3, the diagram is elliptic. It resembles that of a globular protein [121,122,124,128], while being distinct from that of duplex DNA [129]. We propose that the similarity of the pressure–temperature stability phase diagram of a G-quadruplex and a globular protein reflects their shared structural and volumetric features. In particular, both G-quadruplexes and globular proteins are compact and characterized by compressible intramolecular voids. The order-disorder transitions of both structures are accompanied by an increase in expansibility, ΔE, and reductions in volume, ΔV, and compressibility, ΔK_T.

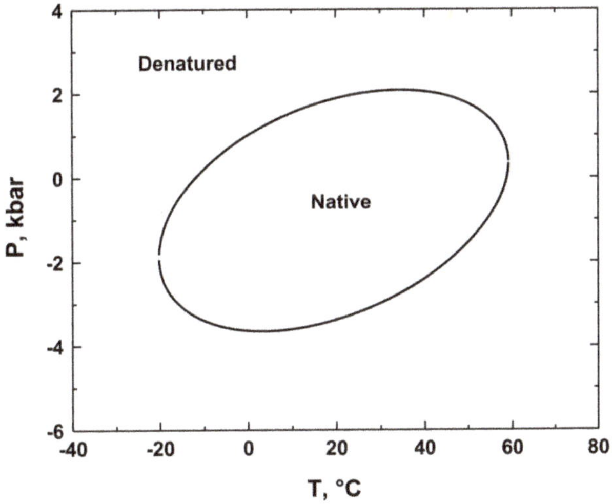

Figure 3. The pressure-temperature phase diagram for the stability c-MYC G-quadruplex at 50 mM CsCl and 0.1 mM KCl computed with Equation (20) from ref. [99].

Pressure-induced structural changes in nucleic acid structures and the resulting inhibition of genomic processes may contribute to pressure-induced cell death and injury in microorganisms. We have previously suggested that the fine-tuned, differential pressure sensitivity of the duplex, G-quadruplex, and *i*-motif conformations adopted by specific genomic loci may be involved in regulation of genomic processes in barophilic organisms thereby governing their survival at high pressures [57]. The differential stability phase diagram of G-quadruplex and duplex DNA [129] may provide an additional platform for developing this hypothesis.

7. Conclusions

There is only a decade of volumetric studies of G-quadruplex and *i*-motif structures. In some ways, our understanding of the volumetric characteristics of these four-stranded structures is reminiscent of the situation with the volumetric studies of proteins in the 1980s. Despite their scarcity, the volumetric data accumulated so far have established several regularities that are common for each of these four-stranded structures. In particular, all G-quadruplex-to-coil transitions studied to date are accompanied by negative changes in volume, ΔV, and compressibility, ΔK_S, and positive changes in expansibility, ΔE. The few *i*-motif-to-coil transitions studied are accompanied by near zero changes in volume, ΔV, and compressibility, ΔK_S. While it is still difficult to reliably rationalize volumetric observations in terms of intrinsic and hydration contributions, they establish an experimental framework for deriving the pressure–temperature stability diagrams of tetraplex DNA structures. Further studies involving a wide range of G-quadruplex and *i*-motif structures are needed to understand the generality and molecular origins of these results.

Author Contributions: T.V.C. and R.B.M.J. performed research, analyzed data, and wrote the paper. All authors have read and agreed to the published version of the manuscript.

Funding: This work was supported by grants from NSERC to T.V.C. and R.B.M.J.

Institutional Review Board Statement: Not applicable.

Informed Consent Statement: Not applicable.

Data Availability Statement: Not applicable.

Conflicts of Interest: The authors declare no conflict of interests.

References

1. Shafer, R.H.; Smirnov, I. Biological aspects of DNA/RNA quadruplexes. *Biopolymers* **2000**, *56*, 209–227. [CrossRef]
2. Huppert, J.L. Four-stranded nucleic acids: Structure, function and targeting of G-quadruplexes. *Chem. Soc. Rev.* **2008**, *37*, 1375–1384. [CrossRef] [PubMed]
3. Huppert, J.L. Structure, location and interactions of G-quadruplexes. *FEBS J.* **2010**, *277*, 3452–3458. [CrossRef]
4. Day, H.A.; Pavlou, P.; Waller, Z.A. *i*-Motif DNA: Structure, stability and targeting with ligands. *Bioorg. Med. Chem.* **2014**, *22*, 4407–4418. [CrossRef] [PubMed]
5. Benabou, S.; Avino, A.; Eritja, R.; Gonzalez, C.; Gargallo, R. Fundamental aspects of the nucleic acid *i*-motif structures. *RSC Adv.* **2014**, *4*, 26956–26980. [CrossRef]
6. Alba, J.J.; Sadurni, A.; Gargallo, R. Nucleic acid *i*-motif structures in analytical chemistry. *Crit. Rev. Anal. Chem.* **2016**, *46*, 443–454. [CrossRef]
7. Lane, A.N.; Chaires, J.B.; Gray, R.D.; Trent, J.O. Stability and kinetics of G-quadruplex structures. *Nucleic Acids Res.* **2008**, *36*, 5482–5515. [CrossRef] [PubMed]
8. Balasubramanian, S.; Hurley, L.H.; Neidle, S. Targeting G-quadruplexes in gene promoters: A novel anticancer strategy? *Nat. Rev. Drug Discov.* **2011**, *10*, 261–275. [CrossRef]
9. Dolinnaya, N.G.; Ogloblina, A.M.; Yakubovskaya, M.G. Structure, properties, and biological relevance of the DNA and RNA G-quadruplexes: Overview 50 Years after their discovery. *Biochemistry* **2016**, *81*, 1602–1649. [CrossRef]
10. Hansel-Hertsch, R.; Di Antonio, M.; Balasubramanian, S. DNA G-quadruplexes in the human genome: Detection, functions and therapeutic potential. *Nat. Rev. Mol. Cell Biol.* **2017**, *18*, 279–284. [CrossRef]
11. Qin, Y.; Hurley, L.H. Structures, folding patterns, and functions of intramolecular DNA G-quadruplexes found in eukaryotic promoter regions. *Biochimie* **2008**, *90*, 1149–1171. [CrossRef]

12. Sen, D.; Gilbert, W. Formation of parallel four-stranded complexes by guanine-rich motifs in DNA and its implications for meiosis. *Nature* **1988**, *334*, 364–366. [CrossRef]
13. Burge, S.; Parkinson, G.N.; Hazel, P.; Todd, A.K.; Neidle, S. Quadruplex DNA: Sequence, topology and structure. *Nucleic Acids Res.* **2006**, *34*, 5402–5415. [CrossRef]
14. Brooks, T.A.; Kendrick, S.; Hurley, L. Making sense of G-quadruplex and *i*-motif functions in oncogene promoters. *FEBS J.* **2010**, *277*, 3459–3469. [CrossRef] [PubMed]
15. Collie, G.W.; Parkinson, G.N. The application of DNA and RNA G-quadruplexes to therapeutic medicines. *Chem. Soc. Rev.* **2011**, *40*, 5867–5892. [CrossRef] [PubMed]
16. Gehring, K.; Leroy, J.L.; Gueron, M. A Tetrameric DNA structure with protonated cytosine·cytosine base pairs. *Nature* **1993**, *363*, 561–565. [CrossRef]
17. Sun, D.; Hurley, L.H. The importance of negative superhelicity in inducing the formation of G-quadruplex and *i*-motif structures in the c-Myc promoter: Implications for drug targeting and control of gene expression. *J. Med. Chem.* **2009**, *52*, 2863–2874. [CrossRef]
18. Kang, H.J.; Kendrick, S.; Hecht, S.M.; Hurley, L.H. The transcriptional complex between the BCL2 *i*-motif and hnRNP LL is a molecular switch for control of gene expression that can be modulated by small molecules. *J. Am. Chem. Soc.* **2014**, *136*, 4172–4185. [CrossRef] [PubMed]
19. Kendrick, S.; Kang, H.J.; Alam, M.P.; Madathil, M.M.; Agrawal, P.; Gokhale, V.; Yang, D.; Hecht, S.M.; Hurley, L.H. The dynamic character of the BCL2 promoter *i*-motif provides a mechanism for modulation of gene expression by compounds that bind selectively to the alternative DNA hairpin structure. *J. Am. Chem. Soc.* **2014**, *136*, 4161–4171. [CrossRef] [PubMed]
20. Zhou, J.; Wei, C.; Jia, G.; Wang, X.; Feng, Z.; Li, C. Formation of *i*-motif structure at neutral and slightly alkaline pH. *Mol. Biosyst.* **2010**, *6*, 580–586. [CrossRef]
21. Tateishi-Karimata, H.; Sugimoto, N. Chemical biology of non-canonical structures of nucleic acids for therapeutic applications. *Chem. Commun.* **2020**, *56*, 2379–2390. [CrossRef]
22. Spiegel, J.; Adhikari, S.; Balasubramanian, S. The structure and function of DNA G-quadruplexes. *Trends Chem.* **2020**, *2*, 123–136. [CrossRef]
23. Varshney, D.; Spiegel, J.; Zyner, K.; Tannahill, D.; Balasubramanian, S. The regulation and functions of DNA and RNA G-quadruplexes. *Nat. Rev. Mol. Cell Biol.* **2020**, *21*, 459–474. [CrossRef]
24. Bryan, T.M. Mechanisms of DNA replication and repair: Insights from the study of G-quadruplexes. *Molecules* **2019**, *24*, 3439. [CrossRef]
25. Armas, P.; David, A.; Calcaterra, N.B. Transcriptional control by G-quadruplexes: In vivo roles and perspectives for specific intervention. *Transcription* **2017**, *8*, 21–25. [CrossRef]
26. Biffi, G.; Tannahill, D.; McCafferty, J.; Balasubramanian, S. Quantitative visualization of DNA G-quadruplex structures in human cells. *Nat. Chem.* **2013**, *5*, 182–186. [CrossRef] [PubMed]
27. Lam, E.Y.; Beraldi, D.; Tannahill, D.; Balasubramanian, S. G-quadruplex structures are stable detectable in human genomic DNA. *Nat. Commun.* **2013**, *4*, 1796. [CrossRef]
28. Biffi, G.; Di, A.M.; Tannahill, D.; Balasubramanian, S. Visualization and selective chemical targeting of RNA G-quadruplex structures in the cytoplasm of human cells. *Nat. Chem.* **2014**, *6*, 75–80. [CrossRef] [PubMed]
29. Zeraati, M.; Langley, D.B.; Schofield, P.; Moye, A.L.; Rouet, R.; Hughes, W.E.; Bryan, T.M.; Dinger, M.E.; Christ, D. *i*-motif DNA structures are formed in the nuclei of human cells. *Nat. Chem.* **2018**, *10*, 631–637. [CrossRef]
30. Abou Assi, H.; Garavis, M.; Gonzalez, C.; Damha, M.J. *i*-Motif DNA: Structural features and significance to cell biology. *Nucleic Acids Res.* **2018**, *46*, 8038–8056. [CrossRef]
31. Kim, B.G.; Chalikian, T.V. Thermodynamic linkage analysis of pH-induced folding and unfolding transitions of *i*-motifs. *Biophys. Chem.* **2016**, *216*, 19–22. [CrossRef] [PubMed]
32. Chalikian, T.V.; Liu, L.; Macgregor, R.B., Jr. Duplex-tetraplex equilibria in guanine- and cytosine-rich DNA. *Biophys. Chem.* **2020**, *267*, 106473. [CrossRef] [PubMed]
33. Takahashi, S.; Sugimoto, N. Stability prediction of canonical and non-canonical structures of nucleic acids in various molecular environments and cells. *Chem. Soc. Rev.* **2020**, *49*, 8439–8468. [CrossRef] [PubMed]
34. Kim, B.G.; Evans, H.M.; Dubins, D.N.; Chalikian, T.V. Effects of salt on the stability of a G-quadruplex from the human c-MYC promoter. *Biochemistry* **2015**, *54*, 3420–3430. [CrossRef] [PubMed]
35. Kim, B.G.; Long, J.; Dubins, D.N.; Chalikian, T.V. Ionic effects on VEGF G-quadruplex stability. *J. Phys. Chem. B* **2016**, *120*, 4963–4971. [CrossRef] [PubMed]
36. Aslanyan, L.; Ko, J.; Kim, B.G.; Vardanyan, I.; Dalyan, Y.B.; Chalikian, T.V. Effect of urea on G-quadruplex stability. *J. Phys. Chem. B* **2017**, *121*, 6511–6519. [CrossRef]
37. Sugimoto, N. Noncanonical structures and their thermodynamics of DNA and RNA under molecular crowding: Beyond the Watson-Crick double helix. *Int. Rev. Cell Mol. Biol.* **2014**, *307*, 205–273.
38. Nakano, S.; Miyoshi, D.; Sugimoto, N. Effects of molecular crowding on the structures, interactions, and functions of nucleic acids. *Chem. Rev.* **2014**, *114*, 2733–2758. [CrossRef]
39. Boncina, M.; Lah, J.; Prislan, I.; Vesnaver, G. Energetic basis of human telomeric DNA folding into G-quadruplex structures. *J. Am. Chem. Soc.* **2012**, *134*, 9657–9663. [CrossRef]

40. Boncina, M.; Vesnaver, G.; Chaires, J.B.; Lah, J. Unraveling the thermodynamics of the folding and interconversion of human telomere G-quadruplexes. *Angew. Chem. Int. Ed. Engl.* **2016**, *55*, 10340–10344. [CrossRef]
41. Olsen, C.M.; Gmeiner, W.H.; Marky, L.A. Unfolding of G-quadruplexes: Energetic, and ion and water contributions of G-quartet stacking. *J. Phys. Chem. B* **2006**, *110*, 6962–6969. [CrossRef]
42. Kaushik, M.; Suehl, N.; Marky, L.A. Calorimetric unfolding of the bimolecular and i-motif complexes of the human telomere complementary strand, $d(C_3TA_2)_4$. *Biophys. Chem.* **2007**, *126*, 154–164. [CrossRef] [PubMed]
43. Macgregor, R.B., Jr. Effect of hydrostatic pressure on nucleic acids. *Biopolymers* **1998**, *48*, 253–263. [CrossRef]
44. Chalikian, T.V.; Macgregor, R.B. Nucleic acid hydration: A volumetric perspective. *Phys. Life Rev.* **2007**, *4*, 91–115. [CrossRef]
45. Chalikian, T.V.; Sarvazyan, A.P.; Breslauer, K.J. Hydration and partial compressibility of biological compounds. *Biophys. Chem.* **1994**, *51*, 89–107. [CrossRef]
46. Chalikian, T.V.; Breslauer, K.J. Thermodynamic analysis of biomolecules: A volumetric approach. *Curr. Opin. Struct. Biol.* **1998**, *8*, 657–664. [CrossRef]
47. Chalikian, T.V.; Breslauer, K.J. Volumetric properties of nucleic acids. *Biopolymers* **1998**, *48*, 264–280. [CrossRef]
48. Takahashi, S.; Sugimoto, N. Pressure-dependent formation of *i*-motif and G-quadruplex DNA structures. *Phys. Chem. Chem. Phys.* **2015**, *17*, 31004–31010. [CrossRef] [PubMed]
49. Winter, R. Interrogating the structural dynamics and energetics of biomolecular systems with pressure modulation. *Annu. Rev. Biophys.* **2019**, *48*, 441–463. [CrossRef] [PubMed]
50. Chalikian, T.V. Volumetric properties of proteins. *Annu. Rev. Biophys. Biomol. Struct.* **2003**, *32*, 207–235. [CrossRef] [PubMed]
51. Chalikian, T.V. Volumetric measurements in binary solvents: Theory to experiment. *Biophys. Chem.* **2011**, *156*, 3–12. [CrossRef]
52. Cooper, A. Protein fluctuations and the thermodynamic uncertainty principle. *Prog. Biophys. Mol. Biol.* **1984**, *44*, 181–214. [CrossRef]
53. Chen, C.R.; Makhatadze, G.I. Molecular determinants of temperature dependence of protein volume change upon unfolding. *J. Phys. Chem. B* **2017**, *121*, 8300–8310. [CrossRef]
54. Chen, C.R.; Makhatadze, G.I. Molecular determinant of the effects of hydrostatic pressure on protein folding stability. *Nat. Commun.* **2017**, *8*, 14561. [CrossRef] [PubMed]
55. Krobath, H.; Chen, T.; Chan, H.S. Volumetric physics of polypeptide coil-helix transitions. *Biochemistry* **2016**, *55*, 6269–6281. [CrossRef] [PubMed]
56. Kim, B.G.; Shek, Y.L.; Chalikian, T.V. Polyelectrolyte effects in G-quadruplexes. *Biophys.Chem.* **2013**, *184*, 95–100. [CrossRef] [PubMed]
57. Liu, L.; Kim, B.G.; Feroze, U.; Macgregor, R.B., Jr.; Chalikian, T.V. Probing the ionic atmosphere and hydration of the c-MYC *i*-motif. *J. Am. Chem. Soc.* **2018**, *140*, 2229–2238. [CrossRef]
58. Blandamer, M.J.; Davis, M.I.; Douheret, G.; Reis, J.C.R. Apparent molar isentropic compressions and expansions of solutions. *Chem. Soc. Rev.* **2001**, *30*, 8–15. [CrossRef]
59. Desnoyers, J.E.; Philip, P.R. Isothermal compressibilities of aqueous solutions of tetraalkylammonium bromides. *Can. J. Chem.* **1972**, *50*, 1094–1096. [CrossRef]
60. Kharakoz, D.P. Partial molar volumes of molecules of arbitrary shape and the effect of hydrogen bonding with water. *J. Solut. Chem.* **1992**, *21*, 569–595. [CrossRef]
61. Pierotti, R.A. Scaled particle theory of aqueous and non-aqueous solutions. *Chem. Rev.* **1976**, *76*, 717–726. [CrossRef]
62. Chalikian, T.V. On the molecular origins of volumetric data. *J. Phys. Chem. B* **2008**, *112*, 911–917. [CrossRef]
63. Patel, N.; Dubins, D.N.; Pomes, R.; Chalikian, T.V. Parsing partial molar volumes of small molecules: A molecular dynamics study. *J. Phys. Chem. B* **2011**, *115*, 4856–4862. [CrossRef] [PubMed]
64. Chalikian, T.V. Structural thermodynamics of hydration. *J. Phys. Chem. B* **2001**, *105*, 12566–12578. [CrossRef]
65. Lee, S.Y.; Chalikian, T.V. Volumetric properties of solvation in binary solvents. *J. Phys. Chem. B* **2009**, *113*, 2443–2450. [CrossRef]
66. Han, F.; Chalikian, T.V. Hydration changes accompanying nucleic acid intercalation reactions:volumetric characterizations. *J. Am. Chem. Soc.* **2003**, *125*, 7219–7229. [CrossRef] [PubMed]
67. Han, F.; Taulier, N.; Chalikian, T.V. Association of the minor groove binding drug Hoechst 33258 with $d(CGCGAATTCGCG)_2$: Volumetric, calorimetric, and spectroscopic characterizations. *Biochemistry* **2005**, *44*, 9785–9794. [CrossRef] [PubMed]
68. Filfil, R.; Chalikian, T.V. The thermodynamics of protein-protein recognition as characterized by a combination of volumetric and calorimetric techniques: The binding of turkey ovomucoid third domain to α-chymotrypsin. *J. Mol. Biol.* **2003**, *326*, 1271–1288. [CrossRef]
69. Filfil, R.; Chalikian, T.V. Volumetric and spectroscopic characterizations of glucose-hexokinase association. *FEBS Lett.* **2003**, *554*, 351–356. [CrossRef]
70. Son, I.; Shek, Y.L.; Dubins, D.N.; Chalikian, T.V. Volumetric characterization of tri-N-acetylglucosamine binding to lysozyme. *Biochemistry* **2012**, *51*, 5784–5790. [CrossRef]
71. Son, I.; Selvaratnam, R.; Dubins, D.N.; Melacini, G.; Chalikian, T.V. Ultrasonic and densimetric characterization of the association of cyclic AMP with the cAMP-binding domain of the exchange protein EPAC1. *J. Phys. Chem. B* **2013**, *117*, 10779–10784. [CrossRef]
72. Liu, L.; Stepanian, L.; Dubins, D.N.; Chalikian, T.V. Binding of L-argininamide to a DNA aptamer: A volumetric study. *J. Phys. Chem. B* **2018**, *122*, 7647–7653. [CrossRef] [PubMed]

73. Filfil, R.; Chalikian, T.V. Volumetric and spectroscopic characterizations of the native and acid-induced denatured states of staphylococcal nuclease. *J. Mol. Biol.* **2000**, *299*, 827–842. [CrossRef]
74. Taulier, N.; Chalikian, T.V. Characterization of pH-induced transitions of β-lactoglobulin: Ultrasonic, densimetric, and spectroscopic studies. *J. Mol. Biol.* **2001**, *314*, 873–889. [CrossRef] [PubMed]
75. Taulier, N.; Beletskaya, I.V.; Chalikian, T.V. Compressibility changes accompanying conformational transitions of apomyoglobin. *Biopolymers* **2005**, *79*, 218–229. [CrossRef] [PubMed]
76. Taulier, N.; Chalikian, T.V. Hydrophobic hydration in cyclodextrin complexation. *J. Phys. Chem. B* **2006**, *110*, 12222–12224. [CrossRef] [PubMed]
77. Taulier, N.; Chalikian, T.V. γ-Cyclodextrin forms a highly compressible complex with 1-adamantanecarboxylic acid. *J. Phys. Chem. B* **2008**, *112*, 9546–9549. [CrossRef]
78. Chalikian, T.V.; Volker, J.; Anafi, D.; Breslauer, K.J. The native and the heat-induced denatured states of α-chymotrypsinogen A: Thermodynamic and spectroscopic studies. *J. Mol. Biol.* **1997**, *274*, 237–252. [CrossRef] [PubMed]
79. Lin, L.N.; Brandts, J.F.; Brandts, J.M.; Plotnikov, V. Determination of the volumetric properties of proteins and other solutes using pressure perturbation calorimetry. *Anal. Biochem.* **2002**, *302*, 144–160. [CrossRef]
80. Suladze, S.; Kahse, M.; Erwin, N.; Tomazic, D.; Winter, R. Probing volumetric properties of biomolecular systems by pressure perturbation calorimetry (PPC)—The effects of hydration, cosolvents and crowding. *Methods* **2015**, *76*, 67–77.
81. Heerklotz, H. Pressure Perturbation Calorimetry. In *Methods in Molecular Biology*; Dopica, A.M., Ed.; Humana Press, Inc.: Totowa, NJ, USA, 2007; pp. 197–206.
82. Mitra, L.; Smolin, N.; Ravindra, R.; Royer, C.; Winter, R. Pressure perturbation calorimetric studies of the solvation properties and the thermal unfolding of proteins in solution—Experiments and theoretical interpretation. *Phys. Chem. Chem. Phys.* **2006**, *8*, 1249–1265. [CrossRef]
83. Schweiker, K.L.; Makhatadze, G.I. Use of pressure perturbation calorimetry to characterize the volumetric properties of proteins. *Methods Enzymol.* **2009**, *466*, 527–547.
84. Sarvazyan, A.P. Ultrasonic velocimetry of biological compounds. *Annu. Rev. Biophys. Biophys. Chem.* **1991**, *20*, 321–342. [CrossRef]
85. Sarvazian, A.P. Ultrasonic velocimetry of biological compounds. *Mol. Biol.* **1983**, *17*, 916–927. [CrossRef]
86. Owen, B.B.; Simons, H.L. Standard partial molal compressibilities by ultrasonics. 1. Sodium chloride and potassium chloride at 25 °C. *J. Phys. Chem.* **1957**, *61*, 479–482. [CrossRef]
87. Barnartt, S. The velocity of sound in electrolytic solutions. *J. Chem. Phys.* **1952**, *20*, 278–279. [CrossRef]
88. Lerch, M.T.; Horwitz, J.; McCoy, J.; Hubbell, W.L. Circular dichroism and site-directed spin labeling reveal structural and dynamical features of high-pressure states of myoglobin. *Proc. Natl. Acad. Sci. USA* **2013**, *110*, E4714–E4722. [CrossRef] [PubMed]
89. Dellarole, M.; Royer, C.A. High-pressure fluorescence applications. *Methods Mol. Biol.* **2014**, *1076*, 53–74. [PubMed]
90. Akasaka, K. Probing conformational fluctuation of proteins by pressure perturbation. *Chem. Rev.* **2006**, *106*, 1814–1835. [CrossRef] [PubMed]
91. Wu, J.Q.; Macgregor, R.B., Jr. Pressure dependence of the melting temperature of dA·dT polymers. *Biochemistry* **1993**, *32*, 12531–12537. [CrossRef] [PubMed]
92. Fan, H.Y.; Shek, Y.L.; Amiri, A.; Dubins, D.N.; Heerklotz, H.; Macgregor, R.B., Jr.; Chalikian, T.V. Volumetric characterization of sodium-induced G-quadruplex formation. *J. Am. Chem. Soc.* **2011**, *133*, 4518–4526. [CrossRef]
93. Shek, Y.L.; Noudeh, G.D.; Nazari, M.; Heerklotz, H.; Abu-Ghazalah, R.M.; Dubins, D.N.; Chalikian, T.V. Folding thermodynamics of the hybrid-1 type intramolecular human telomeric G-quadruplex. *Biopolymers* **2014**, *101*, 216–227. [CrossRef]
94. Takahashi, S.; Sugimoto, N. Effect of pressure on the stability of G-quadruplex DNA: Thermodynamics under crowding conditions. *Angew. Chem.-Int. Ed.* **2013**, *52*, 13774–13778. [CrossRef] [PubMed]
95. Takahashi, S.; Sugimoto, N. Effect of pressure on thermal stability of G-quadruplex DNA and double-stranded DNA structures. *Molecules* **2013**, *18*, 13297–13319. [CrossRef]
96. Molnar, O.R.; Somkuti, J.; Smeller, L. Negative volume changes of human G-quadruplexes at unfolding. *Heliyon* **2020**, *6*, 6. [CrossRef]
97. Li, Y.Y.; Dubins, D.N.; Le, D.; Leung, K.; Macgregor, R.B., Jr. The role of loops and cation on the volume of unfolding of G-quadruplexes related to HTel. *Biophys. Chem.* **2017**, *231*, 55–63. [CrossRef]
98. Chalikian, T.V.; Macgregor, R.B., Jr. On empirical decomposition of volumetric data. *Biophys. Chem.* **2019**, *246*, 8–15. [CrossRef]
99. Liu, L.; Scott, L.; Tariq, N.; Kume, T.; Dubins, D.N.; Macgregor, R.B., Jr.; Chalikian, T.V. Volumetric interplay between the conformational states adopted by guanine-rich DNA from the c-MYC promoter. *J. Phys. Chem. B* **2021**, *125*, 7406–7416. [CrossRef]
100. Li, K.; Yatsunyk, L.; Neidle, S. Water spines and networks in G-quadruplex structures. *Nucleic Acids Res.* **2021**, *49*, 519–528. [CrossRef] [PubMed]
101. Takahashi, S.; Sugimoto, N. Volumetric contributions of loop regions of G-quadruplex DNA to the formation of the tertiary structure. *Biophys. Chem.* **2017**, *231*, 146–154. [CrossRef] [PubMed]
102. Lepper, C.P.; Williams, M.A.K.; Edwards, P.J.B.; Filichev, V.V.; Jameson, G.B. Effects of pressure and pH on the physical stability of an *i*-motif DNA structure. *Chem. Phys. Chem.* **2019**, *20*, 1567–1571. [CrossRef]
103. Somkuti, J.; Molnar, O.R.; Smeller, L. Revealing unfolding steps and volume changes of human telomeric *i*-motif DNA. *Phys. Chem. Chem. Phys.* **2020**, *22*, 23816–23823. [CrossRef]

104. Rashin, A.A.; Iofin, M.; Honig, B. Internal cavities and buried waters in globular proteins. *Biochemistry* **1986**, *25*, 3619–3625. [CrossRef]
105. Liang, J.; Dill, K.A. Are proteins well-packed? *Biophys. J.* **2001**, *81*, 751–766. [CrossRef]
106. Chalikian, T.V.; Sarvazyan, A.P.; Breslauer, K.J. Partial molar volumes, expansibilities, and compressibilities of α,ω-aminocarboxylic acids in aqueous solutions between 18 and 55 °C. *J. Phys. Chem.* **1993**, *97*, 13017–13026. [CrossRef]
107. Chalikian, T.V.; Sarvazyan, A.P.; Funck, T.; Breslauer, K.J. Partial molar volumes, expansibilities, and compressibilities of oligoglycines in aqueous solutions at 18–55 °C. *Biopolymers* **1994**, *34*, 541–553. [CrossRef]
108. Lee, A.; Chalikian, T.V. Volumetric characterization of the hydration properties of heterocyclic bases and nucleosides. *Biophys. Chem.* **2001**, *92*, 209–227. [CrossRef]
109. Kharakoz, D.P. Volumetric properties of proteins and their analogs in diluted water solutions. 1. Partial volumes of amino acids at 15–55 °C. *Biophys. Chem.* **1989**, *34*, 115–125. [CrossRef]
110. Hedwig, G.R.; Hastie, J.D.; Høiland, H. Thermodynamic properties of peptide solutions. 14. Partial molar expansibilities and isothermal compressibilities of some glycyl dipeptides in aqueous solution. *J. Solut. Chem.* **1996**, *25*, 615–633. [CrossRef]
111. Hedwig, G.R.; Jameson, G.B.; Høiland, H. The partial molar heat capacity, expansion, isentropic, and isothermal compressions of thymidine in aqueous solution at T=298.15 K. *J. Chem. Thermodyn.* **2011**, *43*, 1936–1941. [CrossRef]
112. Chalikian, T.V. Ultrasonic and densimetric characterizations of the hydration properties of polar groups in monosaccharides. *J. Phys. Chem. B* **1998**, *102*, 6921–6926. [CrossRef]
113. Lee, S.; Tikhomirova, A.; Shalvardjian, N.; Chalikian, T.V. Partial molar volumes and adiabatic compressibilities of unfolded protein states. *Biophys. Chem.* **2008**, *134*, 185–199. [CrossRef]
114. Chalikian, T.V.; Totrov, M.; Abagyan, R.; Breslauer, K.J. The hydration of globular proteins as derived from volume and compressibility measurements: Cross correlating thermodynamic and structural data. *J. Mol. Biol.* **1996**, *260*, 588–603. [CrossRef]
115. Kharakoz, D.P. Protein compressibility, dynamics, and pressure. *Biophys. J.* **2000**, *79*, 511–525. [CrossRef]
116. Taulier, N.; Chalikian, T.V. Compressibility of protein transitions. *Biochim. Biophys. Acta* **2002**, *1595*, 48–70. [CrossRef]
117. Chalikian, T.V.; Sarvazyan, A.P.; Plum, G.E.; Breslauer, K.J. Influence of base composition, base sequence, and duplex structure on DNA hydration: Apparent molar volumes and apparent molar adiabatic compressibilities of synthetic and natural DNA duplexes at 25 °C. *Biochemistry* **1994**, *33*, 2394–2401. [CrossRef]
118. Tikhomirova, A.; Chalikian, T.V. Probing hydration of monovalent cations condensed around polymeric nucleic acids. *J. Mol. Biol.* **2004**, *341*, 551–563. [CrossRef]
119. Chalikian, T.V.; Volker, J.; Srinivasan, A.R.; Olson, W.K.; Breslauer, K.J. The hydration of nucleic acid duplexes as assessed by a combination of volumetric and structural techniques. *Biopolymers* **1999**, *50*, 459–471. [CrossRef]
120. Kharakoz, D.P. Volumetric properties of proteins and their analogs in diluted water solutions. 2. Partial adiabatic compressibilities of amino acids at 15–70 °C. *J. Phys. Chem.* **1991**, *95*, 5634–5642. [CrossRef]
121. Doster, W.; Friedrich, J. Pressure-temperature phase diagrams of proteinsC. In *Protein Folding Handbook*; Buchner, J., Kiefhaber, T., Eds.; Wiley-V C H Verlag Gmbh: Weinheim, Germany, 2005; pp. 99–126.
122. Hawley, S.A. Reversible pressure-temperature denaturation of chymotrypsinogen. *Biochemistry* **1971**, *10*, 2436–2442. [CrossRef]
123. Ravindra, R.; Winter, R. On the temperature-pressure free-energy landscape of proteins. *Chem. Phys. Chem.* **2003**, *4*, 359–365. [CrossRef] [PubMed]
124. Winter, R.; Lopes, D.; Grudzielanek, S.; Vogtt, K. Towards an understanding of the temperature/pressure configurational and free-energy landscape of biomolecules. *J. Non-Equilib. Thermodyn.* **2007**, *32*, 41–97. [CrossRef]
125. Daniel, I.; Oger, P.; Winter, R. Origins of life and biochemistry under high-pressure conditions. *Chem. Soc. Rev.* **2006**, *35*, 858–875. [CrossRef]
126. Luong, T.Q.; Kapoor, S.; Winter, R. Pressure-a gateway to fundamental insights into protein solvation, dynamics, and function. *Chem. Phys. Chem.* **2015**, *16*, 3555–3571. [CrossRef]
127. Majhi, P.R.; Qi, J.Y.; Tang, C.F.; Shafer, R.H. Heat capacity changes associated with guanine quadruplex formation: An isothermal titration calorimetry study. *Biopolymers* **2008**, *89*, 302–309. [CrossRef]
128. Scharnagl, C.; Reif, M.; Friedrich, J. Stability of proteins: Temperature, pressure and the role of the solvent. *Biochim. Biophys. Acta* **2005**, *1749*, 187–213. [CrossRef]
129. Dubins, D.N.; Lee, A.; Macgregor, R.B., Jr.; Chalikian, T.V. On the stability of double stranded nucleic acids. *J. Am. Chem. Soc.* **2001**, *123*, 9254–9259. [CrossRef]

biology

Review

Molecular Responses to High Hydrostatic Pressure in Eukaryotes: Genetic Insights from Studies on *Saccharomyces cerevisiae*

Fumiyoshi Abe

Department of Chemistry and Biological Science, College of Science and Engineering, Aoyama Gakuin University, Sagamihara 252-5258, Japan; abef@chem.aoyama.ac.jp; Tel.: +81-42-759-6233; Fax: +81-42-759-6511

Simple Summary: High hydrostatic pressure generally has an adverse effect on the biological systems of organisms inhabiting lands or shallow sea regions. Deep-sea piezophiles that prefer high hydrostatic pressure for growth have garnered considerable scientific attention. However, the underlying molecular mechanisms of their adaptation to high pressure remains unclear owing to the challenges of culturing and manipulating the genome of piezophiles. Humans also experience high hydrostatic pressure during exercise. A long-term stay in space can cause muscle weakness in astronauts. Thus, the human body indubitably senses mechanical stresses such as hydrostatic pressure and gravity. Nonetheless, the mechanisms underlying biological responses to high pressures are not clearly understood. This review summarizes the occurrence and significance of high-pressure effects in eukaryotic cells and how the cell responds to increasing pressure by particularly focusing on the physiology of *S. cerevisiae* at the molecular level.

Abstract: High hydrostatic pressure is common mechanical stress in nature and is also experienced by the human body. Organisms in the Challenger Deep of the Mariana Trench are habitually exposed to pressures up to 110 MPa. Human joints are intermittently exposed to hydrostatic pressures of 3–10 MPa. Pressures less than 50 MPa do not deform or kill the cells. However, high pressure can have various effects on the cell's biological processes. Although *Saccharomyces cerevisiae* is not a deep-sea piezophile, it can be used to elucidate the molecular mechanism underlying the cell's responses to high pressures by applying basic knowledge of the effects of pressure on industrial processes involving microorganisms. We have explored the genes associated with the growth of *S. cerevisiae* under high pressure by employing functional genomic strategies and transcriptomics analysis and indicated a strong association between high-pressure signaling and the cell's response to nutrient availability. This review summarizes the occurrence and significance of high-pressure effects on complex metabolic and genetic networks in eukaryotic cells and how the cell responds to increasing pressure by particularly focusing on the physiology of *S. cerevisiae* at the molecular level. Mechanosensation in humans has also been discussed.

Keywords: yeast; *Saccharomyces cerevisiae*; high-pressure response; genetic manipulation; transcriptomics; piezophysiology

Citation: Abe, F. Molecular Responses to High Hydrostatic Pressure in Eukaryotes: Genetic Insights from Studies on *Saccharomyces cerevisiae*. *Biology* **2021**, *10*, 1305. https://doi.org/10.3390/biology10121305

Academic Editors: Dmitri Davydov and Christiane Jung

Received: 19 October 2021
Accepted: 6 December 2021
Published: 9 December 2021

1. General Effects of High Hydrostatic Pressure on Biological Systems

While high hydrostatic pressure is a commonly known characteristic of deep-sea environments, the human body also experiences high pressure. However, it is important to distinguish between the isostatic pressure acting equally in all directions and uniaxial stress. While deep-sea organisms are constantly exposed to the isostatic pressure, uniaxial (or directional) pressure can act on human bones. This review primarily focuses on biological responses to isostatic hydrostatic pressure. A hydrostatic pressure of 10 MPa or higher generally has an adverse effect on the biological systems of organisms inhabiting lands or shallow sea regions [1,2]. Hydrostatic pressure increases by 0.1 MPa (0.1 MPa = 1 bar =

0.9869 atm; for clarity, "MPa" is used throughout) for every 10-m depth. Therefore, deep-sea organisms are exposed to a high pressure of 110 MPa in Challenger Deep, which is the deepest point in the Marina Trench (10,900 m). Deep-sea microorganisms or piezophiles that prefer high hydrostatic pressure for growth have garnered considerable scientific attention [2–5]. However, the molecular mechanism underlying the high-pressure adaptation has not been elucidated in piezophiles because of the difficulties in their cultivation and genetic manipulation (e.g., gene disruption, overexpression, or mutagenesis). Humans also experience high hydrostatic pressure when hip joints are exposed to a pressure of 18 MPa during exercise [6]; the back of the teeth is also exposed to the same levels of pressure. A long-term stay in space can cause muscle weakness in astronauts. Thus, the human body indubitably senses mechanical stresses such as hydrostatic pressure and gravity. Nonetheless, the mechanisms underlying biological responses to high pressures are not clearly understood. Figure 1 illustrates pressure ranges, research fields, and the main subjects in high-pressure bioscience and biotechnology.

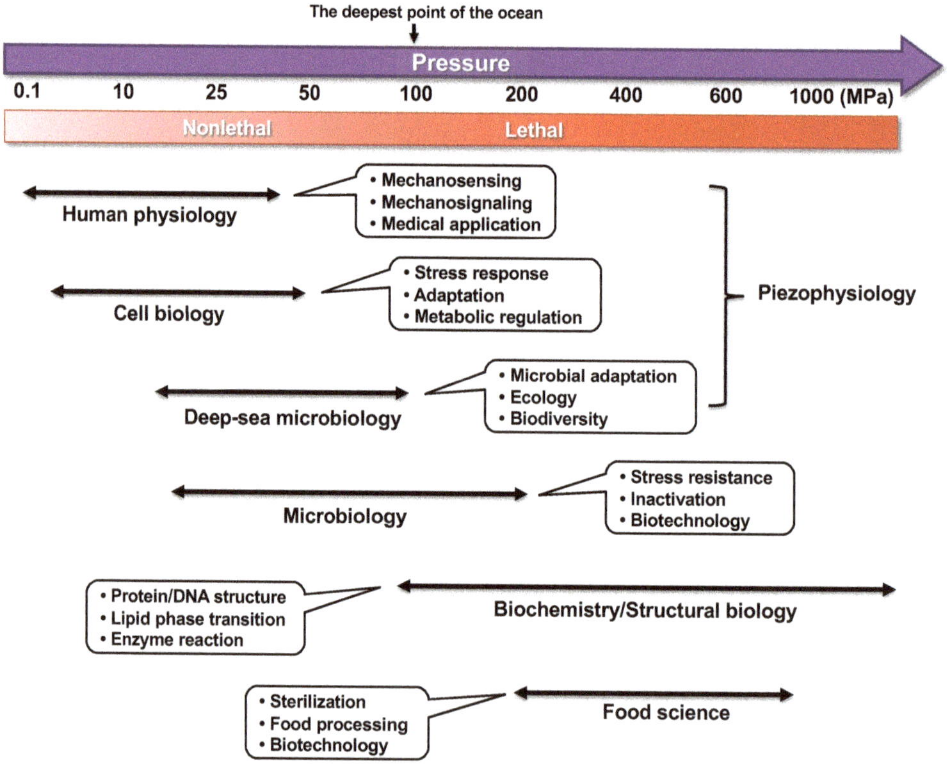

Figure 1. Pressure ranges, research fields, and main subjects in high-pressure bioscience and biotechnology. Thin double-headed arrows indicate approximate pressure ranges for corresponding research. The lethality of organisms under high pressure greatly depends on the species and duration of applied pressure and temperature.

Approximate pressure ranges affecting various biological processes are listed in Table 1 [7]. Generally, microorganisms can survive at high hydrostatic pressures in the range of several dozen MPa; a pressure higher than 200 MPa is lethal to most microorganisms but not to spores of *Clostridium* species, which are resistant to pressures greater than 400 MPa. The non-thermal sterilization of food materials using ultra-high pressure has been studied previously [8,9]. The effects of high pressure depend on the magnitude, pressurizing periods, temperature, pH, oxygen availability, and nutrient composition, which are complex and difficult to interpret. Oxygen supply is one of the limiting factors to cultivating aerobic organisms in a closed hydrostatic chamber. Yeast species isolated from mud samples obtained through submersible explorations with SHINKAI 6500 at the Japan Trench (~6500 m depth) were strictly aerobic, probably because of the oxygen-rich environment and scarcity of fermentable sugars such as glucose in the deep-sea. *Saccharomyces cerevisiae* is a facultative anaerobe, which makes it a useful model organism for studying the effects of high hydrostatic pressure. The *S. cerevisiae* genome encodes 6611 genes (*Saccharomyces* Genome Database, Genome Snapshot: https://www.yeastgenome.org/genomesnapshot; accessed on 8 December 2021). Global functional screening using a *S. cerevisiae* gene knockout mutant library revealed many unexpected genes and intracellular pathways that are associated with environmental stress resistance [10–12]. Figure 2 illustrates the bioinformatic tools employed to elucidate the mechanisms of high-pressure responses and adaptation in *S. cerevisiae*, as a model organism.

Table 1. Approximate pressure ranges affecting various biological processes.

Cellular Function	Inhibitory/Effective Pressure (MPa<)
Nutrient uptake	10
Cell division	20
Alcohol fermentation	15–20
Membrane protein function	25–50
DNA replication	25–50
RNA transcription	50–100
Protein synthesis	50
Microbial death	100–200
Protein oligomerization	50–100
Soluble enzyme activity	100
Protein tertiary structure	200–1000
DNA double strand formation	1000

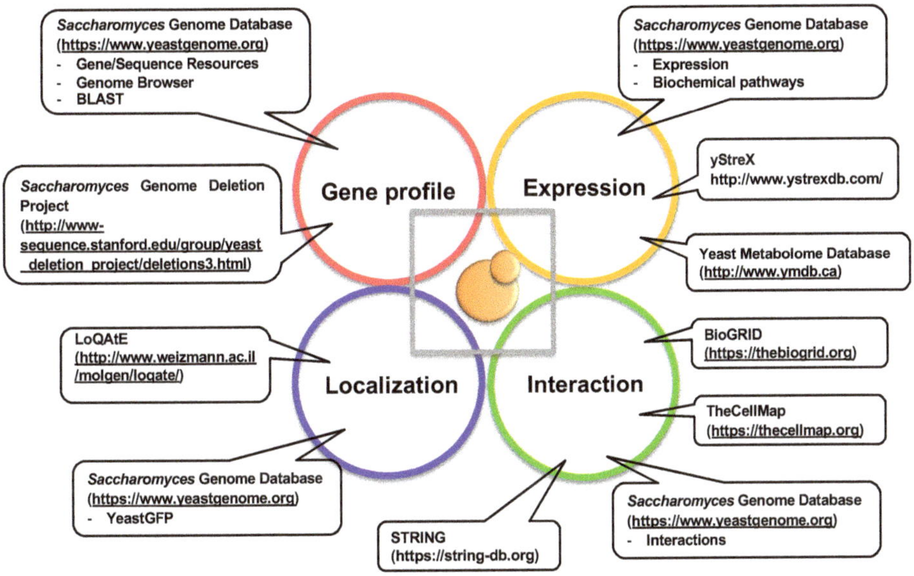

Figure 2. Bioinformatic tools for studying *S. cerevisiae* as a model to elucidate the mechanisms of high-pressure responses and adaptation.

In any reaction, the application of pressure yields a fundamental physical parameter, the volume change. The following two equations describe the effect of hydrostatic pressure on equilibrium A $\rightleftharpoons$ B and reaction A $\rightarrow$ B, respectively:

$$(\partial \ln K/\partial p)_T = -\Delta V/RT \quad (1)$$

$$(\partial \ln k/\partial p)_T = -\Delta V^{\neq}/RT \quad (2)$$

where K is the equilibrium constant, k is the rate constant, p is the pressure (MPa), T is the absolute temperature (K), R is the gas constant (mL·MPa·K^{-1}·mol^{-1}), ΔV is the difference between final and initial volumes in the entire system at equilibrium (reaction volume) including the solute and the solvent, and $\Delta V^{\neq}$ is the apparent volume change in activation (activation volume), representing the difference between the volumes of the ground and transition states. The effects of high pressure depend on the sign and amplitude of the change in volume associated with any reaction; thus, an increase in volume promotes inhibition of the reaction due to a pressure increase, and vice versa. While temperature accelerates any reaction, per the Arrhenius equation, pressure accelerates, inhibits, or does not affect reactions depending on the ΔV and $\Delta V^{\neq}$ values. Although the thermodynamic law is straightforward, estimating whether the expression of individual genes and levels of proteins increase or decrease when living cells are exposed to high pressure is difficult. Nevertheless, many informative studies have reported the biophysical effects of high pressure on biological machinery. In general, a pressure approximately greater than 100 MPa dissociates multimeric proteins as the hydration of charged groups and exposure of nonpolar groups to water is usually accompanied by negative volume changes [13,14]. Therefore, dissociated forms of proteins are formed in the aqueous solution under high pressure. Pressures greater than 60 MPa cause dissociation of ribosome subunits in *Escherichia coli* (at least in part), thereby limiting their growth [13]. Furthermore, the level of eukaryotic elongation factor-2 is decreased under continuous high-pressure culture at 30 MPa in HeLa carcinoma and T/C28a4 chondrocyte cell lines, suggesting that, at least in part, downregulated elongation factor-2 is attributed to the attenuation of protein synthesis under high pressure [15].

A deep-sea bacterium *Moritella profunda* optimally grows under 20–24 MPa at 6 °C under a laboratory condition [16] and is, thus, a psychrophillic piezophile. Interestingly, the dihydrofolate reductase of this bacterium is optimally active at 50 MPa and its secondary structure is stable up to 80 °C [17]. Therefore, a microbial growth profile does not always reflect intracellular enzymatic properties. Indeed, numerous studies have revealed that many deep-sea animal proteins intrinsically exhibit less sensitivity to high pressure than their orthologs from shallow species. Presumably, these differences reduce volume changes occurring in reactions [18]. For example, the formation of cytoskeletal actin filaments is more resistant to high pressure in deep-sea fish species than in their shallow sea counterparts [19]. The acquisition of this pressure tolerance in actin occurs, in part, due to the presence of more salt-bridges between amino acids associated with ATP-binding and structural stability [19]. It has been well-documented that trimethylamine *N*-oxide (TMAO) is the key osmolyte in marine fish, which can effectively counteract the inhibitory effects induced by high pressure on numerous proteins. Accordingly, TMAO content in marine fish increases with depth of capture (see Reviews: [20–22]). In fact, recent whole genome sequencing of a snailfish from the Yap Trench (~7000 m depth) revealed the presence of five copies of a gene encoding a flavin-containing monooxygenase-3 that catalyzes trimethylamine (TMA) to TMAO. In the fish, TMA can be supplied from gut bacteria [23].

Although high pressure induces the unfolding of protein monomers [14,24,25], the effect elicited by pressure is highly dependent on the actual objects and temperature within the range of a few hundred MPa to 1 GPa. Meanwhile, GFP and heat shock proteins are stable even above 1 GPa [26,27]. During protein unfolding, water molecules penetrate the cavities within the proteins and nonpolar groups are exposed to the solvent [28]. Consequently, proteins form aggregates within the cell that are harmful to cells.

The phase transition of lipid bilayers in biological systems is highly sensitive to high pressure. High pressure and low temperature reorder acyl chains of phospholipids, making the membrane stiffer [29,30]. In dipalmitoylphosphatidylcholine lipid bilayers, the temperature for the transition (T_m) from the ripple gel (P_{β}') phase to the liquid crystalline (L_{α}) phase increases by 24 °C with an increase in pressure of 100 MPa [31]. Although a clear phase transition is not observed in natural membranes in living cells, high pressures indubitably harden the membranes, which in turn affects the functionality and structure of transmembrane proteins. The occurrence and response of *S. cerevisiae* cells to high pressure are described in the following sections.

2. Effects of High Pressure on Cultured Human Cells and Tissues

The meniscus is a "C" shaped cartilage-like tissue located inside and outside of the knee joint that absorbs shock and stabilizes the knee joint. However, intense physical exercise and aging can damage the meniscus. The force applied to the meniscus is anisotropic and is complicated by the addition of shear stress, thus making molecular quantitative analysis of the cellular responses difficult. Hydrostatic pressure can regulate the metabolic activities of meniscal cells. For instance, the static application of 4 MPa pressure for 4 h suppresses the transcription of MMP-1 and MMP-13 genes in human meniscal cells in alginate beads [32]. In contrast, cyclic hydrostatic pressure at 1 Hz upregulates genes encoding type I collagen, TIMP-1, and TIMP-2. Meanwhile, upon explant, rabbit meniscal cells increase the transcription of genes encoding MMP-1, MMP-3, TIMPs, NOS2, COX2, IL-1β, and IL-6 [33]. However, the cyclic application of pressure of 1 MPa at 0.5 Hz for 4 h blocked the culture-induced increases in catabolic gene expression. Collectively, these studies indicate that mechanical loading on the meniscus can modulate the physiology of meniscal cells at the transcriptional level to maintain homeostasis in the meniscal tissue during culture [33].

Osteoarthritis is a disease in which the cartilage between the joint bones deteriorates and causes pain, swelling, and ultimately joint deformation. As per statistics, 10 million people of more than 50 years of age in Japan experience knee pain due to knee osteoarthritis. Attempts have been made to solve these problems using regenerative medicine based on cells cultured under high pressure. A pressure of 1 to 15 MPa was used to differentiate between the mesenchymal stem cells isolated from the human body and chondrocytes, which were reviewed by Elder et al. [34] and Pattappa et al. [35]. They tried to determine how the applied pressure leads to the upregulation of specific genes inside the cell. Identifying the sensor molecule that first senses hydrostatic pressure in the cell was difficult. Various candidates for sensor proteins in the induction of chondrogenesis, such as estrogen receptors, voltage-gated ion channels, G-protein-coupled receptors, integrin α10β1, and Ca^{2+} signaling pathways via TRPV4 channels have been reported. Nevertheless, the molecular basis of pressure-induced activation has not been established [35]. As unique applications in medical engineering, hydrostatic pressures at levels much higher than those found in physiological conditions were used to disinfect bone, tendons, and cartilage. The administration of short-term high pressure at 600 MPa to resected bone segments immediately after surgery offers an alternative to the conventional cancerous bone treatment. Under this condition, normal and malignant cells are irreversibly damaged, thereby efficiently blocking the outgrowth of cells from cancerous bone and cartilage segments (see Review [36]). Moreover, high hydrostatic pressure treatment at 480 MPa for 10 min has been applied to devitalize human cartilage with the goal of inducing subsequent cultivation of chondrocytes and mesenchymal stem cells on the devitalized tissue [37]. Meanwhile, the treatment of skin tissues at a moderate pressure of 50 MPa for more than 36 h induces cell death via apoptosis. Subsequent in vivo grafting of the apoptosis-induced inactivated skin was successful. This method is thought to have an advantage over inducing complete cell death via necrosis, as apoptotic cells do not generally promote inflammation [38]. Future progress can be expected for feasible applications of high pressure in medical engineering.

3. Effects of Lethal Levels of High Pressure on Yeast Survival

Figure 3 illustrates the occurrences and responses of *S. cerevisiae* cells upon exposure to various levels of hydrostatic pressure. In a pioneering study, Rosin and Zimmerman reported that when a pressure of 96.6 MPa is applied for 4 h, the occurrence of cytoplasmic petite mutants increases, which are characterized by a small colony size and respiration deficiency and reflect the high-pressure sensitivity of mitochondrial functions [39]. Pressures in the range of 100–150 MPa cause disruption of the spindle pole bodies and microtubules [40], and those of 200–250 MPa induce tetraploids and homozygous diploids [41]. A moderate heat treatment (e.g., 42 °C for 30 min) dramatically increases the survival rate after a subsequent heat-mediated toxic treatment (e.g., 50 °C for 10 min). Among heat shock proteins (Hsps), the molecular chaperone Hsp104 plays a primal role in this acquired heat tolerance mechanism by facilitating the unfolding of the denatured intracellular proteins [42]. This moderate heat treatment enhances cell survival against lethal levels of high pressure at 140–180 MPa with a 100–1000-fold increase in viability [43]. After 140 MPa pressure treatment, Hsp104 associate with insoluble protein aggregates, suggesting the contribution of Hsp104 contributes for the unfolding of high pressure-induced denatured proteins [44,45]. The *hsp104*Δ mutant did not acquire heat-inducible high-pressure tolerance (hereafter referred to as piezotolerance; [44]. Iwahashi et al. reported that piezo-tolerant mutants surviving at 180 MPa for 1 h (25 °C) also display resistance to 1% H_2O_2 for 60 min (0 °C) [46]. Moreover, Palhano et al. reported that treatment of cells with a moderate concentration of H_2O_2 (0.4 mM [0.0012%], 45 min) or 6% ethanol can increase the piezotolerance of yeast cells at 220 MPa for 30 min [47]. H_2O_2 is known to induce many antioxidant genes, including *GSH1* (which encodes γ-glutamylcysteine synthetase, an enzyme in glutathione (GSH) biosynthesis). The addition of GSH (>1 mM) increases piezotolerance in *S. cerevisiae* [47]. Meanwhile, ethanol stress upregulates genes involved in energy metabolism, protein destination, and stress tolerance including the cytoplasmic catalase T (Ctt1) and mitochondrial superoxide dismutase Sod2. *CTT1* and *SOD2* are also upregulated by high pressure [48]. A deletion mutant for *COX1* encoding the subunit I of cytochrome *c* oxidase in mitochondria is also sensitive to pressure at 200 MPa [49]. Taken together, these findings indicate that high hydrostatic pressure of approximately 200 MPa is likely to exert oxidative stresses in yeast cells, and the cellular defense systems against high pressure, at least in part, converge on oxidative stress responses for "cell survival." Consistently, our recent study indicated that the scavenging activity of superoxide anion $O_2^{\bullet-}$ by superoxide dismutase 1 (Sod1) is required for "cell growth" under a moderate growth-permissive pressure at 25 MPa [50]. Moreover, high pressure promoted the accumulation of $O_2^{\bullet-}$ in the mitochondrial inner space and the cytoplasm. Meanwhile, mutations in Sod1 that compromise the scavenging activity (or *CCS1* deletion), encoding a molecular chaperone that delivers copper to Sod1, cause deficient growth under 25 MPa [50].

Pressure pre-treatment at a sublethal level (50 MPa for 1 h) increases the viability of cells at 200 MPa [51]. This acquired piezotolerance via moderate pressure treatment is governed by two transcription factors, namely, Msn2 and Msn4, which are induced by various stresses. The loss of both *MSN2* and *MSN4* genes results in susceptibility to high pressure [51]. *HSP12* is a well-known target of Msn2/Msn4. In fact, the application of a pressure of 50 MPa increases the *HSP12* transcript level in wild-type *S. cerevisiae* cells but does not in the *msn2*Δ*msn4*Δ mutant [51]. However, the single deletion of *HSP12* did not decrease cell viability at 125 MPa for 1 h [52]. Therefore, a certain set of genes, under the control of Msn2/Msn4, could be required for the development of piezotolerance in yeast. Other genes highly upregulated by pressure at 25 MPa, such as the *DAN/TIR* family [53], that encode cell wall mannoproteins are not under the control of Msn2/Msn4 (see below). How high pressure regulates Msn2 and Msn4 after the transcription of their downstream genes remains unknown. Trehalose is a nonreducing disaccharide that protects proteins, membranes, and other macromolecules against various stresses. Trehalose also plays a role in the piezotolerance of yeast by preventing the formation of protein aggregates and promoting the refolding of Hsp104. Trehalose is hydrolyzed by the neutral trehalase Nth1, generating two glucose molecules from one trehalose molecule. Yeast mutants lacking Nth1 are susceptible to high pressures [45]. Neutral trehalase is required for recovering from the damage after high-pressure treatments, whereas it is dispensable for cell survival under high pressure. Accordingly, the recovery process from pressure-induced damage in yeast requires glucose at atmospheric pressure.

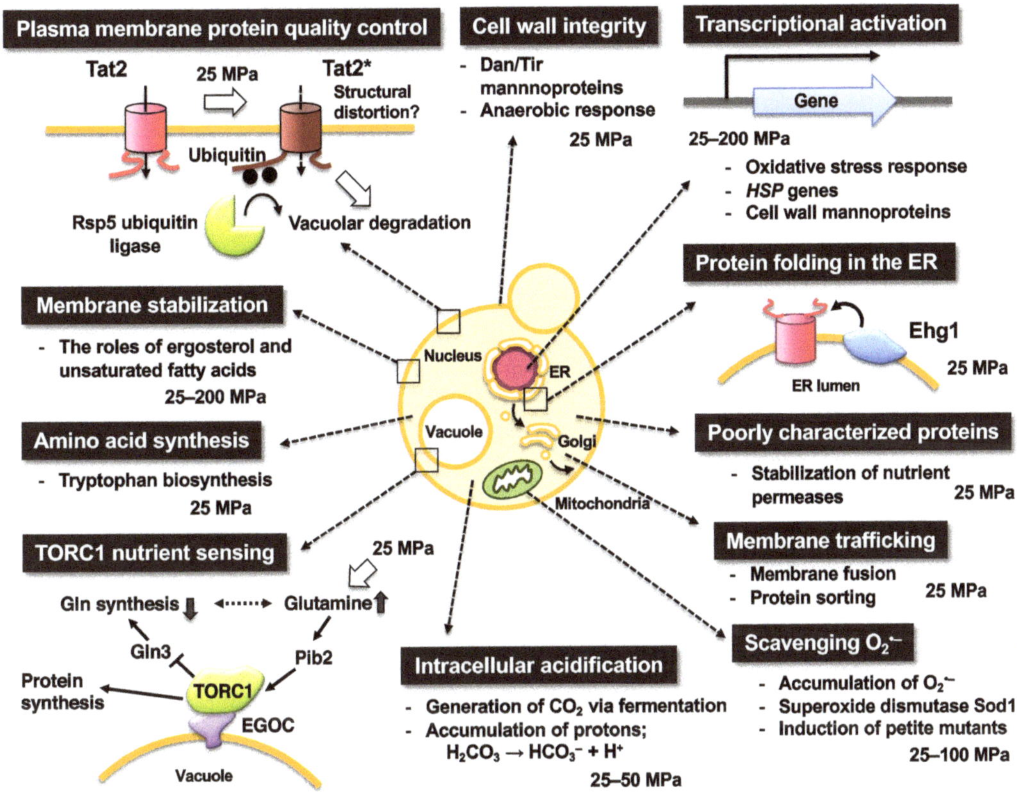

Figure 3. Occurrences and significance of intracellular changes in yeast responding to high hydrostatic pressure. Note that the figure only depicts limited aspects of the effects of high pressure on cellular functions in *S. cerevisiae*.

The composition of fatty acids affects the survival of the cell under lethal pressure of 150–200 MPa. A deletion mutant of *OLE1* encoding a membrane-bound Δ9 desaturase was cultured in a medium supplemented with various fatty acids such as palmitoleic acid (C16:1), oleic acid (C18:1), linoleic acid (C18:2), and linolenic acid (C18:3). Subsequently, the cells were exposed to pressures of 150–200 MPa for 30 min. The effect of increasing cell viability was in the order of linolenic acid > linoleic acid > oleic acid > palmitoleic acid. Therefore, a higher proportion of unsaturated fatty acids is likely to contribute to maintaining appropriate membrane fluidity under high pressure and reduced membrane fluidity would be fatal under high pressure [54]. However, reduced membrane fluidity is not the sole reason for cell death at 150–200 MPa because low temperatures (0–4 °C) are not lethal for the cells.

4. Tryptophan Uptake Is Crucial for Yeast Physiology under High Pressure

The hydrostatic pressure of 15 to 25 MPa is relatively mild for microorganisms and most of them can grow despite their decreased growth rate. The growth properties of experimental yeast strains differ greatly under high pressure and are dependent on the strain's requirement for tryptophan from the external medium. Experimental *S. cerevisiae* strains usually exhibit nutrient auxotrophic markers (e.g., *ade2, ura3, his3, lys3, leu2,* and *trp1*) for plasmid selection, that is, these strains require some elements (e.g., adenine, uracil, histidine, lysine, leucine, and tryptophan) for growth from their external medium. The auxotrophic characteristics of experimental yeast strains are similar to animals, including humans, because they also require histidine, lysine, leucine, and tryptophan from their diet. Tryptophan auxotrophs (Trp^-) are highly sensitive to high pressures. Trp^- cannot grow under 15–25 MPa, whereas tryptophan prototrophs (Trp^+) that can synthesize tryptophan, can grow under the same level of pressure [55,56]. Trp^- strains also exhibit growth deficiency at low temperatures of 10–15 °C, which is consistent with an earlier report [57]. The high-pressure sensitivity is attributed to properties specific to tryptophan uptake, which in *S. cerevisiae* is mediated by the tryptophan permeases Tat1 and Tat2: (i) the transport activity of Tat1 and Tat2 is readily impaired if the membrane is ordered either by high pressure or low temperature; and (ii) Tat1 and Tat2 undergo degradation via ubiquitination under high pressure (see below). Excessive addition of tryptophan or overexpression of *TAT1* or *TAT2* enables Trp^- cells to grow under 25 MPa [55,56]. Accordingly, *S. cerevisiae* can grow at pressures of up to 25 MPa if tryptophan is available in the external medium.

5. High Pressure Induces Degradation of Tryptophan Permeases via Ubiquitination

Ubiquitin is a small protein consisting of 76 amino acid residues and is highly conserved among eukaryotes. Ubiquitin covalently binds to the lysine residue of the target protein to be degraded via the ubiquitin-activating enzyme (E1), ubiquitin-conjugating enzyme (E2), and ubiquitin ligase (E3). The ubiquitinated protein is then transported to the 26S proteasome or vacuole (lysosome in animal cells) for degradation [58,59]. Deficiency in the ubiquitin system causes human diseases such as developmental anomalies, cancer, or neurological disorders; thus, clearance of unwanted proteins by ubiquitination is crucial. Hydrostatic pressure leads to the structural perturbation of biological membranes, which directly or indirectly affects the membrane proteins. As mentioned above, Trp^- strains are sensitive to moderate pressures of 15–25 MPa. Our research group has isolated many mutant strains that acquired the ability to grow under high pressure from the tryptophan-requiring strain YPH499 (a strain that cannot grow at 25 MPa) [56]. Genetic analysis showed that one of these mutations, *HPG1*, occurs in the catalytic domain of the E3 enzyme Rsp5 (Figure 3). E3 plays an important role in the target recognition, and Tat2 is a substrate for Rsp5 ubiquitin ligase. Therefore, Tat2 levels were high in the plasma membrane of the *HPG1* mutant, allowing sufficient tryptophan uptake by the cell, whereas Tat2 was degraded in the wild-type strain. *HPG2* mutation sites are located within the cytoplasmic tails of Tat2 [60], which are accompanied by the loss of negative charge within the cytoplasmic tail. Therefore, the negatively charged amino acid residues in the cytoplasmic tails may be required for Tat2 to interact with the Rsp5 complex via ionic interactions. However, how the denatured states of Tat1 and Tat2 can be structurally characterized and how denatured proteins are recognized by the Rsp5 complex remain to be elucidated.

6. Transcriptional Analysis of Genes Responsive to High Pressures

The yeast genome consists of approximately 12 million base pairs that encode 6611 genes. Among them, the functions of 5229 genes are known or predicted, whereas the rest are poorly characterized (*Saccharomyces* Genome Database). In addition to house-keeping genes that are essential for survival (such as energy metabolism and cell division), many genes are transcriptionally induced when the cells are exposed to critical situations such as heat or oxidative stress. Transcriptionally induced genes are necessary for establishing a cellular defense system in adverse conditions. DNA microarray hybridization and the more recent RNA-Seq techniques are widely used to comprehensively investigate the transcriptional level in response to environmental changes. Under the pressure of 30 MPa and a temperature of 25 °C, which allows for the growth of tryptophan prototrophs, 366 genes were upregulated by more than 2-fold, and 253 genes were downregulated by more than 2-fold [61]. According to the functional categories of the MIPS database, homology data, and yeast genome, the highly upregulated genes were essential for cell cycle, DNA processing, cell rescue, defense and virulence, and metabolism. Heat shock-responsive genes including *HSP12* and *HSP104* are induced by high pressure during acquired piezotolerance [61]. In our DNA microarray analysis, gene expression was compared under conditions of atmospheric pressure (0.1 MPa, 24 °C), high pressure (25 MPa, 24 °C), and low temperature (0.1, 15 °C), and found that the *DAN/TIR* family genes that encode mannoprotein of the cell wall were highly upregulated. Cells pre-exposed to high pressure or low temperature acquired tolerance when treated with moderate concentrations of SDS and zymolyase or a lethal level of high pressure because mannoproteins maintain cell wall integrity (125 MPa for 1 h) [53]. The *DAN/TIR* family genes are significantly induced under hypoxic conditions [62]. Therefore, intracellular signaling pathways responsive to high pressure, low temperature, and hypoxia might interact to establish defense systems.

7. Global Functional Analysis of Genes Required for Growth under High Pressure

Among the 6611 genes encoded by the *S. cerevisiae* genome, the single deletion of approximately 4800 genes is not lethal under normal culture conditions. These genes are considered to contribute to efficient cell growth or survival under hostile environmental conditions; therefore, some of them are functionally redundant. PCR-based systematic deletion of genes was performed (http://www-sequence.stanford.edu/group/yeast_deletion_project/project_desc.html#intro; accessed on 8 December 2021) [63], and deletion (gene knockout) libraries are available for purchase.

Using the deletion library, mutations causing hypersensitivity to high pressure (25 MPa and 24 °C) or low temperature (0.1 MPa and 15 °C) were identified within 4828 non-essential genes. To the best of my knowledge, this is the only study to perform a large-scale screening of the yeast deletion library to identify genes required for growth under a moderate high pressure. This analysis revealed 84 genes, of which 75 were found to be required for growth at 25 MPa and 24 °C and 57 were found to be required for growth at 0.1 MPa and 15 °C [64,65]. There was a marked overlap of 48 genes, implying that various biological functions have common roles allowing cell growth under high pressure and low temperature [64]. These 84 genes were classified into biological processes using STRING, a tool for functional enrichment analyses (https://string-db.org; accessed on 8 December 2021) (Table 2) [66]. Interestingly, there are several distinct clusters in physical or functional protein-protein interactions among the 84 proteins predicted on STRING (Figure 4). Therefore, these specific cellular functions must be highly important for growth under high pressure and low temperature. The 84 deletion mutants displayed variable sensitivity toward high pressure and low temperature. Consistent with earlier observations of growth deficiency in Trp^- strains [55,56], aromatic amino acids are crucial for high-pressure and low-temperature growth. Indeed, it has also been reported that mutants defective in tryptophan biosynthesis are cold sensitive [57]. Three mutants lacking one of the redundant ribosomal subunits displayed sensitivity to high pressure and low temperature (Figure 4). This is consistent with well-known knowledge that *E. coli* and *S. cerevisiae* mutants with defective ribosome assembly are cold sensitive [67–70]. The lack of Ccr4 and Pop2 (which comprise the Ccr4-Not transcriptional regulator [71]), is known to cause marked cold sensitivity; however, the underlying mechanism remains unknown [72]. The deletion of these genes also causes high-pressure sensitivity (Figure 4). Despite the determination of the transcriptional regulator, it is difficult to identify which target genes, of the Ccr4-Not complex, are responsible for high-pressure growth as numerous genes are under the control of this regulator. Although a global screening was performed to identify genes required for tolerance to freeze–thaw stress [73], no overlapping genes required for growth under cold or high-pressure environments [64], were identified. Therefore, a distinctive set of genes support these physiological characteristics of yeast. Deletion of genes involved in the later steps of ergosterol biosynthesis promoted the accumulation of sterol derivatives in cells [74]. Such mutations cause sensitivity to high pressure and low temperature [64]. Thus, ergosterol maintains membrane property by opposing the hardening of the membrane caused by high pressure and low temperature.

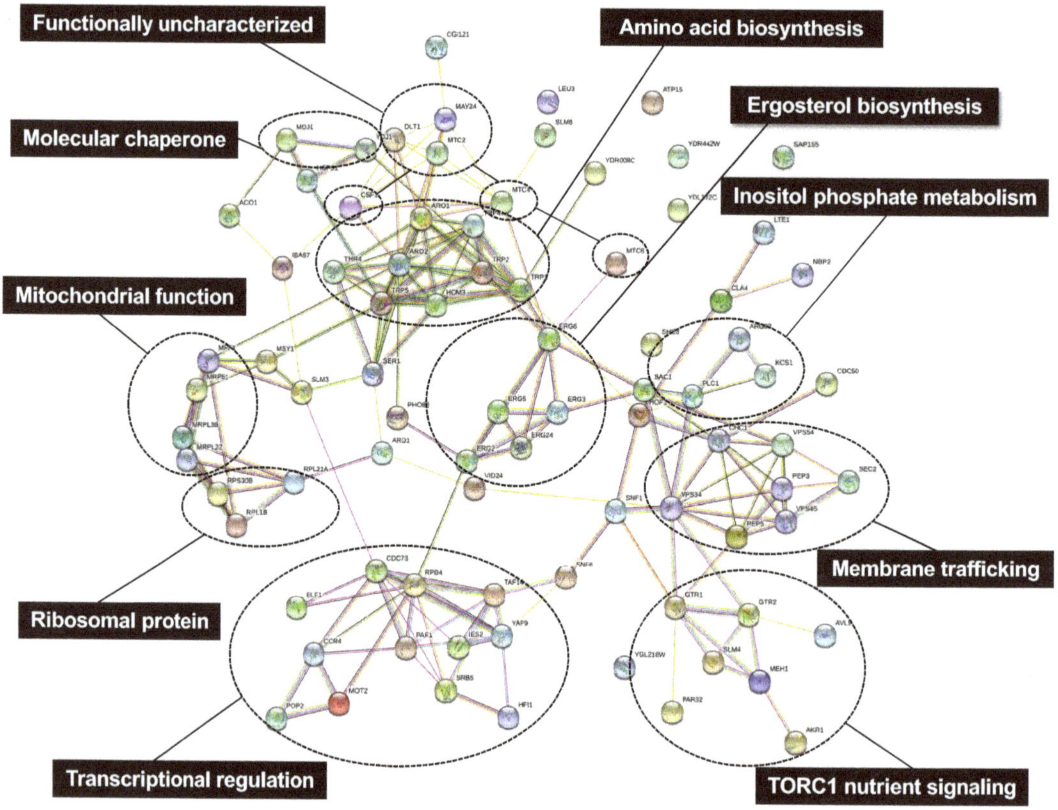

Figure 4. Prediction of protein-protein interactions among the 84 proteins encoded by high-pressure (25 MPa, 24 °C) and/or low-temperature (0.1 MPa, 15 °C) growth genes on STRING including direct (physical) and indirect (functional) associations (https://string-db.org; accessed on 8 December 2021).

Table 2. Biological processes (gene ontology) for proteins required for growth under high pressure and/or low temperature.

Term Description	Observed Gene Count	Background Gene Count	Strength
Lysosome organization	3	3	1.9
Tryptophan biosynthetic process	4	6	1.73
Inositol phosphate biosynthetic process	3	5	1.68
Aromatic amino acid family biosynthetic process	6	24	1.3
Ergosterol biosynthetic process	5	25	1.2
Alcohol biosynthetic process	8	54	1.07
Positive regulation of transcription elongation from RNA polymerase II promoter	6	46	1.02

Table 2. *Cont.*

Term Description	Observed Gene Count	Background Gene Count	Strength
Organic hydroxy compound biosynthetic process	9	76	0.97
Transcription elongation from RNA polymerase II promoter	6	55	0.94
Cellular amino acid biosynthetic process	10	131	0.78
Small molecule biosynthetic process	19	324	0.67
Carboxylic acid biosynthetic process	11	186	0.67
Cellular amino acid metabolic process	12	246	0.59
Positive regulation of cellular biosynthetic process	16	424	0.48
Organic cyclic compound biosynthetic process	30	931	0.41
Small molecule metabolic process	21	693	0.38
Aromatic compound biosynthetic process	25	871	0.36
Organic substance biosynthetic process	46	1810	0.31
Cellular biosynthetic process	44	1764	0.3
Cellular nitrogen compound biosynthetic process	31	1261	0.29

The 84 genes required for *Saccharomyces cerevisiae* cell growth under high pressure (15 MPa, 24 °C) and/or low temperature (0.1 MPa, 15 °C) were classified into biological processes using STRING, a tool for functional enrichment analyses (https://string-db.org; accessed on 8 December 2021). The observed gene count indicates how many proteins in the network are associated with a particular term. The background gene count indicates how many proteins in total (in the network and in the background) have this term assigned. The strength indicates Log_{10} (observed/expected), which describes how large the enrichment effect is.

8. High Pressure Activates a Nutrient Sensor Protein Kinase Complex TORC1

The aforementioned global screening methods revealed that the deletion of genes encoding the EGO complex (*EGO1, EGO3, GTR1,* and *GTR2*) [64,75] results in severe growth deficiency under high pressure and low temperature (Figures 3 and 4). The EGO complex is required to tether the target of rapamycin complex 1 (TORC1). TOR is an evolutionarily serine/threonine kinase in eukaryotes. It regulates the cellular homeostasis by coordinating anabolic and catabolic processes when nutrients are present [76–80]. TORC1 promotes cell growth by activating synthesis of proteins and ribosomes in the presence of favorable nutrients [81]. However, when the cells are starved or exposed to lethal stresses, TORC1 signaling is repressed, which leads to the downregulation of protein synthesis and effectively arrests cell growth [81–84]. A pressure of 25 MPa stimulated TORC1 to promote the phosphorylation of a downstream effector protein such as Sch9 [85]. This stimulation depends on the intracellular glutamine sensor protein, Pib2. Mutants with deleted EGOC complex have an aberrant increase in glutamine levels. Therefore, the EGOC–TORC1 complex plays a critical role in maintaining an appropriate glutamine level under high pressure by downregulating the *de novo* synthesis of glutamine [85]. Although the mechanism by which high pressure causes glutamate accumulation is unclear, these findings provide a unique framework for understanding metabolic adaptation to high pressure. Few reports in other organisms have addressed the amino acid requirement for growth under high pressure. One such report by Catio et al. demonstrated that piezo–hyperthermophilic archaeon *Thermococcus barophilus* requires only three amino acids (glutamate, cysteine, and tyrosine) for growth under atmospheric pressure at 85 °C in peptone replacement, whereas this organism required 17 amino acids (other than alanine, glutamine, and proline) for growth under 40 MPa [86]. Since the strain exhibits uptake activity of amino acids at 40 MPa, the increased requirement for amino acids cannot be explained by attenuation of substrate transport systems by high pressure. Instead, the authors suggested that there is a metabolic shift between atmospheric pressure and high pressure [86].

9. Identification of Novel *S. cerevisiae* Genes Required for Growth under High Pressure

Among the 84 gene deletion mutants that display growth deficiency under high hydrostatic pressure and/or low temperature, 24 deletion mutants can be reversed by the introduction of four plasmids (*LEU2, HIS3, LYS2,* and *URA3*) together that allow the growth at 25 MPa, thereby suggesting a close association between the genes and nutrient uptake [87]. Most highly ranked genes associated with high-pressure growth, including *MAY24*, are poorly characterized. May24 is localized in the endoplasmic reticulum (ER) membrane. Therefore, the gene is designated as *EHG1* (ER-associated high-pressure growth gene 1) [87]. The deletion of *EHG1* caused decreases in nutrient transport rates and reduced nutrient permease levels when the cells were cultured at 25 MPa. Thus, Ehg1 is required for the stability and functionality of permeases under high pressure (Figures 3 and 4) [65]. Ehg1 physically interacted with the histidine permease Hip1, leucine permease Bap2, and uracil permease Fur4. By functioning as a novel chaperone that facilitates coping with high-pressure-induced perturbations, Ehg1 could exhibit a stabilizing effect on nutrient permeases when they are present in the ER [87]. The acquisition of nutrients is one of the crucial biological processes in organisms under normal or harsh environmental conditions. The poorly characterized proteins including Ehg1 play a role in ensuring nutrient uptake via stabilizing the permeases present in the plasma membrane.

10. Conclusions

The use of genetic databases and functional genomic screening of *S. cerevisiae* can improve our fundamental understanding of the effects of high hydrostatic pressure on living cells. Many yeast strains belonging to the genera *Candida* and *Debaryomyces* are found in deep-sea environments and share many common genes with *S. cerevisiae*, which is not found in deep-sea environments. This review summarizes the mechanisms and biological processes associated with high-pressure adaptation in eukaryotes, especially yeasts.

Hydrostatic pressure is a thermodynamic variable that solely affects the equilibrium or the rate associated with any chemical reactions, not introducing any composing elements into the experimental system. The system reverts to its original state after decompression; hence, hydrostatic pressure can be utilized as a cleaning tool to modulate intracellular biochemical processes and may be applied for the production of any useful substances while saving energy. In the studies on "piezophysiology," high hydrostatic pressure is used as a variable to elucidate biological processes accompanying considerable structural changes in living cells. However, we continue to know very little about the effects of high pressure on complex intracellular networks or how to deal with cellular responses to high pressure. A mechanistic understanding of the effects of high pressure on proteins, membranes, and small intracellular molecules is necessary to understand the complete mechanism of cellular responses to high pressure. Advanced transcriptomics, proteomics, and metabolomics studies of yeast under high pressure will be helpful in the selection of yeast strains, media, temperature, and holding time.

Funding: This work was supported by a grant from the Japan Society for the Promotion of Science (No. 18K05397 to F. Abe), and a fund from Aoyama Gakuin University (Aoyama Vision 2019–2021).

Institutional Review Board Statement: Not applicable.

Informed Consent Statement: Not applicable.

Data Availability Statement: Not applicable.

Acknowledgments: I thank members of F.A. laboratory for performing research; the Japan Society of High Pressure Science and Technology for permission of adapting Figure 1 from Ref. [65].

Conflicts of Interest: The author declares no conflict of interests.

References

1. Abe, F.; Kato, C.; Horikoshi, K. Pressure-regulated metabolism in microorganisms. *Trends Microbiol.* **1999**, *7*, 447–453. [CrossRef]
2. Bartlett, D.H. Pressure effects on in vivo microbial processes. *Biochim. Biophys. Acta* **2002**, *1595*, 367–381. [CrossRef]
3. Yayanos, A.A. Microbiology to 10,500 m in the deep sea. *Annu. Rev. Microbiol.* **1995**, *49*, 777–805. [CrossRef] [PubMed]
4. Abe, F.; Horikoshi, K. The biotechnological potential of piezophiles. *Trends Biotechnol.* **2001**, *19*, 102–108. [CrossRef]
5. Oger, P.M.; Jebbar, M. The many ways of coping with pressure. *Res. Microbiol.* **2010**, *161*, 799–809. [CrossRef] [PubMed]

6. Muir, H. The chondrocyte, architect of cartilage. Biomechanics, structure, function and molecular biology of cartilage matrix macromolecules. *Bioessays* **1995**, *17*, 1039–1048. [CrossRef]
7. Abe, F. Exploration of the effects of high hydrostatic pressure on microbial growth, physiology and survival: Perspectives from piezophysiology. *Biosci. Biotechnol. Biochem.* **2007**, *71*, 2347–2357. [CrossRef] [PubMed]
8. Aertsen, A.; Meersman, F.; Hendrickx, M.E.; Vogel, R.F.; Michiels, C.W. Biotechnology under high pressure: Applications and implications. *Trends Biotechnol.* **2009**, *27*, 434–441. [CrossRef]
9. Lenz, C.A.; Vogel, R.F. Pressure-Based Strategy for the Inactivation of Spores. *Subcell. Biochem.* **2015**, *72*, 469–537.
10. Coelho, P.S.; Kumar, A.; Snyder, M. Genome-wide mutant collections: Toolboxes for functional genomics. *Curr. Opin. Microbiol.* **2000**, *3*, 309–315. [CrossRef]
11. Vidan, S.; Snyder, M. Large-scale mutagenesis: Yeast genetics in the genome era. *Curr. Opin. Biotechnol.* **2001**, *12*, 28–34. [CrossRef]
12. Nislow, C.; Wong, L.H.; Lee, A.H.; Giaever, G. Functional Profiling Using the Saccharomyces Genome Deletion Project Collections. *Cold Spring Harb. Protoc.* **2016**, *2016*, pdb-prot088039. [CrossRef] [PubMed]
13. Gross, M.; Jaenicke, R. Proteins under pressure. The influence of high hydrostatic pressure on structure, function and assembly of proteins and protein complexes. *Eur. J. Biochem.* **1994**, *221*, 617–630. [CrossRef] [PubMed]
14. Meersman, F.; Smeller, L.; Heremans, K. Protein stability and dynamics in the pressure-temperature plane. *Biochim. Biophys. Acta* **2006**, *1764*, 346–354. [CrossRef]
15. Elo, M.A.; Karjalainen, H.M.; Sironen, R.K.; Valmu, L.; Redpath, N.T.; Browne, G.J.; Kalkkinen, N.; Helminen, H.J.; Lammi, M.J. High hydrostatic pressure inhibits the biosynthesis of eukaryotic elongation factor-2. *J. Cell. Biochem.* **2005**, *94*, 497–507. [CrossRef] [PubMed]
16. Xu, Y.; Nogi, Y.; Kato, C.; Liang, Z.; Ruger, H.J.; De Kegel, D.; Glansdorff, N. *Moritella profunda* sp. nov. and *Moritella abyssi* sp. nov., two psychropiezophilic organisms isolated from deep Atlantic sediments. *Int. J. Syst. Evol. Microbiol.* **2003**, *53*, 533–538. [CrossRef]
17. Ohmae, E.; Murakami, C.; Tate, S.; Gekko, K.; Hata, K.; Akasaka, K.; Kato, C. Pressure dependence of activity and stability of dihydrofolate reductases of the deep-sea bacterium *Moritella profunda* and *Escherichia coli*. *Biochim. Biophys. Acta* **2012**, *1824*, 511–519. [CrossRef] [PubMed]
18. Somero, G.N. Protein adaptations to temperature and pressure: Complementary roles of adaptive changes in amino acid sequence and internal milieu. *Comp. Biochem. Physiol. B. Biochem. Mol. Biol.* **2003**, *136*, 577–591. [CrossRef]
19. Morita, T. Structure-based analysis of high pressure adaptation of alpha-actin. *J. Biol. Chem.* **2003**, *278*, 28060–28066. [CrossRef]
20. Yancey, P.H.; Blake, W.R.; Conley, J. Unusual organic osmolytes in deep-sea animals: Adaptations to hydrostatic pressure and other perturbants. *Comp. Biochem. Physiol. A. Mol. Integr. Physiol.* **2002**, *133*, 667–676. [CrossRef]
21. Yancey, P.H.; Siebenaller, J.F. Co-evolution of proteins and solutions: Protein adaptation versus cytoprotective micromolecules and their roles in marine organisms. *J. Exp. Biol.* **2015**, *218*, 1880–1896. [CrossRef]
22. Yancey, P.H. Cellular responses in marine animals to hydrostatic pressure. *J. Exp. Zool. A. Ecol. Integr. Physiol.* **2020**, *333*, 398–420. [CrossRef] [PubMed]
23. Mu, Y.; Bian, C.; Liu, R.; Wang, Y.; Shao, G.; Li, J.; Qiu, Y.; He, T.; Li, W.; Ao, J.; et al. Whole genome sequencing of a snailfish from the Yap Trench (~7000 m) clarifies the molecular mechanisms underlying adaptation to the deep sea. *PLoS Genet.* **2021**, *17*, e1009530. [CrossRef]
24. Fourme, R.; Girard, E.; Akasaka, K. High-pressure macromolecular crystallography and NMR: Status, achievements and prospects. *Curr. Opin. Struct. Biol.* **2012**, *22*, 636–642. [CrossRef] [PubMed]
25. Akasaka, K.; Kitahara, R.; Kamatari, Y.O. Exploring the folding energy landscape with pressure. *Arch. Biochem. Biophys.* **2013**, *531*, 110–115. [CrossRef] [PubMed]
26. Scheyhing, C.H.; Meersman, F.; Ehrmann, M.A.; Heremans, K.; Vogel, R.F. Temperature-pressure stability of green fluorescent protein: A Fourier transform infrared spectroscopy study. *Biopolymers* **2002**, *65*, 244–253. [CrossRef] [PubMed]
27. Tolgyesi, E.; Bode, C.S.; Smelleri, L.; Kim, D.R.; Kim, K.K.; Heremans, K.; Fidy, J. Pressure activation of the chaperone function of small heat shock proteins. *Cell. Mol. Biol. (Noisy-le-Grand)* **2004**, *50*, 361–369.
28. Gekko, K. Compressibility gives new insight into protein dynamics and enzyme function. *Biochim. Biophys. Acta* **2002**, *1595*, 382–386. [CrossRef]
29. Winter, R. Synchrotron X-ray and neutron small-angle scattering of lyotropic lipid mesophases, model biomembranes and proteins in solution at high pressure. *Biochim. Biophys. Acta* **2002**, *1595*, 160–184. [CrossRef]
30. Matsuki, H.; Goto, M.; Tada, K.; Tamai, N. Thermotropic and barotropic phase behavior of phosphatidylcholine bilayers. *Int. J. Mol. Sci.* **2013**, *14*, 2282–2302. [CrossRef]
31. Ichimori, H.; Hata, T.; Matsuki, H.; Kaneshina, S. Barotropic phase transitions and pressure-induced interdigitation on bilayer membranes of phospholipids with varying acyl chain lengths. *Biochim. Biophys. Acta* **1998**, *1414*, 165–174. [CrossRef]
32. Suzuki, T.; Toyoda, T.; Suzuki, H.; Hisamori, N.; Matsumoto, H.; Toyama, Y. Hydrostatic pressure modulates mRNA expressions for matrix proteins in human meniscal cells. *Biorheology* **2006**, *43*, 611–622. [PubMed]
33. Natsu-Ume, T.; Majima, T.; Reno, C.; Shrive, N.G.; Frank, C.B.; Hart, D.A. Menisci of the rabbit knee require mechanical loading to maintain homeostasis: Cyclic hydrostatic compression in vitro prevents derepression of catabolic genes. *J. Orthop. Sci.* **2005**, *10*, 396–405. [CrossRef] [PubMed]

34. Elder, B.D.; Athanasiou, K.A. Hydrostatic pressure in articular cartilage tissue engineering: From chondrocytes to tissue regeneration. *Tissue Eng. Part B. Rev.* **2009**, *15*, 43–53. [CrossRef]
35. Pattappa, G.; Zellner, J.; Johnstone, B.; Docheva, D.; Angele, P. Cells under pressure—The relationship between hydrostatic pressure and mesenchymal stem cell chondrogenesis. *Eur. Cell. Mater.* **2019**, *37*, 360–381. [CrossRef]
36. Diehl, P.; Schauwecker, J.; Mittelmeier, W.; Schmitt, M. High hydrostatic pressure, a novel approach in orthopedic surgical oncology to disinfect bone, tendons and cartilage. *Anticancer Res.* **2008**, *28*, 3877–3883.
37. Hiemer, B.; Genz, B.; Jonitz-Heincke, A.; Pasold, J.; Wree, A.; Dommerich, S.; Bader, R. Devitalisation of human cartilage by high hydrostatic pressure treatment: Subsequent cultivation of chondrocytes and mesenchymal stem cells on the devitalised tissue. *Sci. Rep.* **2016**, *6*, 33747. [CrossRef]
38. Le, T.M.; Morimoto, N.; Ly, N.T.M.; Mitsui, T.; Notodihardjo, S.C.; Munisso, M.C.; Kakudo, N.; Moriyama, H.; Yamaoka, T.; Kusumoto, K. Hydrostatic pressure can induce apoptosis of the skin. *Sci. Rep.* **2020**, *10*, 17594. [CrossRef] [PubMed]
39. Rosin, M.P.; Zimmerman, A.M. The induction of cytoplasmic petite mutants of Saccharomyces cerevisiae by hydrostatic pressure. *J. Cell. Sci.* **1977**, *26*, 373–385. [CrossRef]
40. Kobori, H.; Sato, M.; Tameike, A.; Hamada, K.; Shimada, S.; Osumi, M. Ultrastructural effects of pressure stress to the nucleus in *Saccharomyces cerevisiae*: A study by immunoelectron microscopy using frozen thin sections. *FEMS Microbiol. Lett.* **1995**, *132*, 253–258. [CrossRef]
41. Hamada, K.; Nakatomi, Y.; Shimada, S. Direct induction of tetraploids or homozygous diploids in the industrial yeast *Saccharomyces cerevisiae* by hydrostatic pressure. *Curr. Genet.* **1992**, *22*, 371–376. [CrossRef] [PubMed]
42. Glover, J.R.; Lindquist, S. Hsp104, Hsp70, and Hsp40: A novel chaperone system that rescues previously aggregated proteins. *Cell* **1998**, *94*, 73–82. [CrossRef]
43. Iwahashi, H.; Kaul, S.C.; Obuchi, K.; Komatsu, Y. Induction of barotolerance by heat shock treatment in yeast. *FEMS Microbiol. Lett.* **1991**, *64*, 325–328. [CrossRef] [PubMed]
44. Iwahashi, H.; Obuchi, K.; Fujii, S.; Komatsu, Y. Effect of temperature on the role of Hsp104 and trehalose in barotolerance of *Saccharomyces cerevisiae*. *FEBS Lett.* **1997**, *416*, 1–5. [CrossRef]
45. Iwahashi, H.; Nwaka, S.; Obuchi, K. Evidence for contribution of neutral trehalase in barotolerance of *Saccharomyces cerevisiae*. *Appl. Environ. Microbiol.* **2000**, *66*, 5182–5185. [CrossRef] [PubMed]
46. Iwahashi, H.; Fujii, S.; Obuchi, K.; Kaul, S.C.; Sato, A.; Komatsu, Y. Hydrostatic pressure is like high temperature and oxidative stress in the damage it causes to yeast. *FEMS Microbiol. Lett.* **1993**, *108*, 53–57. [CrossRef]
47. Palhano, F.L.; Orlando, M.T.; Fernandes, P.M. Induction of baroresistance by hydrogen peroxide, ethanol and cold-shock in *Saccharomyces cerevisiae*. *FEMS Microbiol. Lett.* **2004**, *233*, 139–145. [CrossRef] [PubMed]
48. Fernandes, P.M.; Domitrovic, T.; Kao, C.M.; Kurtenbach, E. Genomic expression pattern in *Saccharomyces cerevisiae* cells in response to high hydrostatic pressure. *FEBS Lett.* **2004**, *556*, 153–160. [CrossRef]
49. Nomura, K.; Iwahashi, H.; Iguchi, A.; Shigematsu, T. Barosensitivity in *Saccharomyces cerevisiae* is Closely Associated with a Deletion of the COX1 Gene. *J. Food Sci.* **2015**, *80*, M1051-9. [CrossRef] [PubMed]
50. Funada, C.; Tanino, N.; Fukaya, M.; Mikajiri, Y.; Nishiguchi, M.; Otake, M.; Nakasuji, H.; Kawahito, R.; Abe, F. *SOD1* mutations cause hypersensitivity to high-pressure-induced oxidative stress in *Saccharomyces cerevisiae*. *Biochim. Biophys. Acta Gen. Subj.* **2021**, *1866*, 130049. [CrossRef] [PubMed]
51. Domitrovic, T.; Fernandes, C.M.; Boy-Marcotte, E.; Kurtenbach, E. High hydrostatic pressure activates gene expression through Msn2/4 stress transcription factors which are involved in the acquired tolerance by mild pressure precondition in *Saccharomyces cerevisiae*. *FEBS Lett.* **2006**, *580*, 6033–6038. [CrossRef] [PubMed]
52. Miura, T.; Minegishi, H.; Usami, R.; Abe, F. Systematic analysis of *HSP* gene expression and effects on cell growth and survival at high hydrostatic pressure in *Saccharomyces cerevisiae*. *Extremophiles* **2006**, *10*, 279–284. [CrossRef] [PubMed]
53. Abe, F. Induction of *DAN/TIR* yeast cell wall mannoprotein genes in response to high hydrostatic pressure and low temperature. *FEBS Lett.* **2007**, *581*, 4993–4998. [CrossRef] [PubMed]
54. de Freitas, J.M.; Bravim, F.; Buss, D.S.; Lemos, E.M.; Fernandes, A.A.; Fernandes, P.M. Influence of cellular fatty acid composition on the response of *Saccharomyces cerevisiae* to hydrostatic pressure stress. *FEMS Yeast Res.* **2012**, *12*, 871–878. [CrossRef]
55. Abe, F.; Horikoshi, K. Tryptophan permease gene *TAT2* confers high-pressure growth in *Saccharomyces cerevisiae*. *Mol. Cell. Biol.* **2000**, *20*, 8093–8102. [CrossRef]
56. Abe, F.; Iida, H. Pressure-induced differential regulation of the two tryptophan permeases Tat1 and Tat2 by ubiquitin ligase Rsp5 and its binding proteins, Bul1 and Bul2. *Mol. Cell Biol.* **2003**, *23*, 7566–7584. [CrossRef]
57. Chen, X.H.; Xiao, Z.; Fitzgerald-Hayes, M. SCM2, a tryptophan permease in *Saccharomyces cerevisiae*, is important for cell growth. *Mol. Gen. Genet.* **1994**, *244*, 260–268. [CrossRef] [PubMed]
58. Hershko, A.; Ciechanover, A. The ubiquitin system. *Annu. Rev. Biochem.* **1998**, *67*, 425–479. [CrossRef]
59. Rotin, D.; Kumar, S. Physiological functions of the HECT family of ubiquitin ligases. *Nat. Rev. Mol. Cell Biol.* **2009**, *10*, 398–409. [CrossRef] [PubMed]
60. Nagayama, A.; Kato, C.; Abe, F. The *N*- and *C*-terminal mutations in tryptophan permease Tat2 confer cell growth in *Saccharomyces cerevisiae* under high-pressure and low-temperature conditions. *Extremophiles* **2004**, *8*, 143–149. [CrossRef]
61. Iwahashi, H.; Odani, M.; Ishidou, E.; Kitagawa, E. Adaptation of *Saccharomyces cerevisiae* to high hydrostatic pressure causing growth inhibition. *FEBS Lett.* **2005**, *579*, 2847–2852. [CrossRef]

62. Abramova, N.; Sertil, O.; Mehta, S.; Lowry, C.V. Reciprocal regulation of anaerobic and aerobic cell wall mannoprotein gene expression in *Saccharomyces cerevisiae*. *J. Bacteriol.* **2001**, *183*, 2881–2887. [CrossRef]
63. Giaever, G.; Chu, A.M.; Ni, L.; Connelly, C.; Riles, L.; Veronneau, S.; Dow, S.; Lucau-Danila, A.; Anderson, K.; Andre, B.; et al. Functional profiling of the *Saccharomyces cerevisiae* genome. *Nature* **2002**, *418*, 387–391. [CrossRef]
64. Abe, F.; Minegishi, H. Global screening of genes essential for growth in high-pressure and cold environments: Searching for basic adaptive strategies using a yeast deletion library. *Genetics* **2008**, *178*, 851–872. [CrossRef] [PubMed]
65. Abe, F. The effects of high hydrostatic pressure on the complex intermolecular networks in a living cell. *Rev. High Press. Sci. Technol.* **2021**, *31*, 54–65. [CrossRef]
66. Szklarczyk, D.; Gable, A.L.; Nastou, K.C.; Lyon, D.; Kirsch, R.; Pyysalo, S.; Doncheva, N.T.; Legeay, M.; Fang, T.; Bork, P.; et al. The STRING database in 2021: Customizable protein-protein networks, and functional characterization of user-uploaded gene/measurement sets. *Nucleic Acids Res.* **2021**, *49*, D605–D612. [CrossRef] [PubMed]
67. Friedman, H.; Lu, P.; Rich, A. Ribosomal subunits produced by cold sensitive initiation of protein synthesis. *Nature* **1969**, *223*, 909–913. [CrossRef] [PubMed]
68. Bryant, R.E.; Sypherd, P.S. Genetic analysis of cold-sensitive ribosome maturation mutants of *Escherichia coli*. *J. Bacteriol.* **1974**, *117*, 1082–1092. [CrossRef] [PubMed]
69. Singh, A.; Manney, T.R. Genetic analysis of mutations affecting growth of Saccharomyces cerevisiae at low temperature. *Genetics* **1974**, *77*, 651–659. [CrossRef] [PubMed]
70. Ursic, D.; Davies, J. A cold-sensitive mutant of *Saccharomyces cerevisiae* defective in ribosome processing. *Mol. Gen. Genet.* **1979**, *175*, 313–323. [CrossRef]
71. Tucker, M.; Valencia-Sanchez, M.A.; Staples, R.R.; Chen, J.; Denis, C.L.; Parker, R. The transcription factor associated Ccr4 and Caf1 proteins are components of the major cytoplasmic mRNA deadenylase in *Saccharomyces cerevisiae*. *Cell* **2001**, *104*, 377–386. [CrossRef]
72. Hata, H.; Mitsui, H.; Liu, H.; Bai, Y.; Denis, C.L.; Shimizu, Y.; Sakai, A. Dhh1p, a putative RNA helicase, associates with the general transcription factors Pop2p and Ccr4p from *Saccharomyces cerevisiae*. *Genetics* **1998**, *148*, 571–579. [CrossRef]
73. Ando, A.; Nakamura, T.; Murata, Y.; Takagi, H.; Shima, J. Identification and classification of genes required for tolerance to freeze-thaw stress revealed by genome-wide screening of *Saccharomyces cerevisiae* deletion strains. *FEMS Yeast Res.* **2007**, *7*, 244–253. [CrossRef]
74. Guan, X.L.; Souza, C.M.; Pichler, H.; Dewhurst, G.; Schaad, O.; Kajiwara, K.; Wakabayashi, H.; Ivanova, T.; Castillon, G.A.; Piccolis, M.; et al. Functional interactions between sphingolipids and sterols in biological membranes regulating cell physiology. *Mol. Biol. Cell* **2009**, *20*, 2083–2095. [CrossRef]
75. Dubouloz, F.; Deloche, O.; Wanke, V.; Cameroni, E.; De Virgilio, C. The TOR and EGO protein complexes orchestrate microautophagy in yeast. *Mol. Cell* **2005**, *19*, 15–26. [CrossRef]
76. Heitman, J.; Movva, N.R.; Hall, M.N. Targets for cell cycle arrest by the immunosuppressant rapamycin in yeast. *Science* **1991**, *253*, 905–909. [CrossRef]
77. Dokudovskaya, S.; Rout, M.P. SEA you later alli-GATOR– a dynamic regulator of the TORC1 stress response pathway. *J. Cell. Sci.* **2015**, *128*, 2219–2228. [CrossRef] [PubMed]
78. Powis, K.; De Virgilio, C. Conserved regulators of Rag GTPases orchestrate amino acid-dependent TORC1 signaling. *Cell Discov.* **2016**, *2*, 15049. [CrossRef]
79. Lim, C.Y.; Zoncu, R. The lysosome as a command-and-control center for cellular metabolism. *J. Cell Biol.* **2016**, *214*, 653–664. [CrossRef] [PubMed]
80. Gonzalez, A.; Hall, M.N. Nutrient sensing and TOR signaling in yeast and mammals. *EMBO J.* **2017**, *36*, 397–408. [CrossRef] [PubMed]
81. Urban, J.; Soulard, A.; Huber, A.; Lippman, S.; Mukhopadhyay, D.; Deloche, O.; Wanke, V.; Anrather, D.; Ammerer, G.; Riezman, H.; et al. Sch9 is a major target of TORC1 in Saccharomyces cerevisiae. *Mol. Cell* **2007**, *26*, 663–674. [CrossRef]
82. Powers, T.; Walter, P. Regulation of ribosome biogenesis by the rapamycin-sensitive TOR-signaling pathway in *Saccharomyces cerevisiae*. *Mol. Biol. Cell* **1999**, *10*, 987–1000. [CrossRef]
83. Gasch, A.P.; Spellman, P.T.; Kao, C.M.; Carmel-Harel, O.; Eisen, M.B.; Storz, G.; Botstein, D.; Brown, P.O. Genomic expression programs in the response of yeast cells to environmental changes. *Mol. Biol. Cell* **2000**, *11*, 4241–4257. [CrossRef]
84. Brauer, M.J.; Huttenhower, C.; Airoldi, E.M.; Rosenstein, R.; Matese, J.C.; Gresham, D.; Boer, V.M.; Troyanskaya, O.G.; Botstein, D. Coordination of growth rate, cell cycle, stress response, and metabolic activity in yeast. *Mol. Biol. Cell* **2008**, *19*, 352–367. [CrossRef]
85. Uemura, S.; Mochizuki, T.; Amemiya, K.; Kurosaka, G.; Yazawa, M.; Nakamoto, K.; Ishikawa, Y.; Izawa, S.; Abe, F. Amino acid homeostatic control by TORC1 in *Saccharomyces cerevisiae* under high hydrostatic pressure. *J. Cell. Sci.* **2020**, *133*, 10.1242/jcs.245555. [CrossRef]
86. Cario, A.; Lormieres, F.; Xiang, X.; Oger, P. High hydrostatic pressure increases amino acid requirements in the piezo-hyperthermophilic archaeon Thermococcus barophilus. *Res. Microbiol.* **2015**, *166*, 710–716. [CrossRef]
87. Kurosaka, G.; Uemura, S.; Mochizuki, T.; Kozaki, Y.; Hozumi, A.; Suwa, S.; Ishii, R.; Kato, Y.; Imura, S.; Ishida, N.; et al. A novel ER membrane protein Ehg1/May24 plays a critical role in maintaining multiple nutrient permeases in yeast under high-pressure perturbation. *Sci. Rep.* **2019**, *9*, 18341. [CrossRef]

MDPI
St. Alban-Anlage 66
4052 Basel
Switzerland
Tel. +41 61 683 77 34
Fax +41 61 302 89 18
www.mdpi.com

Biology Editorial Office
E-mail: biology@mdpi.com
www.mdpi.com/journal/biology

www.ingramcontent.com/pod-product-compliance
Lightning Source LLC
LaVergne TN
LVHW070623100526
838202LV00012B/709